# MEASUREMENT OF NURSING OUTCOMES

## VOLUME TWO

**Ora L. Strickland, Ph.D., R.N., F.A.A.N.**, is a professor in the School of Nursing of the University of Maryland at Baltimore where she is also Project Director of the Measurement of Clinical and Educational Nursing Outcomes project. Dr. Strickland earned a doctoral degree in child development and family relations from the University of North Carolina, Greensboro. She took a master's degree in maternal and child health nursing from Boston University, and received a bachelor's degree in nursing from North Carolina Agricultural and Technical State University.

As a nationally known specialist in nursing research, measurement, evaluation, maternal and child health, and parenting, Dr. Strickland is frequently called on as a consultant by universities, health care agencies, community organizations, and governmental agencies. She has presented more than 100 public lectures, speeches, and workshops, and her research has been featured in newspapers and on radio and television. Dr. Strickland is on the editorial boards of several professional journals.

**Carolyn F. Waltz, R.N., Ph.D., F.A.A.N.**, is a professor and coordinator of evaluation at the University of Maryland School of Nursing and is program director of the Measurement of Clinical and Educational Nursing Outcomes grant funded by the Division of Nursing. She is also program director of the Accreditation Outcomes Project of the National League for Nursing, which is funded by the Helene Fuld Health Trust Fund. She received her B.S. and M.S. degrees from the University of Maryland and her Ph.D. from the University of Delaware. Dr. Waltz has published numerous books and articles on measurement, nursing outcomes, and evaluation. To date, she has served as consultant to more than 100 universities and institutions nationally and internationally regarding topics such as measurement, program evaluation, and nursing outcomes.

# MEASUREMENT OF NURSING OUTCOMES

## Volume Two
## Measuring Nursing Performance:
### Practice, Education, and Research

**Ora L. Strickland**
R.N., Ph.D., F.A.A.N.
**Carolyn F. Waltz**
R.N., Ph.D., F.A.A.N.
*Editors*

SPRINGER PUBLISHING COMPANY
New York

Springer Publishing Company, Inc.
536 Broadway
New York, NY 10012

88  89  90  91  92  /  5  4  3  2  1

LIBRARY OF CONGRESS
Library of Congress Cataloging-in-Publication Data

Measurement of nursing outcomes/Carolyn F. Waltz, Ora L. Strickland,
  editors.
      p.      cm.
    Includes bibliographies and indexes.
    Contents: v. 1. Measuring client outcomes – v. 2. Measuring
nursing performance.
    ISBN 0-8261-5271-6 (v. 1). ISBN 0-8261-5272-4 (v. 2)
    ISBN 0-8261-5270-8 (2 vol. set)
    1. Nursing audit.  2. Nursing – Standards.  I. Waltz, Carolyn
Feher.  II. Strickland, Ora.
    [DNLM: 1. Nursing – methods.  2. Nursing – standards.
3. Personnel Management. WY 16 M484]
RT85.5.M434  1988
362.1'73'068 – dc19
DNLM/DLC                                                    88-19961
for Library of Congress                                          CIP

Printed in the United States of America

# CONTENTS

## Part III   MEASURING EDUCATIONAL OUTCOMES

# CONTRIBUTORS

Paulette Freeman Adams, R.N.,
Ed.D.
Assistant Dean, Undergraduate
Program
University of Louisville
School of Nursing
Louisville, Kentucky

Jean M. Arnold, R.N., Ed.D.
Associate Professor
College of Nursing
Rutgers-The State University
Newark, New Jersey

Eloise M. Balasco, R.N., M.S.N.
The Children's Hospital
Boston, Massachusetts

Elizabeth A. Barrett, R.N., Ph.D.
Associate Professor of Nursing
Hunter-Bellevue
Hunter College
The City University of New York
and Private Practice
New York, New York

Anne S. Black, R.N., M.S.N.
The Children's Hospital
Boston, Massachusetts

Doris Blaney, R.N., Ed.D.,
F.A.A.N.
Professor and Assistant Dean
Indiana University-Northwest Campus
School of Nursing
Gary, Indiana

Felicitas A. dela Cruz, R.N., M.A.
California State University
Los Angeles, California

Karen E. Dennis, R.N., Ph.D.
Nursing Program Director
General Clinical Research Center
Nursing Research Director
Department of Nursing
Francis Scott Key Medical Center
Johns Hopkins Medical Institution
Baltimore, Maryland

Mary E. Duffy, R.N., Ph.D.
Associate Professor
The University of Texas
Science Center at Houston
Austin, Texas

Linda Holbrook Freeman, R.N.,
M.S.N.
Assistant Dean, Continuing Education
University of Louisville
School of Nursing
Louisville, Kentuky

Margaret E. Gredler, Ph.D.
Associate Professor
College of Education
University of South Carolina
Columbia, South Carolina

Blossom Gullickson, R.N., M.S.
Assistant Professor
St. Olaf College
Department of Nursing
Northfield, Minnesota

Nan D. Hechenberger, Ph.D.
Dean and Professor
University of Maryland
School of Nursing
Baltimore, Maryland

Kathryn S. Hegedus, R.N.,
D.N.Sc.
Director, Staff Development and
Research
The Children's Hospital
Boston, Massachusetts

Charles J. Hobson, Ph.D.
Indiana University-Northwest
Campus
School of Nursing
Gary, Indiana

Angeline M. Jacobs, R.N., M.S.
Program Evaluator
California State University
Los Angeles, California

**Helen M. Jenkins, R.N., Ph.D.**
Assistant Professor
George Mason University
Fairfax, Virginia

**Joan M. Johnson, R.N., Ph.D.**
Assistant Professor
College of Nursing
University of Wisconsin-Oshkosh
Oshkosh, Wisconsin

**Margaret R. Kostopoulos, R.N., M.S.N., C.N.A.**
Assistant Director of Nursing Services
AMI Doctors' Hospital of Prince
  George's County
Lanham, Maryland

**Ursel Krumme, R.N., M.A.**
Associate Professor
Seattle University
School of Nursing
Seattle, Washington

**Therese G. Lawler, R.N., Ed.D.**
Professor of Nursing
East Carolina University
Greenville, North Carolina

**Jean A. Massey, R.N., Ph.D., C.C.R.N.**
Assistant Professor
College of Nursing
University of South Carolina
Columbia, South Carolina

**Barbara Clark Mims, R.N., M.S.N., C.C.R.N.**
Nurse Internship Coordinator
Parkland Memorial Hospital
Dallas, Texas

**Doris E. Nicholas, R.N., Ph.D.**
Associate Professor
Howard University
College of Nursing
Washington, D.C.

**Karen Kelly Schutzenhofer, R.N., Ed.D.**
Assistant Dean and Assistant Professor
School of Nursing
University of Missouri-St. Louis

**E. Ann Sheridan, R.N., Ed.D.**
University of Massachusetts
School of Health Sciences
Division of Nursing
Amherst, Massachusetts

**Bonnie Ketchum Smola, R.N., Ph.D.**
Professor, Nursing
University of Dubuque
Dubuque, Iowa

**Jacqueline Stemple, R.N., Ed.D.**
Associate Professor and Chairperson
Sophomore Academic Unit
West Virginia University
Morgantown, West Virginia

**Cheryl B. Stetler, R.N., Ph.D.**
Nurse Researcher
New England Medical Center
  Hospitals
Department of Nursing
Boston, Massachusetts

**Donna Ketchum Story, R.N., Ph.D.**
Associate Professor
Luther College
Decorah, Iowa

**Gladys Torres, R.N., Ed.D.**
Assistant Professor
Health Science Center
Brooklyn College of Nursing
State University of New York
Brooklyn, New York

**Sandra Millon Underwood, R.N., M.S.N.**
Assistant Professor
Chicago State University
Chicago, Illinois

**DeAnn M. Young, R.N., M.S.**
California State University
Los Angeles, California

# PART I
# Measuring Professionalism

# 1

# Measuring Professional Autonomy in Nurses

## Karen Kelly Schutzenhofer

*This chapter discusses the Schutzenhofer Profesional Nursing Autonomy Scale, a measure of professional autonomy in nurses.*

This study focuses on the development of an instrument to measure the professional autonomy of nurses. While nursing strives toward professionalization, there is consensus that it is not yet a full-fledged profession. Stuart (1981), in a paper on the professionalization of nursing, applied Moore's (1970) Scale of Professionalism to nursing. She noted that while nursing generally meets five of the criteria (occupation, calling, organization, educational program, and service orientation), it falls short on the criterion of autonomy. In recent years much effort has been directed at increasing the autonomy of individual nurses through education and changing the work environment, since the autonomy of the whole of nursing is dependent on the autonomy of individual practitioners. Some researchers have had to rely on general measures of work-related autonomy or measures of personal autonomy because the appropriate instrument was not available. These efforts require instruments that measure this characteristic of professional behavior. Such was the goal of this study.

For purposes of this study, professional autonomy was defined as "the practice of one's occupation in accordance with one's education, with members of that occupation governing, defining, and controlling their own activities in the absence of external controls" (Barber, 1965; Engel, 1970; Maas & Jacox, 1977; Moore, 1970).

## CONCEPTUAL BASIS FOR THE STUDY

It is evident that the fate of nursing has been molded by the predominance of women in its ranks, and feminist theory has provided the basis for this study. As stated by the late JoAnn Asyley (1976):

The role of nursing in the health field is the epitome of women's role in American society. Not accorded full professional status or an opportunity to obtain it, the nurse is viewed as a working female who is not expected to make a life long commitment to her career. (p. 125)

From the beginning of modern nursing in the 19th century, the nurse's role was seen as simply an extension of a woman's expected role as caregiver and nurturer. Thus, developing nursing roles of those early days were defined in terms of the stereotyped feminine behaviors of the time: submissiveness, dependency, and deference to authority (Kalisch & Kalisch, 1982; Lowery-Palmer, 1982), behaviors inconsistent with autonomy. Even contemporary nursing continues to be influenced by similar stereotyping in the socialization experienced by the majority of its members, both as women and as nurses.

## Themes in the Autonomy of Women

In an earlier paper (Schutzenhofer, 1983), this author noted several themes evident in the study of autonomy in women. Generally, these themes related to forces that limited the development and exercise of autonomy by women. Several of these will be discussed here.

The first of these, which limits the study of the status of autonomy in women, is the poor fit of current models of adult development to the experiences of women. From Freud to Levinson and other contemporary theorists, much research in adult development has focused on the male, generalizing these findings to the female without consideration of possible differences in their developmental experiences (Kahnweller & Johnson, 1980; Pinch, 1981). When such differences are acknowledged, they are sometimes equated with being lesser or somehow inferior to the experiences of men, without simply being recognized as different without any kind of value assigned (Barnett, Baruch, Dibner, & Parlea, 1976; Chesler, 1973; Pinch, 1981; Sochen, 1979). Since some theories view only men as normally autonomous and assertive and women as normally passive and submissive, a double standard of development and relatively little valid research on the autonomy of women exist (Chesler, 1973; Pinch, 1981).

From the nursery, where we were wrapped in pink or blue blankets, throughout the rest of our lives, women and men have experienced different socializations, the second theme. Two examples demonstrate the limiting effect this can have on the autonomy of women. Nurturance has been traditionally viewed as a female characteristic. In the name of nurturance, women have too often been socialized to put others before self (Chesler, 1973; Chodorow, 1974; O'Neil & Bush, 1978; Sochen, 1979). This other-centeredness influences the way women value and view relationships in contrast to men, with women experiencing a strong sense of responsibility in their relationships (Chesler, 1973; Chodorow, 1974; Gilligan, 1977; 1979). While there is value in this other-centeredness, it can frequently result in women's equating their own wants with selfishness and to consider acting on these wants as wrong (Chodorow, 1974; Gilligan, 1977, 1979). Thus, some women tend to equate goodness with self-sacrifice, a trend noted in nurses who work extra shifts, skip their meals and breaks, and tolerate terrible working conditions in the name of nurturance and duty to their patients.

Also related to these socialization experiences is identity formation. Whereas American men tend to be identified through their work, women's identities are often defined relationally: someone's wife, mother, sister, and so on. Women have been traditionally without such an occupational identity (Bardwick & Douvan, 1972; Chodorow, 1974; Miller, 1976). It may be very diffficult for a woman to act out various aspects of her life without external constraints when her very identity is defined externally. Perhaps this is why some nurses describe themselves as "only a nurse," just as some homemakers describe themselves as "only a housewife."

Another, and one of the most powerful themes that may limit autonomy in women, is that of legal constraints that permeate the socialization of women. Influenced by religious and social values, laws at all levels of government have contributed to differences in the autonomy of men and women (Grissum & Spengler, 1976). Women have at times been viewed as the property of their husbands and denied certain rights guaranteed to men: the rights to vote, to hold property, to have credit in their own names, and to retain after marriage the names given them at birth. Allthough these laws have slowly changed, the attitudes that support traditional constraints change even more slowly. Some of these attitudes seem to underlie the attempts of groups outside nursing to control education and practice through legislative changes.

Another theme noted is the relationship of autonomy to decision making. Heath (1968) linked decision-making skills to autonomy in mature adults. Women in traditional homemaker roles have had both legal and social limitations on their decision-making opportunities, not only in the public sphere but in the home as well (Barnett et al., 1976; Chesler, 1973; Dowling, 1981; Harway & Astin, 1977; Knapp, 1981; O'Neil & Bush, 1978). Traditionally, decorating the home has been considered a woman's domain of decision making, but the law often gave only her husband the right to decide where that home would be (Grissum & Spengler, 1976). Gilligan (1977), in her study on moral decision making among women, quoted a well-educated, middle-adult woman with three adolescent daughters, who illustrated the effects of these constraints on decision-making skills:

> As a women, I feel I never understood that I was a person, that I can make decisions and have a right to make decisions. I always felt that I belonged to my father or my husband. . . I still let things happen, than to make choices, although I know all about choices. (p. 487)

The constraints on decision making in nursing, although often artificial and arbitrary, have been accepted too frequently by nurses who lacked sufficient experience in decision making to challenge the system.

## Limiting Forces within Nursing

In addition to those themes just identified that apply to women in general, themes or forces unique to nursing have further impaired the development and exercise of professional autonomy by nurses. Paternalism, on the part of both physicians and hospital administrators, was identified by Ashley (1976) as a force limiting the autonomy of nurses and nursing from its earliest days. Ashley's work documents the efforts of both physicians and hospital administrators to control both the education and the practice of nurses to prevent nursing from becoming independent of medicine. Paternalism continues to be evidenced in the efforts of medicine and other groups to limit the scope of practice of nurses, especially nurse midwives and nurse practitioners.

While the long-term impact of paternalism cannot be minimized, other limitations on professional autonomy in nursing lie within the profession itself. The passivity of nurses who accept without protest efforts to constrain their practice help's to perpetuate the failure of nursing to achieve full professional status.

The other-centeredness previously noted in relation to women in general has strong implications for nurses. Being all things to all people is still accepted by some nurses, who also try to be pharmacists, occupational therapists, and janitors in an effort to meet the needs of not only their patients but the employing institution as well (Welch, 1980).

The work environment of nurses also tends to limit their autonomy. Hospital policies that constrain the practice of nurses, the indifference of administrators to nurses' ideas and needs, and inadequate staffing are examples of environmental forces that can influence the development and exercise of professional autonomy, forces fostered by the reluctance of nurses to demand change (Davis, Kramer, & Strauss, 1975; Lysaught, 1981; Maas & Jacox, 1977; Wandelt, Pierce, & Widdowson, 1981).

Nursing education is another powerful force that has impaired the autonomy of nurses. The regimentation of students, the tangled web of educational programs that lead to nursing licensure, and the rigidity of learning experiences have all been cited as faults of nursing education that limit students' opportunities to act autonomously (Ashley, 1976, 1980; Cohen, 1981; Leininger, 1970; Welch, 1980). Thus, some nurses have never recognized their failure to develop a sense of professional autonomy, and they practice in a constricted and purely technical nursing role (Grissum & Spengler, 1976).

## DEVELOPING THE SCHUTZENHOFER PROFESSIONAL AUTONOMY SCALE: METHODOLOGY AND RESULTS

As previously noted, recent efforts to increase the autonomy of nurses demand instruments that measure this characteristic. One such instrument has been in use for over a decade. The Pankratz & Pankratz Scale

(1974) is not without certain measurement problems. This 47-item instrument has three subscales that actually measure three interrelated variables: nursing autonomy, patient rights, and rejection of the traditional nursing role. Additionally, the variable of nursing autonomy is linked with the advocacy role. Of the 26 items that comprise the autonomy/advocacy subscale, 10 deal with advocacy, and 6 items of the 26 are also co-measures of either patient rights or rejection of the traditional nursing role. Hence, both the overall scale and even the autonomy subscale are of limited usefulness in measuring professional nursing autonomy.

The wording of several items in the scale further limits its measurement usefulness. One item in the autonomy subscale reads: "I should have the right to know why a change is necessary before it is accepted." The unnecessary qualifier "should" clouds the exact meaning of the item, shifting the emphasis of the item to whether the nurse deserves a certain right from what appears to be the main focus of the item, involvement of the nurse in institutional change. Additionally, the nature of the change proposed is ambiguous. A nurse might respond differently to an item that deals with institutional change regarding meal times in the cafeteria than to an item dealing with changes in personnel policies or in patient care procedures. Another item reads: "I rarely ask a patient a personal question." Nursing histories are replete with questions about patients' menstrual cycles, elimination patterns, dietary habits, and family background. In any context these would be considered personal questions, and therefore, few nurses in clinical practice could agree with the item, unless the nurse simply lacks the opportunity to ask such questions during the course of patient contact. However, if the item seeks to measure the nurse's attitude about asking questions of a personal or sensitive nature, then a more precisely worded item might be more effective in achieving that intent.

The use of a 5-point Likert scale (strongly agree, agree, undecided, disagree, and strongly disagree) presents another potential problem of measurement. Can one be assured that a respondent who is undecided on selected items is more autonomous than a respondent who disagrees, as the scoring of some items would imply? Furthermore, there is no indication that the items in the autonomy subscale represent behaviors that reflect a range of autonomous activity. Without any effort to weight the items in the autonomy subscale, it appears that all items represent behaviors that are equally autonomous. Thus, a nurse who is very autonomous according to the Pankratz and Pankratz Scale (1974) in effect carries out greater numbers of autonomous behaviors than a less autonomous nurse. This seems to oversimplify the measurement of professional autonomy.

With these problems in mind, this study was aimed at developing an instrument that measured only professional autonomy. The process of item development focused on the generation of clearly worded items that reflected only the concept of professional autonomy. Additionally, a means of measurement was sought that recognized that some behaviors are more autonomous than others.

The instrument that was developed in this study, the Schutzenhofer Professional Nursing Autonomy Scale (SPNAS), is the product of a two-stage effort. The initial 12-item scale developed in Stage 1 proved not to meet the standards for the statistical methods utilized. A revised, 30-item scale was developed in the second stage of the study after a change in methodology.

## Stage 1: Item Development

The original 12-item professional autonomy scale was developed from a pool of 29 items drawn from the nursing literature and from a survey of deans and selected directors of nursing service and clinical specialists at major hospitals in the St.Louis area. Shaw and Wright (1967) recommend the use of content experts in the development of scale items to strengthen the content validity of the items. Therefore, the nursing literature was consulted for examples of autonomous behavior, since the ideas of these authors had passed the rigors of peer review. Additionally, selected nursing leaders in the metropolitan area were polled for their expertise in line with Shaw and Wright's recommendation.

Some items offered by the panel of nursing leaders were immediately rejected because they were specific to certain clinical specialties. Items included in the scale had to be applicable across clinical specialties. Some were similar to other items and were not included in the initial pool. Twenty-nine items were submitted to a panel of doctorally prepared nursing faculty for review and ranking. Some items were rejected because they were viewed as addressing additional variables, such as ethics, or nursing issues and trends, such as nursing diagnoses, with which many nurses may be unfamiliar.

The remaining 20 items were rated by the panel of nursing faculty who rated them as reflecting low, medium, or high levels of professional autonomy. The Statistical Package for the Social Sciences SPSS (Nie, Bent & Hull, 1975) used to analyze these data limited a scale to 12 items. Thus, four items from each of the three rating categories were included in the instrument. Selected items represented the highest levels of interrater agreement within each category, with each item demonstrating interrater agreement of .80 or higher. The items included in both stages of instrument development dealt only with the variable of professional autonomy, were not specific to any one clinical area, and described situations in which the nurse must act autonomously to some degree.

## Administration and Scoring

The tool is a self-report paper-and-pencil instrument that consists of 35 items of which only 30 are scored. The respondents use a 4-point scale to indicate the likelihood of their carrying out the actions described in the items in the instrument (Table 1.1). The instrument is scored by weighting items on a scale of 1 to 3 (low to high) based on the adjusted ratings of the respondents in the second stage of the study. Scores can range from 60 to 240 and are based on the summation of weighted item scores.

Five additional items were added to the scale as experimental items but are not included in the scoring (see Table 1.2 for examples). These experimental items should be compared with selected scale items as an additional measure of reliability. The experimental items represent the same categories of nursing action as the instrument items but reflect dependent, deferent, or self-effacing outcomes. Examples of experimental items were "assume all blame for any conflicts I have with physicians"; "administer a medication to which a patient reports an allergy if the physician will assume responsibility for my actions."

Comments from respondents indicated some problems with the clarity of some of the experimental items included on the measure. These problems will be dealt with during further use of the instrument. Despite problems with the wording, data analysis revealed an $r$ of .58. Additional reliability studies are being conducted.

**TABLE 1.1 Rating Scale for Responding to Professional Autonomy Items**

1 = Very unlikely of me to act in this manner
2 = Unlikely of me to act in this manner
3 = Likely of me to act in this manner
4 = Very likely of me to act in this manner

**TABLE 1.2 Examples of Scale Items and Experimental Items**

S: Report incidents of physician harassment to the appropriate manager or administrator.
E: Assume all blame for any conflicts I have with physicians.
S: Assume complete responsibility for my own professional actions without expecting to be protected by the physician or hospital in the case of a malpractice suit.
E: Administer a medication to which a patient reports an allergy if the physician will assume responsibility for my actions.

## The Samples

The original scale was tested on two groups of registered nurses (RNs). Only female RNs were included in both stages of instrument development since female socialization is considered an important factor in the development and exercise of professional autonomy, as identified in the conceptual framework of the study. A convenience sample of 68 RN and BSN students in a degree-completion program was the first group tested. When the responses of the first group of respondents proved nonscalable (see Data Analysis below), the instrument was then submitted to a second sample. This second group, which provided 133 usable responses, was obtained from a computerized random sample of 250 RNs who lived in the St.Louis area.

The typical respondent in the RN-BSN group was 28.8 years old, not currently married, and employed at least part-time. She had been graduated from a diploma program 5.9 years earlier, had worked 5.5 years in nursing, and held no degree of any kind. The typical respondent from the random sample was 35.7 years old, married, a diploma graduate of 12.1 years earlier, and not currently enrolled in school. She held no degree of any kind and had worked for 10.5 years in nursing.

## Data Analysis

Respondents in both groups during this first stage of the study replied to the 12-item scale with agree-disagree. In a theoretically perfect Guttman Scale, respondents would all agree with the least difficult item and disagree with the most difficult item, in this case the least autonomous act to the most autonomous act (Nie et al., 1975). The critical statistic of Guttman Scale analysis is Rep, the coefficient of reproducidility. This is a proportion that can range from 0 to 1 (Nie et al., 1975). A Rep of .90 was the minimally acceptable level for proof of scalability for this study. A Rep of .81 was obtained from the RN-BSN student group and a Rep of .82 was obtained in the analysis of the data from the random sample RN group. Both statistics fell below the acceptable level.

A major weakness of the Guttman Technique is that an instrument may prove scalable with one group but not with another from the same population (Nie et al., 1975). The differential rankings by these two groups illustrated this weakness. While both Reps approached the acceptable level for scalability, both fell short, and the rank order of the items differed for the two groups.

## Stage 2

Because of the problems inherent in Guttman technique, the methodology was changed in the second stage of the study. The scale was expanded to 30 items to improve the reliability of the scale. Five items were revised for clarity, stemming from the comments made by respondents in the first stage. Six additional items were added from the original pool of 29, and 12 new items were developed by a group of nursing faculty. The items were again rated, as in the first stage, by doctorally prepared nursing faculty to develop a range of items by tentative level of autonomy, thus ensuring a range of autonomous behavior.

## The Sample

This revised scale was mailed to a random sample of 500 female RNs in the state of Missouri who had indicated, on the latest survey of RNs by the state board of nursing, that they were employed. One hundred nineteen usable responses were received (response rate of 23.8%). The typical respondent in this sample was 38.2 years old, married, and a diploma program graduate of 16 years earlier. She was not currently in school and held no degree. She had worked 14.0 years as an RN. The demographic questionnaire included an item on current employment, and only data from nurses reporting current employment were used; this was done to ensure familiarity with contemporary nursing practice and issues. Anecdotal comments from some unemployed respondents in the random sample of Stage 1 indicated a lack of familiarity with terms such as independent practice, nursing research, and nursing orders.

The respondents were asked how autonomous a nurse had to be in order to carry out the situations by rating the items on a scale of 1 to 5, moving from very low to very high levels of professional autonomy. Those participating in this stage of the study were provided with the working definition of professional autonomy noted earlier in this chapter. Anecdotal comments from a number of respondents in the first stage indicated that they had little or no understanding of the concept of professional autonomy. Since this group was serving as a panel of nursing experts in rating these items, it was essential that they understood the concept of professional autonomy.

## Data Analysis

Data analysis was completed using Cronbach's alpha as a measure of internal consistency of responses. An alpha of .92 was obtained, indicating a high level of reliability of the responses. It was noted that there was a tendency of the respondents not to rate items as a 1 or a 2 (the lower levels of autonomy). The most obvious explanation of this event is that few respondents viewed any of the items as representing the lower levels of professional autonomy. However, more than 40 of the respondents wrote comments on the instrument indicating that a rating of 3 reflected what any RN would do, thus inclusive of lower levels of autonomy. Because of this pattern of responses and the comments, data were reanalyzed using a 3-point scale, collapsing the original ratings of 1, 2, and 3 into the new rating of 1, with the original ratings of 4 and 5 now equivalent to 2 and 3, respectively. This analysis yielded an alpha of .91.

If, under the original 5-point rating scale, the items had grouped perfectly into five discrete categories of six items each, with six items receiving a rating of 1, six items rated a 2, and so on, the mean score of the ratings by the random sample of nurses should have been 90. However, the real mean score for these ratings was 115. With the rating scale revised to a 3-point system, ideally the 30 items would have now fallen into three categories of 10 items each, with 10 items rated as a 1, 10 as a 2, and 10 as a 3. Under this approach, the mean score of ratings should have been 60, and the actual mean was 60.81. The mean of the ratings was a useful statistic only in determining the evenness of distribution of items by their rated level of autonomy.

Content validity of the scale, as previously noted, is addressed through the use of nursing experts and the nursing literature for the generation of the items (Shaw & Wright, 1967). Anecdotal comments generated by the respondents in both stages of the study aided in editing the items for clarity but also demonstrated the appropriateness of the items to the topic of the instrument. Internal reliability of the scale was established through the alpha scores of .91 and .92. Initial efforts to determine reliability of the instrument in use are addressed below.

## Testing of the Instrument

Reliability data were obtained by using a test-retest approach with a convenience sample of 58 RN-BSN students (a different cohort from the original sample in the first stage of the study). The instrument was administered twice, at a 4-week interval. Respondents were mostly female ($N = 55$), married, and diploma graduates. The mean age was 31.6 years. The typical respondent had graduated from a diploma program 8 years earlier but held no degree and was currently employed as a staff nurse on a medical/surgical unit, having worked for 6.3 years since graduation. Correlation of the two sets of responses yielded an $r$ of .79.

## DISCUSSION

Future use of the Schutzenhofer Professional Nursing Autonomy Scale by the author includes a longitudinal study of RNs in a BSN completion program and a study of RNs to identify correlates of professional autonomy. Additional research on the professional autonomy of RNs needs to be directed at identifying personal and behavioral characteristics of RNs that are related to both high and low levels of autonomous behaviors. Recognition of such characteristics can aid in furthering the development of both individual practitioners and the profession as a whole. Identification of these characteristics could assist in the selection of candidates for nursing education programs. Education programs, including staff development, could engage teaching methodologies that foster the development of those characteristics that are learned behaviors. Other research might seek to measure the effectiveness of educational efforts to increase the professional autonomy of RNs.

## REFERENCES

Ashley, J. (1976). *Hospitals, paternalism, and the role of the nurse.* New York: Teacher's College Press.

Ashley, J. (1980). Power in structured misogyny: Implications for the politics of care. *Advances in Nursing Science, 2*(3), 3-22.

Barber, B. (1965). Some problems in the sociology of the professions. In K. S. Lynn (Ed.), *The professions in America* (pp. 15-34). Boston: Houghton-Mifflin.

Bardwick, J. M., & Douvan, E. (1972). Ambivalence: The socialization of women. In J. M. Bardwick (Ed.), *Readings on the psychology of women* (pp. 52-58). New York: Harper & Row.

Barnett, R. C., Baruch, G. D., Dibner, S., & Parlea, M. B. (1976). *Will the real middle-aged woman please stand up? Toward an understanding of adult development in women.* New York: Eastern Psychologhcal Association. (ERIC Document Reproduction Services No. ED 130 215).

Chesler, P. (1973). *Women and madness.* New York: Avon Books.

Chodorow, N. (1974). Family structure and feminine personality. In M. Zimbalist, A. Rosaldo, & L. Lamphere (Eds.), *Woman, culture and society* (pp. 43-46). Stanford, Ca: Stanford University Press.

Cohen, M. E. (1981). *The nurse's quest for a new professional identity.* Menlo Park, CA: Addison-Wesley.

Davis, M. Z., Kramer, M., & Strauss, A. L. (1975). *Nurses in practice: A perspective on work environments.* St. Louis: C. V. Mosby.

Dowling, C. (1981). *The Cinderella complex: Women's hidden fear of independence.* New York: Summit Books.

Engel, G. V. (1970). Professional autonomy and the bureaucratic organization. *Administrative Science Quarterly, 30*, 12-21.

Gilligan, C. (1977). In a different voice: Women's conception of self and of morality. *Harvard Educational Review, 47*, 481-517.

Gilligan, C. (1979). Woman's place in man's life cycle. *Harvard Educational Review, 49*, 431-446.

Grissum, M., & Spengler, C. (1976). *Woman power and health care.* Boston: Little, Brown.

Harway, M., & Astin, H. S. (1977). *Sex discrimination in career counseling and education.* New York: Praeger.

Heath, D. H. (1968). *Growing up in college.* San Francisco: Jossey-Bass.

Kahnweller, J. B., & Johnson, P. L. (1980). A midlife developmental profile of the returning woman student. *Journal of College Student Personnel, 21*,414-419.

Kalisch, B. J., & Kalisch, P. A. (1982). An analysis of the sources of physician-nurse conflict. In J. Muff (Ed.), *Socialization, sexism and stereotyping: Women's issues in nursing* (pp. 221-233). St. Louis: C. V. Mosby.

Knapp, M. S. (1981). Response to a neglected need: Resocializing dependent women. *Lifelong Learning/The Adult Years, 28*(10), 12-13; 25.

Leininger, M. M. (1970). *Nursing and anthropology: Two worlds to blend.* New York: John Wiley.

Lowery-Palmer, A. (1982). The cultural basis of political behavior in two groups: Nurses and political activists. In J. Muff (ED.), *Socialization, sexism,* and stereotyping: Women's issues in nursing (pp. 189-209). St.Louis: C. V. Mosby.

Lysaught, J. P. (1981). *Action in affirmation: Toward an unambiguous profession of nursing*. New York: McGraw-Hill.

Maas, M., & Jacox, A. K. (1977). *Guidelines for nurse autonomy/patient welfare*. New York: Appleton-Century-Crofts.

Moore, W. E. (1970). *The professions: Roles and rules*. New York: Russell Sage Foundation.

Miller, J. B. (1976). *Toward a new psychology of women*. Boston: Beacon Press.

Nie, N., Bent, D. H., & Hull, C. H. (1975). *SPSS: Statistical Package for the Social Sciences* (2nd ed.). New York: McGraw-Hill.

O'Neil, J. M., & Bush, B. E. (1978). Psychosocial factors affecting career development of adult women. In D. P. Garner (Ed.), *The career educator:Vol. 2: The adult learner, the world of work, and career education* (pp. 70-90). Dubuque, IA: Kendall/Hunt.

Pankratz, L., & Pankratz, D. (1974). Nursing autonomy and patient rights: development of a nursing attitude scale. *Journal of Health and Social Behavior, 15*, 211-216.

Pinch, W. J. (1981). Feminine attributes in a masculine world. *Nursing Outlook, 29*, 596-599.

Schutzenhofer, K. K. (1983). The development of autonomy in adult women. *Journal of Psychosocial Nursing and Mental Health Services, 21*(4), 25-30.

Shaw, M. E., & Wright, J. M. (1967). *Scales for the measurement of attitudes*. New York: McGraw-Hill.

Sochen, J. (1979). The "new, new" woman. In D. H. Salene & M. D. Jacobson (Eds.), *Managing the lifecycle. Conference proceedings and commissioned papers*. Evanstone, IL: Northwestern University. (ERIC Document Reproduction Service No. ED 181 189).

Stuart, F. W. (1981). How professionalized is nursing? *Image, 12*, 18-23.

Wandelt, M. A., Pierce, P. M., & Widdowson, R. R. (1981). Why nurses leave nursing and what can be done about it. *American Journal of Nursing, 81*, 72-77.

Welch, M. J. (1980). Dysfunctional parenting of a profession. *Nursing Outlook, 28*, 724-727.

# Schutzenhofer Professional Nursing Autonomy Scale

The following items describe situations in which a nurse must take some action that requires the exercise of professional nursing judgment. You are asked to respond to each item according to how likely you would be to carry out the action in each item. Please respond to *each item* even if you have not encountered such a situation before. Use the following scale in responding to the items.

1 = Very unlikely of me to act in this manner
2 = Unlikely of me to act in this manner
3 = Likely of me to act in this manner
4 = Very likely of me to act in this manner

Circle the number after each situation that best describes how you would act as a nurse. There are no right or wrong answers.

Code Number _____

| | Very unlikely | Unlikely | Likely | Very likely | Do not mark in this space |
|---|---|---|---|---|---|
| 1. Develop a career plan for myself and regularly review it for achievement of steps in the plan. | 1 | 2 | 3 | 4 | _____ |
| 2. Consider entry into independent nursing practice with the appropriate education and experience. | 1 | 2 | 3 | 4 | _____ |
| 3. Voice opposition to any medical order to discharge a patient without an opportunity for nursing follow-up if my teaching plan for the patient is not completed. | 1 | 2 | 3 | 4 | _____ |
| 4. Initiate clinical research to investigate a recurrent clinical nursing problem. | 1 | 2 | 3 | 4 | _____ |
| 5. Refuse to administer a contraindicated drug despite the physician's insistence that the drug be given. | 1 | 2 | 3 | 4 | _____ |
| 6. Consult with the patient's physician if the patient is not responding to the treatment plan. | 1 | 2 | 3 | 4 | _____ |
| 7. Depend upon the profession of nursing and not on physicians for the ultimate determination of what I do as a nurse. | 1 | 2 | 3 | 4 | _____ |
| 8. Evaluate the hospitalized patient's need for home nursing care and determine the need for such a referral without a medical order. | 1 | 2 | 3 | 4 | _____ |
| 9. Accept a temporary assignment to a unit even if I lack the education and experience to work in that unit. | 1 | 2 | 3 | 4 | _____ |

10. Propose changes in my job description to my super-
    visor in order to develop the position further.        1    2    3    4    _____
11. Answer the patient's questions about a new medica-
    tion or a change in medication before administering
    a drug, whether or not this has been done previ-
    ously by the physician.                                 1    2    3    4    _____
12. Institute nursing rounds.                               1    2    3    4    _____
13. Withhold a medicine that is contraindicated for a
    patient despite pressure from nursing peers to carry
    our the medical order.                                  1    2    3    4    _____
14. Consult with other nurses when a patient is not
    responding to the plan of nursing care.                 1    2    3    4    _____
15. Routinely implement innovations in patient care iden-
    tified in the current nursing literature.               1    2    3    4    _____
16. Initiate a request for a psychiatric consult with the
    patient's physician if my assessment of the patient
    indicates such a need.                                  1    2    3    4    _____
17. Promote innovative nursing activities, like follow-up
    phone calls to recently discharged patients, to evalu-
    ate the effectiveness of patient teaching.              1    2    3    4    _____
18. Assess the patient's level of understanding concern-
    ing a diagnostic procedure and its risks before con-
    sulting with the patients physician if a patient has
    questions about the risks of the procedure.             1    2    3    4    _____
19. Assume complete responsibility for my own profes-
    sional actions without expecting to be protected by
    the physician or hospital in the case of a malpractice
    suit.                                                   1    2    3    4    _____
20. Develop effective communication channels in my
    employing institution for nurses' input regarding the
    policies that affect patient care.                      1    2    3    4    _____
21. Make appropriate in-house referrals to social service
    and dietary only after obtaining a medical order.       1    2    3    4    _____
22. Develop and refine assessment tools appropriate to
    my area of clinical practice.                           1    2    3    4    _____
23. Record in the chart the data from my physical
    assessment of the patient to use in planning and
    implementing nursing care.                              1    2    3    4    _____
24. Initiate discharge planning concerning the nursing
    care of the patient, even in the absence of medical
    discharge planning.                                     1    2    3    4    _____
25. Report incidents of physician harassment to the
    appropriate manager or administrator.                   1    2    3    4    _____
26. Offer input to administrators concerning the design
    of a new nursing unit or the purchase of new equip-
    ment to be used by nurses.                              1    2    3    4    _____
27. Complete a psychosocial assessment on each patient
    and use this data in formulating nursing care.          1    2    3    4    _____
28. Adapt assessment tools from other disciplines to use
    in my clinical area.                                    1    2    3    4    _____

29. Carry out patient care procedures utilizing my professional judgment to meet the individual patient's needs even when this means deviating from the "cookbook" description in the hospital procedure manual.                                              1    2    3    4 _____
30. Decline a temporary reassignment to a specialty unit when I lack the education and experience to carry out the demands of the assignment.                    1    2    3    4 _____
31. Initiate referrals to social service and dietary at the patient's request.                                       1    2    3    4 _____
32. Assess needs of patient for home nursing care only under order of physician.                               1    2    3    4 _____
33. Write nursing orders to increase the frequency of vital signs of a patient whose condition is deteriorating even in the absence of a medical order to increase the frequency of such monitoring.            1    2    3    4 _____
34. Administer a medication to which a patient reports an allergy if the physician will assume responsibility for my actions.                                         1    2    3    4 _____
35. Assume all blame for any conflicts or problems I have with physicians.                                       1    2    3    4 _____

## SCORING INSTRUCTIONS FOR THE SCHUTZENHOFER PROFESSIONAL NURSING AUTONOMY SCALE

Of the 35 items in the instrument, only 30 are scored. Five items (Nos. 9, 21, 32, 34, 35) are nonscored items that are used in comparison with five scale items for continuing measure of internal consistency. You may omit these items when using the scale. If you include these items in your use of the scale, please send the results to me (either the raw data or the correlation scores). The items that are compared are listed below:

| Experimental Items | Scale Items |
| --- | --- |
| 9 | 30 |
| 21 | 31 |
| 32 | 8 |
| 34 | 19 |
| 35 | 25 |

The table below gives the weight for each scale item. A weight of 1 indicates a low level of autonomy; a weight of 3 reflects a high level.

| Item | Weight | Item | Weight | Item | Weight |
|------|--------|------|--------|------|--------|
| 1    | 3      | 12   | 3      | 23   | 2      |
| 2    | 3      | 13   | 3      | 24   | 1      |
| 3    | 3      | 14   | 2      | 25   | 2      |
| 4    | 3      | 15   | 1      | 26   | 2      |
| 5    | 3      | 16   | 1      | 27   | 1      |
| 6    | 3      | 17   | 2      | 28   | 1      |
| 7    | 2      | 18   | 1      | 29   | 2      |
| 8    | 1      | 19   | 3      | 30   | 3      |
| 10   | 1      | 20   | 2      | 31   | 1      |
| 11   | 2      | 22   | 2      | 33   | 1      |

Multiply the respondent's score on each item by the weight of the item. Total these adjusted scores. Scores can range from 60 to 240 with the following breakdown for approximate levels of autonomy:

  60 to 120 = lower level of professional autonomy
  121 to 180 = mid level of professional autonomy
  181 to 240 = higher level of professional autonomy

Questions regarding scoring should be sent to Karen Kelly Schutzenhofer, R.N., Ed.D., Assistant Dean, School of Nursing, University of Missouri-St. Louis, 8001 Natural Bridge Road, St. Louis, MO 63121.

# 2

# Measuring Nursing Care Role Orientation

*Jacqueline Stemple*

*This chapter discusses the Nursing Care Role Orientation Scale, a measure of orientation to the nursing care role on the part of nurses.*

## PURPOSE

The purpose of the study was to further develop an instrument to measure nursing care role orientation.

## CONCEPTUAL BASIS

The framework for the Nursing Care Role Orientation Scale is based on a synthesis of nursing theory derived through the analysis of the writings of several nursing theorists (Harmer, 1922; Harmer & Henderson, 1955; Kinlein, 1977; Nightingale, 1859; Orem, 1971, 1980; Smith, 1979). The characteristics of a profession, as suggested by Lysaught (1981), was also used, as well as the conceptual framework of one school of nursing. As nursing moves in the direction of an unambigious profession, it is necessary to develop an instrument that measures nursing care role orientation based on a sound nursing theoretical framework.

An additional indication of the need to measure the nursing care role orientation of nurses is the fact that there has been as increase in the number of publications in nursing journals dealing with the concept of self-care, from three articles located via Med-line search in 1977 to more than 150 articles located in a fall 1983 Med-line search. No such instrument was available despite the marked increase in the number of publications on self-care since 1977.

The contribution of John J. Paterson, Ed.D, Professor of Educational Psychology, West Virginia University, in the instrument development is acknowledged.

The nursing role orientation tool was initially developed from one specific graduate curriculum that embodied a strong self-care philosophical base. The philosophy of the school included this statement about nursing: "Specifically, the purpose of nursing is to assist clients, wherever they are, in the performance of those activities contributing to optimal health (or a peaceful death) that the clients would normally initiate and perform unaided if they had the necessary strength, knowledge, and motivation" (WVUSN, 1984). This statement can be recognized as based on Henderson's (1978) well-known definition of nursing. The tool was further tested for generalizability on a population of associate-degree and baccalaureate-degree students. It was believed that there are major concepts in the curriculum that are similar across schools. Stemple (1981) used factor analytic techniques to determine the factors underlying nursing role orientation. The factors identified were nurse/client, research, collaboration, and independent nursing practice.

The nurse/client dimension includes items that reflect a positive orientation toward health promotion. Since the early 1960s nursing education has emphasized the importance of health promotion in nursing curriculum development. However, as late as 1964, Simmons and Henderson reported that the role of nurse as teacher was controversial, and yet as early as 1859 Nightingale recognized and addressed the need for greater knowledge in maintaining one's health. The factor of nurse/client included items thought to measure knowledge, health/illness, decision making, and action.

The second factor of nursing care role orientation is research. In a practice discipline such as nursing, theory, research, and practice are interrelated and interdependent. Theory may be created and initiated in practice, tested in research, and returned to practice for further development. The Nursing Development Conference Group (NDCG) 1973 emphasized the importance of the synthesis of theory, practice, and research.

> To theorize is to create a conceptual framework to some purpose. A concept of nursing has concrete referents, it deals with the real world where nursing is practiced but it frees thought and expression from the domination of that real world. If the concept is too static and over verbalized, however, it will make inadequate reference to actual nursing situations. A static concept of nursing, then, must continue to become dynamic in the fields of research and practice. (p.23)

Henderson (1966) stated: "When a nurse operated under a definition of nursing that specified an area in which she is preeminently qualified, she automatically imposes on herself the responsibility for designing the methods she uses in her area of expertise" p.32. Based on the review of the literature on the interrelationship and interdependence of research, theory, and practice, it was concluded that research is an important element in nursing care role orientation.

The third factor of nursing care role orientation is collaboration. Observation as a basic tool was discussed by Nightingale (1859, pp. 69-70), and collaboration was suggested as a means of improving health care. The nurse should have "the power of laying clearly and shortly the factors from which she derives her opinion" p.69. As stated by Henderson 1966, "The final test of each health worker is how effectively he or she can work collaboratively with other health and welfare workers in the community who serve the client and his family" p.67.

The fourth factor of nursing care role orientation is autonomy or independent nursing practice. Henderson (1966, 1978) conceptualized nursing from a self-care perspective and emphasized the independent nature of nursing. She suggested that the nurse should be the authority on basic nursing care, that is, helping the client with activities of daily living or providing conditions to make it possible for the client to perform them unaided. Kinlein 1977, who established an independent nursing practice in 1971, stated: "Nursing is assisting the person in his self-care practices in regard to his state of health" pp. 23-24.

Taking into consideration the types of nursing related to sickness and health, Nightingale 1859 presented a clear autonomous role for the nurse and also advocated greater consumer responsibility for the consumer's own health. Lysaught (1981) reported that "progress in clinical authority and judgment has been made" (p.23). Analysis of the above writings provided support for the autonomy dimension of nursing care role orientation.

These factors are similar to four of the six characteristics of a profession as described by Lysaught (1981). Strong level of committment is related to nurse/client; unique body of knowledge and skill is related to research; acknowledged social worth and contribution may be related to collaboration; and discretionary authority and judgment are related to independent nursing practice or autonomy. Results of the initial instrument validation studies led to the development of an instrument that needed further refinement.

## PILOT INSTRUMENT DEVELOPMENT

The Nursing Role Orientation Scale was initially developed with a sample of 312 nursing students enrolled in the 1978 fall semester at a southeastern university. The original scale consisted of 20 items. Each item was structured in a modified Likert scale format to elicit views on a particular nursing concept.

The item content selected was based on the literature review of past and current concepts of nursing related to nursing care role. In addition, a selected university school of nursing's conceptual framework was reviewed, and the self-care component of this conceptual framework was reflected in some of the items. The scale was reviewed for content validity by five members of the graduate faculty of the selected university, all of whom believed in the self-care concept of nursing.

Using the data from the 312 nursing students, five factors were determined from the Varimax rotation. The five factors accounted for a total of 51% of the variance. Of the 20 items, 6 were found to measure directly the concept of nurse/client, 3 to measure independent nursing practice, 4 to measure the importance of research to nursing practice, 5 to measure collaboration, and 2 to measure the importance of professional growth.

Analysis of the data also consisted of computing item-total correlations. Of the 20 items in the original scale, 6 were deleted due to low item-total correlation. Ten of the items were retained in their original form, four were modified slightly, and three new items were written. The revised instrument was a 17-item scale designed to measure factors comprising a nursing care role orientation.

The revised 17-item scale was used in study 2 with 77 nursing students in the fall of 1979. Examination of the six-factor solution from the sample resulted in the decision to extract only the four factors that seemed to be interpretable. Factor analysis using those four factors accounted for 54% of the total variance. The four factors were research, collaboration, nurse/client, and autonomy. The internal consistency coefficient for the 17-item scale (coefficient alpha) was .80. Since (1) sample size was small ($N = 77$); (2) factors were not as conceptualized; and (3) the internal consistency of the total instrument was .80, it was decided to collect data from a third group of students to better determine the dimensions and psychometric properties of nursing care role orientation.

A third study was conducted in the spring of 1980 to continue the development of the 17-item instrument designed to assess nursing students' orientation to the nursing care role. The sample of the third study consisted of nursing students enrolled in the last year of their educational program. The total possible sample consisted of 403 nursing students, representing 11 schools of nursing, 235 associate-degree students, and 168 baccalaureate-degree students.

The minimum eigenvalue was set at 1.0. The factor analysis on the data from the third study yielded five factors for the nursing care role orientation scale, which accounted for 51% of the variance. Examination of the five-factor solution resulted in the decision to extract the four interpretable factors. Factor analysis using those four factors accounted for 45% of the variance. The four rotated factors with loadings of 30 or greater were named nurse/client, research, collaboration, and autonomy.

The item-total correlations performed on the study data for the 17-item scale ranged from .26 to .62, with 10 of the 17 items having a coefficient above .40. The internal consistency (coefficient alpha) for the 17-item test was .71. The coefficient alpha for the nurse/client scale (sum of seven items) was .70; for the research scale (sum of three items), .62;

for the collaboration scale (sum of three items), .45; and for the independent scale (sum of four items), .28.

As hypothesized, as the educational level of the nursing student increased, an orientation toward the nursing care role also increased. It was assumed that the subjects had been taught to have greater orientation toward the nursing care role; therefore, these results supported the validity of the construct (Stemple, 1981).

The instrument was revised for this fourth and final study. Seven new items were written, seven were revised, and ten of the original items were retained.

# METHODOLOGY

## Sample

The population consisted of all registered professional nurses in a southeastern state who had earned an associate degree (AD), baccalaureate degree (BSN), or masters degree in nursing (MSN). The total population included nurses with AD, 3, 910; ESN, 1, 492; and MSN, 231. A stratified sample of 827 registered professional nurses was selected, using a systematic sampling procedure. Of the 827 nurses there were 300 AD, 296 BSN, and 231 MSN graduates. The total response rate was 241, or 29%. For the AD the response rate was 53 or 18%, for the BSN, 78 or 26%, and for the MSN, 100 or 48%.

## Procedure

Each subject was mailed the Nursing Care Role Orientation Scale, two additional instruments that were used in a broader study, and a self-addressed stamped envelope. The subjects were requested to return the questionnaires within 2 weeks. A follow-up letter was mailed to nonrespondents 1 month after the first mailing in order to increase the response rate. Each subject was assured of the confidentiality of the data and that the data would not be used in any way to identify specific individuals.

## Administration and Scoring

The Nursing Care Role Orientation Scale is a 24-item norm-referenced instrument with a modified Likert scale format. The items are rated from 1 to 5, with a score of 5 representing a greater nursing care role orientation. The total possible score is 120. So that response bias might be decreased, some of the items were written in reverse order and were recoded before the data were analyzed.

# RESULTS

## Reliability

Cronbach's coefficient alpha was used to estimate the internal consistency of the instrument. The alpha standard was .70, an acceptable reliability estimate for exploratory scales (Nunnally, 1978). The total score of the Nursing Care Role Orientation Scale ranged from 72 to 117, with a mean of 96.8 and standard deviation of 10. The item-total correlations ranged from .11 to .68, with 19 of the 24 items having a coefficient above .40. Items 1, 10, 18, and 23 had coefficients below .30. See Table 2.1. When these items were deleted, the coefficient alpha for the 20-item scale was .87. The coefficient alpha for the 24-item scale was .83.

## Content Validity

The scale was reviewed for content validity by four school of nursing faculty members from a southeastern university. Two of the faculty were from the undergraduate program and two from the graduate program. Each faculty member was asked to select the competency from the respective program that the item best reflected. There was agreement on 15 of the 24 items, or 54% agreement, between the two undergraduate faculty members on the content reflected in the item. There was agreement on 19 of the 24 items, or 79% agreement, between the two graduate program faculty members on the concept reflected in the item.

## Construct Validity

To determine construct validity three hypotheses were tested. As hypothesized, there was a significant difference between each educational level; as the education of the nurse increased, an orientation toward nursing care role orientation increased. It was assumed that the subjects had been taught to have greater orientation toward nursing care role; therefore, these results supported the validity of the construct. A two-sample $t$-test was used to test two of the hypotheses.

### Hypothesis 1

There would be a significant difference in the nursing care role orientation scores achieved by nurses with an AD and those with a BSN in nursing. The mean score of the 45 AD graduates was 88; the mean for the 64 BSN graduates was 94. The hypothesis was supported by the data with a $t$-value of $-2.98$ ($df = 107$) at the .003 level of significance. See Table 2.2.

**TABLE 2.1 Means, Standard Deviations, and Item Total Correlations for Nursing Care Role Orientation Scale Items (*N* = 235)**

| Abbreviated item content | Mean | SD | Item-total Correlation |
|---|---|---|---|
| 1. Health care for the client (community, family, individual) in most situations is most efficiently performed | 4.4 | .83 | .17 |
| 2. The nursing care goals of Client X are determined mostly by | 4.2 | .86 | .49 |
| 3. Nursing is best defined at what point on following continuum | 3.6 | .80 | .51 |
| 4. The quality of health care for the client is increased through the nurses' | 3.8 | .88 | .51 |
| 5. It is more important to nursing that the nurse | 4.3 | .85 | .68 |
| 6. The assessment of the client's problem should begin with | 3.9 | 1.17 | .53 |
| 7. Most nursing practices should be based | 3.8 | .87 | .36 |
| 8. Nursing practice is best described by the nurses's | 3.8 | .97 | .57 |
| 9. The client in most situations if given an understanding of his health state | 3.5 | 1.19 | .49 |
| 10. Most individual's contacts with a nurse for nursing care should be | 4.2 | .90 | .29 |
| 11. The strategies for meeting the health goals of the client is best done by | 3.7 | 1.00 | .47 |
| 12. Most of the nurse-client interactions should be based on | 4.3 | .78 | .55 |
| 13. The primary data source for health assessment of the client should be obtained from the clients | 4.2 | .91 | .58 |
| 14. The health history of the client should be directed toward | 3.9 | .94 | .62 |
| 15. The identification of health goals of the client is best done by | 4.0 | .95 | .62 |
| 16. The quality of nursing care is increased more through | 3.5 | .98 | .55 |
| 17. The nurse's purpose in performing a physical exam should be to gain data to | 4.1 | .95 | .48 |
| 18. The effective program on nutrition for the client could best be developed through | 4.3 | .77 | .11 |
| 19. The obligation of the nurse should be to which of the following | 4.5 | .75 | .55 |
| 20. The life style data should be used | 4.6 | .69 | .46 |
| 21. The specific dimensions of nursing care and the specific dimensions of medical care are very | 3.6 | 1.18 | .55 |
| 22. The blood pressure data should be used | 3.4 | .97 | .56 |
| 23. The effect program on drug abuse for the client could be best developed through | 3.4 | 1.02 | .21 |
| 24. The best nursing care is determined by nurse and | 4.1 | .97 | .61 |

**TABLE 2.2** Two-Sample *t*-Test on Nursing Care
Role between AD and BSN Graduates (*N* = 109)

| Variable | *N* | Mean | SD | *t* | *df* | *p* |
|----------|-----|------|-----|-------|-----|------|
| AD | 45 | 88 | 7.8 | −2.98 | 107 | .003 |
| BSN | 64 | 94 | 10 | | | |

**TABLE 2.3** Two-Sample *t*-Test on Nursing Care
Role between BSN and MSN Graduates
(*N* = 160)

| Variable | *N* | Mean | SD | *t* | *df* | *p* |
|----------|-----|------|-----|-------|-----|-------|
| BSN | 64 | 94 | 10 | −4.84 | 158 | .0001 |
| MSN | 96 | 101 | 8 | | | |

## Hypothesis 2

There would be a significant difference in the nursing care role orientation scores achieved by nurses with a BSN and those with an MSN in nursing. The 64 BSN graduates had a mean score of 94, in comparison to a mean of 101 for the 96 MSN graduates. Therefore, the second research hypothesis was also supported by the data. The *t*-value was −4.84 (*df* = 158) at the .0001 level of significance. See Table 2.3.

The factor analysis procedure was used to test the third hypothesis.

## Hypothesis 3

The four factors of professional role orientation are collaboration, research, nurse/client, and autonomy. The research hypothesis was not supported by the data. The four interpretable factors were (a) autonomy/research, which included items 2, 3, 5, 7, 8, 10, 12, 16, 19, and 20 with factor loadings ranging from .35 to .66; (b) nurse/client, which consisted of items 6, 13, 14, 17, 21, and 22, with factor loadings ranging from .47 to .68; (c) health goals/care, which was composed of items 9, 11, 15, and 24, with factor loadings ranging from .46 to .67; and (d) collaboration, which included items 1, 4, 18, and 23, with factor loadings ranging from .37 to .70.

Although the research hypothesis was not supported, the factor analysis lends some support for the construct validity of the instrument.

The 24-item Nursing Care Role Orientation Scale was subjected to a principal component factor analysis. The factor analysis yielded eight factors with eigenvalues greater than 1, which accounted for 60% of the variance. The eight factors were not interpretable. A second factor analysis using four factors accounted for 42% of the variance. The four rotated factors with loadings of 30 greater were autonomy/research nurse/client, health goals/care, and collaboration. The coefficient alpha for the autonomy/research scale (sum of 10 items) was .75; for the nurse/client scale (sum of six items), .60; for the health goals/care scale (sum of four items), .80; and for the collaboration scale (sum of four items), .34. The first rotated factor, research/autonomy, consisted of five autonomy independent-practice items, three research items, and two nurse/client items. The second rotated factor, nurse/client, consisted of four nurse/ client items and two autonomy, or independent-practice, items. The third rotated factor, health goals/care, consisted of one nurse/client item, two collaboration items, and one autonomy, or independent-practice, item. Fourteen items obtained, factor loadings as conceptualized. Each of the factors had at least one 0 loading as recommended by Nunnally (1978).

## CONCLUSION AND LIMITATIONS

It was concluded that the 24-item Nursing Care Role Orientation Scale had reasonable estimates of content and construct validity and a reasonable reliability estimate of .83. Two of the four factors, nurse/client and collaboration, were as conceptualized. One of the factors consisted of items reflective of the additional two factors conceptualized. This was the autonomy/research factor. One factor was not as conceptualized and seemed to reflect a health goals/care component. Two of the four subscales have reasonable estimates of internal consistency; two of the subscales need further development. A limitation of the study was the low response rate. However, it is interesting to note that as the educational level of the nurse increased, the response rate increased.

## RECOMMENDATIONS AND NURSING IMPLICATIONS

As with any instrument in an early developmental stage, the Nursing Care Role Orientation Scale must be used with caution and discretion. Four of the items need to be revised due to the low item-total correlations. These are items 1, 10, 18, and 23. Further development of the scale on a larger regional population of nursing students enrolled in the three nursing educational programs would yield additional information on the factor structure of the instrument. Further analysis of the data, using generalizability theory, would provide additional information on estimates of reliability.

The instrument may be used to determine the level of nursing care role orientation of students as they progress through their educational program. Since the instrument does discriminate between students in AD and BSN programs (Stemple, 1981) and also measures a difference between registered nurses prepared at the AD and the BSN level, the instrument may also be used to evaluate an increase in nursing care role orientation of RN BSN students following a course on role socialization. In addition, the Nursing Care Role Orientation Scale may be used to evaluate continuing education programs on nursing care role for registered nurses to determine if the program is effective in producing an increase in nursing care role orientation.

## REFERENCES

Harmer, B. (1922). *Textbook of the principles and practice of nursing.* New York: Macmillan.

Harmer, B., & Henderson, V. (1955). *Textbook of the principles and practice of nursing.* Macmillan.

Henderson, V. (1966). *The nature of nursing.* New York: Macmillan.

Henderson, V. (1978). The concept of nursing. *Journal of Advanced Nursing, 3,* 113-130.

Kinlein, L. (1977). *Independent nursing practice with clients.* Philadelphia: J. B. Lippincott.

Lysaught, J. P. (1981). *Action in affirmation toward an unambigous profession of nursing.* New York: McGraw-Hill.

Nightingale, F. (1859). *Notes on nursing: What it is and what it is not.* London: Harrison.

Nunnally, J. (1978). *Psychometric theory.* New York: McGraw-Hill.

Nursing Development Conference Group (1973). *Concept formalization in nursing: Process and product.* Boston: Little, Brown.

Orem, V. (1971). *Nursing concepts of practice.* New York: McGraw-Hill.

Orem, V. (1980). *Nursing concepts of practice.* New York: McGraw-Hill.

Simmons, L. W., & Henderson, V. (1954). *Nursing research a survey and assessment.* New York: Appleton-Century Crofts.

Smith, M. C. (1979, October). Proposed metaparadigm for nursing research the theory development. *Image,* pp. 75-79.

Stemple, J. (1981). *Self-care orientations of associate degree and baccalaureate degree students: Test of a causal model.* Unpublished doctoral dissertation, West Virginia University, Morqantown, WV.

West Virginic University School of Nursing (WVUSN). (1984). *Conceptual framework.* Morgantown, WV: West Virginia University.

# Nursing Care Role Orientation Scale

## CONCEPT MEASUREMENT

I am conducting a survey of nurses' preceptions of concepts in nursing. The purpose is to determine the relationship between nurses' conceptualization of nursing from different educational programs and practice settings.

Your participation in the project is voluntary. All information will be kept confidential and will not be used in any way to identify specific individuals. Thank you very much for your cooperation.

Please Circle                                      Please Record:
Highest Academic Degree:   AD   BSN   MSN         Date of Birth _____
Present Practice Setting:   Primary Care   Acute Care   Long-term Care

## Example:

The major function of teaching is to
            assist the student in
            developing skills in criti-
            cal thinking.              1 2 3 4 5     present nursing content.
   1. Indicates you *strongly agree* with
      (assist the student in developing skills in critical thinking is the major function).
   2. Indicates that you *agree* with
      (assist the student in developing skills in critical thinking is the more important function).
   3. Indicates that you *agree* with
      both (assist the student in developing skills in critical thinking and present nursing content are equally important functions).
   4. Indicates that you *agree* with
      (present nursing content as the major function).
   5. Indicates that you *strongly agree* with
      (present nursing content as the major function).

## Directions:

Circle the number that best expresses your view on the following statements.
   1. Health care for the client (community, family, individual) in most situations
      is most efficiently performed
            through health team                      through nursing care
            collaboration.            1 2 3 4 5      only.

2. The nursing care goals of Client X are determined mostly by
   the consideration of client
   needs.                                    1 2 3 4 5    physicians' orders.
3. Nursing is best defined at what point on the following continuum?
   Assisting the client in his                            Administering therapeutic
   self-care practices.                      1 2 3 4 5    measures.
4. The quality of health care for the client is increased through nurses'
   collaboration with the                                 careful attention to their
   nursing team.                             1 2 3 4 5    technical skills.
5. It is more important to nursing that the nurse
   document client                                        record data for physi-
   outcomes.                                 1 2 3 4 5    cian's record.
6. The assessment of the client's problem should begin with
   where the client is in
   understanding.                            1 2 3 4 5    complaints and tests.
7. Most nursing practices should be based upon
   research by others.                       1 2 3 4 5    research by nurses.
8. Nursing practice is best described by the nurse's
   concepts used in practice.    1 2 3 4 5    activities performed.
9. The client in most situations, if given an understanding of his health state,
   can make appropriate                                   still requires judgment
   decisions regarding his                                and advice regarding
   health practices.                         1 2 3 4 5    health practices.
10. Most individuals' contacts with a nurse for nursing care should be
    through the physician.        1 2 3 4 5    direct.
11. The strategies for meeting the health goals of the client is best done by
    collaboration with the                                identifying the nature of
    client.                                   1 2 3 4 5    the health problem.
12. Most of the nurse client interactions should be based on
    client needs.                             1 2 3 4 5    physicians' orders.
13. The primary data source for health assessment of the client should be
    obtained from the client's
    behavior and responses.       1 2 3 4 5    Kardex and chart.
14. The health history of the client should be directed toward
    helping the client identify                           identifying symptoms of
    and express health needs.     1 2 3 4 5    illness.
15. The identification of health goals of the client is best done by
    assessment of nature of                               collaboration with the
    illness.                                  1 2 3 4 5    client.
16. The quality of nursing care is increased more through
    technical skills of nurse.    1 2 3 4 5    nursing research.
17. The nurse's purpose in performing a physical exam should be to gain data to
    assist the the client to
    understand his health                                 diagnose the client's
    state.                                    1 2 3 4 5    illness.
18. The effective program on nutrition for the client could best be developed
    through
    collaboration with the                                use of extensive literature
    nutritionist.                             1 2 3 4 5    review.

19. The obligation of the nurse should be to which of the following?
    Mainly physician.      1 2 3 4 5    Mainly client.
20. The life-style data should be used
    to request the physician           to educate the client
    to discuss causes of heart          about health promotion
    disease.         1 2 3 4 5    activities.
21. The specific dimensions of nursing care and the specific dimensions of medical care are very
    different.        1 2 3 4 5    similar.
22. The blood pressure data should be used
    to educate the client            by the doctor in health
    about change in status.    1 2 3 4 5    assessment.
23. The effective program on drug abuse for the client could be best developed through
    collaboration with the            use of extensive literature
    pharmacist.       1 2 3 4 5    review.
24. The best nursing care is determined by nurse and
    client.        1 2 3 4 5    doctor.

# 3

# Measuring Socialization to the Professional Nursing Role

## Therese G. Lawler

*This chapter discusses a modification of the Corwin's Nursing Role Conception Scale (Professional subscale) and a modification of the Stone Health Care Professional Attitude Inventory, measures of professionalism and socialization to the professional nursing role.*

This chapter explores an area of concern dear to the hearts of all nursing educators – socialization to the professional role. Faculty engage in much dialogue about how essential it is to socialize students to the profession. Nursing program philosophies invariably reflect that basic premise. Nursing curricular objectives are formulated and consistently predicated on a program goal of professional socialization. The National League for Nursing (1978) was quite directive in cautioning nursing faculty to build the curriculum in part around the past, present, and emerging roles of the professional nurse. But does the capability to validly measure professionalism in nursing graduates really exist? What are the specific outcomes of the educational and socialization process in this regard?

These questions are especially pertinent to those involved in working with registered nurses returning for baccalaureate degrees in nursing – particularly in outreach programs. The proliferating preparation of associate degree nurses at the community college level has led to an increasing number of registered nurse students enrolling in baccalaureate degree programs in nursing to further their education. Some of the issues raised by both researchers and faculty relate directly to the socialization of these students. Central to these issues is a quality assurance problem, that is, whether registered nurses in either a discrete curriculum track or in an off-campus program can possibly attain the degree of professional orientation that their counterparts, the generic baccalaureate students, do.

Critical to the effective study of socialization to the professional role is the development, testing, and utilization of valid and reliable instruments. The purpose of this study was to develop a conceptual framework that could serve as a basis for the research on professional nursing socialization, to review the literature on professionalization and the attendant instruments, and to test the reliability and validity of two selected instruments.

## CONCEPTUAL BACKGROUND

The conceptual framework for this study is derived from literature on socialization and professionalism. Hinshaw (1977) states that "socialization is the process of learning new roles and the adaptation to them, and, as such, continual processes by which individuals become members of a social group" (p. 2). The acquisition of the knowledge and skills necessary for the occupational role is one of the most critical socialization processes that adults experience. The interpretation of socialization given by Simpson (1967) is learning the "cultural content" of a role and the acquisition of self-identification. Simpson considers this a sequenced process that includes the goals of proficiency, identification of significant others in the role, and internalization of the role. Therefore, socialization to the professional nursing role provides requisite values and norms for practice.

Houle (1980) asserts that the canons of professionalization, or characteristics of professional behavior, include self-determination, desire to advance learning, ability to solve problems, collective identity, credentialing, legal accountability, ethical practice, provision of service, and public acceptance. Similarly, Dumont (1970) claimed that new professionalism (broadening of the law-medicine-church-university traditionalist view) is more complex, more interesting and more meaningful to modern society. Common principles of neoprofessionalism are consumer orientation, a growing concern with credentialing, an imbued sense of superordinate purpose, possession of an attitude of criticism, impatience with the rate of change, and motivation by compassion.

The National League for Nursing (1984) describes professional nurses (i.e., baccalaureate-prepared nurses) as (1) accountable for their own nursing practice, (2) accepting responsibility for the provision of nursing care through others, (3) accepting the advocacy role in relation to clients, (4) working collaboratively with other health disciplines, and (5) motivated toward continued learning. Professionalization is then multidimensional and behavioral. In this regard, Simpson (1967) describes the professionalization of nursing students as progressing from service orientation to a technical focus of interest and, finally, to a seeking of acceptance as professional colleagues.

## REVIEW OF LITERATURE

Sams (1977) reported at a National League for Nursing (NLN) convention the results of 50 task group discussions on the socialization of baccalaureate students, using a consensus strategy. Facilitators of socialization to the professional role were identified as a growth-focused curriculum design and implementation, feedback mechanisms to reinforce positive professional behaviors, intense practicums to encourage independent decision making, and rewarding collaborative behaviors instead of competitive behavior outcomes. These were felt to be aligned to professionalism and its requisite values and norms.

Smullen (1982), using a perceptual scale, found that registered nurse students perceived changes in themselves during their baccalaureate programs of study as encompassing a heightened awareness of the broad issues facing the nursing profession, the need for cohesive and collaborative goals, the merit of organizational activities, and a growing commitment to lifelong learning and nursing as a career. Again these are consonant with the construct of professionalization.

Jako (1980) measured professional behaviors in a sample of 124 registered nurses in six second-step programs. Results of pre-and posttests showed an increase in mean interest in the seven variables measuring professionalism. These variables were (a) belonging to nursing organizations, (b) reading nursing journals, (c) attending nursing meetings, (d) doing nursing/health research, (e) writing articles relating to nursing/health, (f) being a resource person to other nurses, and (g) being a leader or coordinator in nursing.

Using Valliot's (1962) Professionalization Scale, which measures professional versus traditional orientation in nursing, Richards (1972) found that baccalaureate graduates held a more professional ideal than did their associate-degree and diploma counterparts. Baccalaureate candidates also perceived their instructors' values as more professionally oriented. A comparison study of the professional socialization of senior baccalaureate nursing students was conducted by Lynn in 1981. She employed the Nurses Professional Orientation Scale (NPOS), composed of 60 behaviors designed to measure congruence between student and faculty perception of the nursing role. The work of Lynn, developed by Crocker and Brodie (1974), specifically focused on testing two new scoring methods with concomitant reliability and validity data collected. Lynn dichotomized professional orientation into traditional and nontraditional and found that associate-degree students held a significantly more traditional view of nursing (as measured by the NPOS).

Stone & Knopke (1978) measured professionalization in nursing students at the University of Wisconsin, using the Health Care Professional Attitude Inventory. The instrument was developed to correspond with Dumont's (1970) paradigm of neoprofessionalism. Findings pointed to a significant difference between first- and fourth-year students in regard to consumer control, critical approach, rate of social change, and compassion. The fourth-year nursing students exhibited a more professional attitude.

The work of Corwin (1961) over the past 24 years is well recognized. His seminal study, measuring role conception by nurses in the Midwest, has been replicated and has served as a basis, among others, for Kramer's (1968) research on reality shock and biculturalism. Corwin trichotomized the nursing role into commitment to the hospital bureaucracy, commitment to the nursing profession, and commitment to the patient. His Nursing Role Conception Scale's subscale on professional role conception measures these aspects of the nursing role. Corwin found that baccalaureate-prepared nursing graduates maintained higher professional role conceptions than did nonbaccalareate nurses. These findings have been supported by Davis & Olesen (1964), Kramer (1968), and Pieta (1981).

Only one study has been found that deals with socialization differences between registered nurses returning for a bachelor of science degree in nursing and generic baccalaureate nursing majors. An unpublished study by Hughes, Turpin, and Reed (1982), conducted at the University of Texas at Arlington, measures professional attitudes of graduating senior nursing students as part of the curriculum evaluation plan, using Stone's (Stone & Knopke, 1978) inventory. Pretests and posttests on both generic ($N = 35$) and registered nurse baccalaureate students ($N = 32$) were administered. Results indicated a more positive attitude in registered nurse baccalaureate nursing students on the "consumer control" and "superordinate purpose" subscales. Furthermore, no investigations were discovered that compared the professionalization of off-campus students to those educated in on-campus academic programs.

In a meta-evaluation of the literature on socialization and nursing roles, Conway (1983) asserts that the measurement of socialization has proved problematic at best, since there has been (1) inadequate conceptualization of the construct, (2) heavy reliance on values and norms of faculty as criterion measures, (3) faulty methodology in many instances, and (4) the utilization of tools that have been researcher-generated and for which no reliability and/or validity data have been reported. Variables assessed in the studies reviewed by Conway included role conception, autonomy, ambiguity, and personality characteristics. Conway felt that findings were inconsistent and called for the use of "standard measuring instruments for which construct validity has been established" (p. 153).

## MEASUREMENT PROTOCOL

Two instruments were revised and tested in this investigation. The first was Stone's Health Care Professional Attitude Inventory (Stone & Knopke 1978). This measure purports to capture the variables intrinsic to Dumont's (1970) construct of professionalism (i.e., consumer control, credentialing, critical attitudes, etc.). The inventory contains 36 items calling for responses along a number-anchored Likert scale. Both construct and content validity were addressed in the development of the tool by the use of an expert panel and contrasting groups. Alpha coefficient for reliability on the entire scale was .72 for university nursing students ($N = 274$) in Stone's initial group. No one subsequently using the Inventory has reported additional reliability and validity data. Further information on the original development of the instrument can be found in Ward and Felter (1979).

The second instrument used was the Professional subscale from Corwin's (1961) Nursing Role Conception Scale. There are eight hypothetical situations comprising the subscale, followed by questions that respondents rate on a Likert-type index, assessing role conception and dissonance. Variables addressed in the subscale relate to independence of practice, standards of excellence, membership in professional organizations, credentialing, continued learning, and interest in research. Content validity was addressed in the instrument's development by Corwin and Taves (1962); construct validity was tested by Kramer (1968), who found significant differences in role orientation between groups in expected directions. Ward and Felter (1979) give additional detail on the procedures used to develop the scale. Corwin reports no reliability data in his studies and in personal correspondence.

Together, the two instruments appear to represent those characteristics ascribed to the baccalaureate product by the NLN. Thus, they would be consonant with program objectives and expected outcomes in typical NLN-accredited university schools of nursing. Both instruments are norm-referenced measures and utilize the domain sampling model for item construction. They both are affective, subjective instruments that collect data by self-report. Stone and Corwin granted permission for the use of their tools in this study. Since professionalism as such is a multidimensional construct, it would seem appropriate to employ multiple measures to assess its status in nursing graduates.

Instrument modification and data on reliability and validity of the Stone (Stone & Knopke 1978) inventory and Corwin (1961) scale that were modified for this study are described below.

## MODIFICATION OF TOOL AND CONTENT VALIDITY ASSESSMENT

A panel of nursing experts ($N = 8$) who have taught and/or administered programs for baccalaureate students, including registered nurse students, was selected. This faculty group of content specialists was chosen from individuals who were employed in various university settings in order to diminish program bias. They reviewed the two measures of professionalization in two distinct steps. On the first review, items were judged for clarity, readability, and comprehensiveness, as well as for appropriateness in measuring variables characterizing the professional role. The modification of any questionable item was specifically encouraged as were deletions and construction of new items to measure the domain. On the first round, panel members made changes in some items' form, structure, and meaning on both of the instruments; they felt that the changes enhanced relevance and coherence. Feedback from the panel members also suggested that the Stone inventory was, in their perception, a better measure of professional orientation than the Corwin scale. Added to the changes suggested by the panel were modifications recommended by Ward and Felter (1979) for specific items.

Revisions and changes made in the Stone inventory related to item construction, the ranking scale, and the scoring. Items 4, 7, 8. 14. 20. and 29 had multiple focuses and were edited to address single concepts (this yielded additional items). Items 10, 27, 30, and 32 were considered stylistically flawed or long and were edited. Items 11, 12, 21, 22, and 33 were reworded to use more generally accepted terms for nursing. The 7-point number-anchored scale was modified to a 5-point descriptor-anchored scale both to be more explicit and to allow opscanning by the computer for large samples. A scoring plan was simplified from Stone's original conversion technique from raw to scaled to absolute scores. (Stone's inventory is found at the end of this chapter.) Changes made in the Corwin subscale related solely to item additions and revisions. Items 4, 5, and 6 were edited for current usage and clarity, and in all items the term "registered nurse" was substituted for "graduate nurse." Eight more hypothetical situations were added that were derived from panel suggestions and the nursing literature (see Corwin's scale at the end of the chapter). The following are samples from each instrument that illustrate both original and new items.

From Stone (Stone & Knopke, 1978)

8. Health care professionals such as nurses generally are impersonal and scientifically oriented.
11. At this point in time, the consumers of health care have been adequately involved in the development of health care delivery systems.

From Corwin (1961), modified by Lawler

4. All registered nurses in a hospital spend, on the average, at least six hours a week reading professional journals and taking continuing education courses.
   A. Do you think this should be true of all nurses?
   B. Is this true of nurses that you have observed?
9. The nursing administrators in a large home health agency encourage their staff members to become active members of their professional nursing organizations.

   A. Do you think that this is what all nursing administrators should do?
   B. Is this what you have observed nursing administrators actually doing?

On the second review, the panel judged each item on both tools for relevance to the operationally defined construct of professionalism. A 5-point Likert scale that ranged from Irrelevant to Most relevant was used to record each panelist's view of item relevance. Seventy-five percent agreement (.75) was determined as the criterion for final acceptance of an item. Interrater coefficients of agreement ranged from .75 to 1.0, and all items were accepted with a few minor refinements.

## ADMINISTRATION AND SCORING

The revised Nursing Role Conception Scale and the revised Health Care Professional Attitude Inventory are both administered in the form of questionnaires that allow the respondent to rate each item on a 5-point scale from 1 (strongly agree) to 5 (strongly disagree). Total scores are derived by summing item ratings. For the modified Stone Health Care Professional Attitude Inventory, the higher the score the more professional is the nurse's attitude. The higher the score on the modified Corwin's Professional Role Subscale, the stronger is the perception of either the ideal professional role (A) or the real professional role (B). The difference between the ideal role and the real professional role (A − B) represents the amount of dissonance present.

### Assessment of Reliability and Validity of Modified Instruments

### *Sample*

In order to capture further data on the reliability and validity of the modified Stone and Corwin tools, a sample was drawn from the nursing student population. Subjects for the study were enrolled from three nursing programs in North Carolina. Two programs were in the east, and one was located in the mountains; these were considered demographically comparable regions. Assignment to the sample was made by the nonprobability purposive technique. The nonequivalent groups were composed of the following:

   1. Generic baccalaureate students who were seniors within 2 to 3 weeks of graduation in a large state university program ($N = 25$).
   2. RN baccalaureate students (ADN plus) who were seniors within 2 to 3 weeks of graduation in a small state university outreach program ($N = 18$) (not an RN completion program). For much of the analysis, groups 1 and 2 were collapsed.
   3. Associate degree students who were seniors within 2 to 3 weeks of

graduation from a community college program within the same city as the large university ($N = 36$).

Data were collected from the subjects by use of a standardized format. Each of the student cohorts was administered the instruments in a group setting. Directions were explicit, and the scales were passed out and collected. Subjects were guaranteed that their anonymity would be protected. Administration took place $1^1/_2$ to 2 weeks prior to graduation for all in the sample.

## Construct Validity

This was examined by the use of the contrasted groups approach (Waltz, Strickland, & Lenz, 1984) and the convergent principle. This technique is most appropriate with norm-referenced measures. The underlying theoretical assumption is that certain attridutes are present in varying degrees in different groups. One can then hypothesize which group would score high on the trait in question and which group would score low on an affective measure. For the attribute of nursing professionalism, BSN graduates were contrasted with ADN graduates. If the instrument(s) of interest are valid, they should discriminate significantly between the two groups, with the BSN group scoring higher than the ADN group. Table 3.1 shows the results of tests for the assessment of construct validity. The independent T-test was used to determine differences between the means, and $p < .05$ was set as the level of significance.

**TABLE 3.1 Mean Scores of BSN and ADN Nursing Students and Significance Levels on Corwin/Lawler Scale and Stone Inventory**

| Instrument | Group 1[a]<br>BSN<br>mean | Group 2[b]<br>ADN<br>mean | $t$ Value<br>(pooled)[c] | Significance<br>after $t$-test |
|---|---|---|---|---|
| Corwin | | | | |
|   Role 1 – ideal | 52.8 | 51.4 | 1.08 | NS |
|   Role 2 – actual | 34.6 | 39.8 | −4.12 | .0001 |
|     Total | 87.4 | 91.2 | −2.20 | .03 |
| Stone | | | | |
|   Subscale 1: Consumer<br>    control | 20.8 | 18.9 | 2.66 | .01 |
|   Subscale 2: Credentialism | 22.7 | 21.5 | 2.15 | .04 |
|   Subscale 3: Superordinate<br>    purpose | 21.9 | 20.3 | 0.37 | .02 |
|   Subscale 4: Criticism | 24.0 | 22.8 | 1.86 | NS |
|   Subscale 5: Change<br>    impatience | 19.3 | 16.7 | 4.47 | .0001 |
|   Subscale 6: Compassion | 21.6 | 20.2 | 2.47 | .02 |
|     Total | 130.3 | 120.4 | 3.80 | .0001 |

[a]Group 1 = BSN + RN/BSN ($N = 41$).
[b]Group 2 = ADN ($N = 36$).
[c]$df = 75$.

It is apparent that the modified Corwin scale does not differentiate well between the two groups as far as ideal role (Role 1) is concerned, which should equate with professional orientation. Its validity may be compromised in this regard. The perception of actual role (Role 2), however, was significantly different between the BSN and ADN groups. BSN graduates saw other nurses as exhibiting less professional behaviors than did the ADN graduates; the BSN subjects held a more professionally oriented ideal. This dichotomy is what Corwin termed role deprivation, or better yet, dissonance. This is not consistent with reports of prior studies. It has been reported in prior studies that scores for BSN graduates were higher on both subscores in that they displayed a higher professional role conception and a greater role deprivation.

On the Stone measure there were appreciable and significant differences on five of the six scales and on the total instrument. The only subscale that was not found to discriminate highly between the BSN and ADN graduates was that of critical attitude (Scale 4). Certainly, from the results it would seem that the Stone inventory has good construct validity.

Further validity testing of the measures was accomplished by application of the convergent validity principle. The convergent principle dictates that different instruments that purport to measure the same variable(s) should correlate positively with each other, as should their subscales, if any. Using Pearson product-moment coefficients ($r$), the association between the Stone and Corwin instruments was explored. It is of note that only Role 1, the first subscale of the Corwin tool, was included since it is claimed to be the measure of professional orientation. Table 3.2 displays the convergent analysis.

**TABLE 3.2** Correlation Coefficients between Subscales and Total Scores on the Modified Stone Inventory and Modified Corwin Role 1 (Ideal) as Measures of the Convergent Principle

| Instrument | Corwin Role 1 | Stone Subscale 1 | Subscale 2 | Subscale 3 | Subscale 4 | Subscale 5 | Subscale 6 | Total |
|---|---|---|---|---|---|---|---|---|
| Corwin | | | | | | | | |
| Role 1 | – | .10 | .27 | .18 | .33 | .03 | .32 | .29 |
| Stone | | | | | | | | |
| Subscale 1 | .10 | – | .29 | .35 | .33 | .50 | .54 | .79 |
| Subscale 2 | .27 | .29 | – | .23 | .18 | .25 | .39 | .58 |
| Subscale 3 | .18 | .35 | .23 | – | .08 | .25 | .27 | .55 |
| Subscale 4 | .33 | .33 | .18 | .08 | – | .20 | .36 | .58 |
| Subscale 5 | .03 | .49 | .25 | .25 | .20 | – | .33 | .65 |
| Subscale 6 | .32 | .54 | .39 | .27 | .36 | .33 | – | .74 |
| Total | .29 | .79 | .58 | .55 | .58 | .65 | .73 | – |

The relationships (expressed as correlation coefficients) between and among the subscales on the modified Stone inventory range from .08 to .79, all in the positive direction. There is a particularly strong correlation between each subscale and the total tool. Subscale 3 on the Stone inventory (Superordinate Purpose) exhibits the weakest relationship among the five. Moreover, the correlations between the modified Stone and Role 1 (ideal professional role) of the modifed Corwin, albeit weaker, still are also positive. Certainly, there is sufficient evidence to suggest that there is compliance with the convergent validity principle on the modified Stone inventory but that the modified Corwin scale may be imprecise.

## Reliability

Internal consistency of both instruments (total and subscales) was assessed by Cronbach's alpha coefficient. According to Waltz and associates (1984), an instrument may be said to be internally consistent or homogeneous to the extent that all of its subparts are measuring the same characteristic. Results of this test of reliability are shown in Table 3.3.

The internal consistency reliability coefficients for the modified Corwin Professional subscale are in the .50s range, which is considered minimally acceptable for group level comparisons. Lower reliability coefficients on the modified Stone subscales can probably be accounted for by the small number of items (6-7) that comprise each subscale. Furthermore, it is evident again that Subscale 3 (Superordinate Purpose) proves troublesome. The alpha for the total Stone inventory, however, is .73, indicative of an acceptable level of reliability.

**TABLE 3.3** Cronbach Alphas as Measures of Internal Consistency on the Modified Corwin Scale and the Modified Stone Inventory

| Instrument | Total alpha | BSN | ADN |
|---|---|---|---|
| Corwin | | | |
| Professional subscale | | | |
| Role 1 | .58 | | |
| Role 2 | .69 | | |
| Total | .55 | .59 | .52 |
| Stone | | | |
| Subscale 1 | .60 | | |
| Subscale 2 | .34 | | |
| Subscale 3 | .07 | | |
| Subscale 4 | .33 | | |
| Subscale 5 | .34 | | |
| Subscale 6 | .30 | | |
| Total | .73 | .75 | .51 |

Another method of testing the reliability of a measure is to employ the test-retest technique. This is especially appropriate for affective measures designed to assess characteristics that are relatively stable over time and to assess consistency of performance (Waltz et al., 1984). For this purpose, both the modified Stone and the modified Corwin were administered twice to the generic baccalaureate student group ($N = 23$). The first time was $2^1/_2$ weeks prior to graduation, and the second time was 3 days prior to graduation. Pearson correlation coefficients were derived and were .59 for the modified Corwin Scale and .52 acceptable for test-retest comparisons.

## INTERPRETATIONS AND IMPLICATIONS

It would be well to put the findings of this research into a utilitarian perspective. First, the modified Stone Health Care Professional Attitude Inventory seems valid and reliable as a measure of professional orientation in nursing. The tool discriminates well between different groups who might possess that attribute at varying levels. A panel of nursing experts, furthermore, judged the items on the inventory as relevant to the construct of interest. While reliability was assessed as sound for the entire instrument, it would seem to be judicious to run both item analysis and factor analysis on the subscales (especially Subscale 3) to determine whether there are any flawed items.

Second, the modified Corwin Nursing Role Conception Scale's Professional subscale appears to be useful in measuring professional role deprivation or dissonance (Role 2) between and among different groups of RNs. Its worth, however, is questionable in gauging nursing professionalism as an orientation or level of attribute as evidenced by some validity and reliability problems that persist.

Finally, there remains a need to continue to evaluate the outcomes of nursing education, particularly socialization to the professional role. A parallel need exists to employ standard measures; that means the use of common instruments that will enable the comparison of results across programs and studies. Based on the data accrued from the study reported, a strong recommendation is made to use the Stone inventory as modified for the purpose of further research in this area.

## REFERENCES

Conway, M. E., (1983). Socialization and roles in nursing. In H. H. Werley & J. Fitzpatrick (Eds), *Annucl review of nursing research* (pp. 183-205) New York: Springer Publishing Co.

Corwin, R. G. (1961). Professional employee: *A* study in conflict in nursing roles. *American Journal of Sociology, 66,* 604-615.

Corwin, R. G., & Taves, M. (1962). Some concomitants of bureaucratic and professional conceptions of the nurse role. *Nursing Research, 11,* 223-228.

Crocker, L. M., & Brodie, B. J. (1974). Development of a scale to asses student nurses' views of the professional nursing role. *Journal of Applied Psychology, 59*, 233-235.

Davis, F., & Olesen, V. L. (1964). Baccalaureate students' images of nursing. *Nursing Research, 13,* 8-15.

Dumont, M. (1970). The changing face of professionalism. In L. Netzer (Ed.), *Education, administration and change* (pp. 20-26). New York: Harper & Row.

Hinshaw, A. S. (1977). Socialization and resocialization of nurses for professional nursing practice. In L.Sams (Ed.), *Socialization and resocialization of nurses.* (pp. 1-15). New York: National League for Nursing. (Publication. No. 15-1659).

Houle, C. (1980). *Continuing learning in the professions.* San Francisco: Jossey-Bass.

Hughes, R., Turpin, R., & Reed, S. (1982). *An evaluation of the baccalaureate nursing program.* Unpublished manuscript, University of Texas Arlington, Tx.

Jako, K. (1980). Frontiering: An emergent concept for nursing research. In K. Jako (Ed.), *Researching second step nursing education, proceedings* (pp. 35-45). Rohnert Park, CA. Sonoma State University.

Kramer, M. (1968). Nurse role deprivation: A symptom of needed change. *Social Science and Medicine, 2,* 461-474.

Lynn, M. (1981). The professional socialization of nursing students: A comparison based on type of education, program. In *Proceedings of the American Educational Research Association Conference, Boston, MA, April, 1980.* Washington, DC: AERA.

National League for Nursing. (1978). *Curriculum process for developing or revising baccalaureate nursing programs.* New York: National League for Nursing. (Publication No. 15-1700).

National League for Nursing. (1984). *Criteria for evaluation of baccalaureate and higher degree programs in nursing.* New York: National League for Nursing. (Publication No. 15-1251).

Pieta, B. (1981). A comparison of role conceptions among nursing students and faculty from associate degree, baccalaureate degree, and diploma nursing programs and head nurses. *Proceedings of First Annual SCCEN Research Conference* (pp. 125-128). Austin, TX: Wm. Field.

Richards, M. A. (1972). A study of differences in psychological characteristics of students graduating from three types of basic nursing programs. *Nursing research, 21*(3), 258-261.

Sams, L. (1977). Factors that affect the socialization and resocialization of nurses for professional practice. In L. Sam (Ed.), *Socialization and resocialization of nurses.* (pp. 35-41). New York: National League for Nursing. (Publication No. 15-1659)

Simpson, I. (1967). Patterns of socialization into professions: The case of student nurses. *Sociological inquiry, 37,* 47-54.

Smullen, B. (1982). Second-step education for RN's: The quiet revolution. *Nursing and Health Care, 3*(7), 369-373.

Stone, H., & Knopke, H. (1978). *Data gathering instruments for evaluating educational programs in the health sciences.* Unpublished manuscript. University of Wisconsin, Madison.

Valliot, Sr. M. (1962). *Commitment to nursing.* Philadelphia: J. B. Lippincott.

Waltz, C., Strickland, O., & Lenz, E. (1984). *Measurement in nursing research.* Philadelphia: F. A. Davis.

Ward, M. J., & Felter, M. E. (1979). *Instruments for use in nursing education research.* Boulder, CO: WICHE.

# Corwin's Nursing Role Conception Scale (Modified Professional Subscale)

*Instructions:* This scale consists of a list of 14 hypothetical situations in which a nurse might find herself. You are asked to indicate both:

(A) the extent to which you think the situation should be the *ideal* nursing.
(B) the extent to which you have *observed* the situation in your hospital.

Notice that *two* (2) questions must be answered for *each* situation. Consider the questions of what *ought to be* the case and what *is really* the case separately; try not to let your answer to one question influence your answer to the other question. Give your opinions; there are no "wrong" answers.

Indicate the *degree* to which you agree or disagree with the statement by checking one of the alternative answers, ranging from STRONGLY AGREE, AGREE, UNDECIDED, DISAGREE, to STRONGLY DISAGREE.

*STRONGLY AGREE* indicates that you agree with the statement with *some exceptions.*
*AGREE* indicates that you agree with the statement with *some exceptions.*
*UNDECIDED* indicates that you could either "agree" or "disagree" with the statement with about an equal number of exceptions in either case.
*DISAGREE* indicates that you disagree with the statement with *some exceptions.*
*STRONGLY DISAGREE* indicates that you disagree with the statement with *almost no exceptions.*

## Professional Subscale

| | STRONGLY AGREE | AGREE | UNDECIDED | DISAGREE | STRONGLY DISAGREE |
|---|---|---|---|---|---|

1. One registered nurse tries to put her standards and ideals about good nursing into practice even if hospital rules and procedures prohibit it.
   A. Do you think that this is what registered nurses *should* do?
   B. *Is* this what most nurses that you have observed actually *do* when the occasion arises?
2. One registered nurse does not do anything which she is told to do unless she is satisfied that it is

best for the welfare of the patient.

   A.  Do you think that this is what registered
nurses *should* do?

   B.  *Is* this what most nurses that you have
observed actually *do* when the occasion arises?

3.  All registered nurses in a hospital are active members in professional nursing associations, attending most conferences and meetings of the association.

   A.  Do you think this should be true of all nurses?

   B.  *Is* this true of nurses that you have observed?

4.  All registered nurses in a hospital spend, on the average, at least six hours a week reading professional journals and taking continuing education courses.

   A.  Do you think this should be true of all nurses?

   B.  *Is* this true of nurses that you have observed?

5.  Some nurses try to live up to what they think are the standards of their profession, even if other nurses on the unit or supervisors don't seem to like it.

   A.  Do you think that this is what registered
nurses *should* do?

   B.  *Is* this what nurses that you have observed
actually *do* when the occasion arises?

6.  Some registered nurses believe that they can get along very well without a lot of formal education, such as that required for a B.S.N. or M.S. degree.

   A.  Do you think that this is what registered
nurses *should* do?

   B.  *Is* this what nurses actually *do* believe.

7.  At some hospitals when a registered nurse is considered for promotion, one of the most important factors considered by the supervisor is her knowledge of, and ability to use, judgment about nursing care procedures.

   A.  Do you think this is what supervisors *should*
regard as important?

   B.  *Is* this what head nurses/supervisors actually
*do* regard as important?

8.  Some hospitals try to hire only registered nurses educated in colleges and universities which are equipped to teach the basic theoretical knowledge of nursing science.

   A.  Do you think this is the way it *should* be in
nursing?

   B.  Is this the way things are at your hospital?

9.  The nursing administrators in a large home health agency encourage their staff members to become active members of the professional nursing organizations.

   A.  Do you think that this is what all nursing
       administrators *should* do?
   B.  *Is* this what you observed nursing administra-
       tors actually *doing*?
10. A director of nursing service tells you, "If nursing is
    to attain full professional status in the near future,
    the minimum of a baccalaureate degree should be
    required of all registered nurses."
   A.  Is this the way it *should* be in nursing?
   B.  *Is* this what most nurses you have observed
       *believe*?
11. In a certain hospital, a registered nurse is fully
    responsible/accountable to plan and carry out the
    total nursing care of clients entrusted to her.
   A.  Do you think that this is how it *should* be in
       nursing?
   B.  Is this what most nurses that you have
       observed actually *do* in practice?
12. A nurse testifies before legislators that the respon-
    sibility for setting standards of practice for the
    delivery of nursing services should rest with the
    nursing profession alone.
   A.  Do you think this is how it *should* be in nursing?
   B.  Is this what you have observed nurses *doing*?
13. In one hospital nurses develop clinical practice
    models based on nursing theory for use on specific
    patient units.
   A.  Do you think this *is* important for nurses to do?
   B.  *Is* this true of nurses that you have observed?
14. A nursing friend returning from a workshop claims
    that "once a nurse graduates from nursing school
    she/he bears the sole responsibility to maintain com-
    petence by regularly reading the professional journals
    and attending continuing education programs."
   A.  Do you think this is what registered nurses
       *should* do?
   B.  *Is* this what you have observed nurses actually
       *doing*?

Source: From Professional employee: A study in conflict in nursing roles by R.G. Corwin,
1961, *American Journal of Sociology, 66,* pp. 604-615, Adapted by Permission.


# STONE'S HEALTH CARE PROFESSIONAL ATTITUDE INVENTORY (MODIFIED FOR NURSING)

This inventory contains a series of statements about today's health care professions and health care delivery systems. These statements are not intended to elicit
a right or wrong answer; rather to collect your perceptions of the accuracy and/or
validity of each statement.

   You are requested to read each statement. Then, utilizing the response scale below, indicate the degree to which you agree or disagree with each statement in respect to the health care professions and/or delivery systems.

Health care professionals, for the purpose of this inventory, include all registered nurses who function as a member of the health care team. Health care delivery systems are those mechanisms and strategies designed to facilitate the delivery of health care to the consumer.

### RESPONSE SCALE

Strongly Agree <u>1    2    3    4    5</u> Strongly Disagree

|  | Number from |
|---|---|
| <u>Statements</u> | Response Scale |

1. Current health care delivery systems adequately meet the _____
   needs of society.
2. The potential for a financially secure position is a major rea- _____
   son for pursuing a career in the health care professions.
3. There has been inadequate interaction between health care _____
   professionals and their client public in the development of
   health care delivery systems.
4. Students in the health care disciplines should be expected _____
   to emulate or model the role to their instructors.
5. Students in the health disciplines should incorporate the phi- _____
   losophy of their educational program into their practice.
6. Policies based solely on scientific methodology are most _____
   appropriate for the resolution of society's health care
   problems.
7. The introduction of nurse practitioners, physician's assis- _____
   tants, and paramedical personnel has been of significant
   importance in improving the delivery of health care.
8. Health care professionals such as nurses generally are _____
   impersonal and scientifically oriented.
9. Health care professionals generally fail to show adequate _____
   interest in the health needs of consumers.
10. Criticism of health care practices and procedures by persons _____
    outside the profession is usually acknowledged and acted
    upon by health care professionals.
11. At this point in time, the consumers of health care have _____
    been adequately involved in the development of health care
    delivery systems.
12. Certification of competence upon receipt of the profes- _____
    sional degree is necessary to assure that behavioral sci-
    ences, basic sciences, and health care sciences were part of
    professional education.
13. Education programs for health care professionals spend _____
    more time preparing students for careers in research and/or
    teaching than for careers as practitioners.
14. Education programs for health care professionals have not _____
    been adequately responsive to the identified needs of local
    communities.

15  Health care teams tend to become so busy coordinating care          _____
    that they lose sight of patient needs.

16. Priorities for the user of human and material resources in          _____
    the health care professions are best achieved through cen-
    tralized decision-making.

17. Health care professionals have actively encouraged con-            _____
    sumer participation in current delivery systems.

18. Inefficient use of existing personnel poses a major problem         _____
    for delivering adequate health care.

19. The desire for a position of status should be accorded little       _____
    importance as a reason for pursuing a career in the health
    care professions.

20. In order to alleviate health manpower shortages in certain          _____
    geographical areas, health care professionals should be
    encouraged to deliver health legislation.

21. Special economic interests have too often had a negative           _____
    influence on public health legislation.

22. Education programs for health care professionals are cur-           _____
    rently designed to prepare professionals who will be able to
    appropriately respond to the needs of local communities.

23. Health care professional education programs offering               _____
    certification, e.g., physician assistants, nurse practitioners, etc.,
    are alternatives that will result in more effective health care.

24. Training greater numbers of health care professionals to           _____
    deliver primary care is one alternative that will be beneficial
    in meeting the long-term health needs of society.

25. Health care professionals have been actively promoting             _____
    change in the health care delivery systems for the improve-
    ment of health care for all citizens.

26. Health care is currently available to people at differing          _____
    income levels on a selective basis.

27. Health care professionals have developed adequate self-            _____
    evaluation of procedures and techniques in the delivery of
    health care.

28. Consumer involvement is essential to provide new alterna-          _____
    tives in developing health care delivery systems.

29. Health care providers who work with professionals from            _____
    other disciplines discover a common purpose in providing
    adequate health care for all citizens.

30. Societal class and social distinctions should be of no            _____
    importance in a health care setting.

31. Educational institutions have assumed a central role, not          _____
    only in the education of professionals, but in determining the
    nature and quality of health care and services provided to
    the community.

32. The health care professional such as a nurse should be con-        _____
    cerned solely with clinical practice and not with social
    change in his community.

33. Nursing educators are considered alternate rather than ulti-       _____
    mate sources of information for their students.

34. Consumer-oriented agencies should play a minimal role in establishing standards or criteria to assess the quality of care provided to health care consumers. _____

35. The greatest need for improvement in health care education concerns knowledge and skills about delivery of health care rather then in expanding knowledge about disease. _____

36. The existing forms of health care delivery systems allow professional personnel to efficiently deliver health care services to meet the needs of individual consumers. _____

37. The inability to change the attitudes of people is a greater obstacle to effecting change in the delivery of health care services than a lack of adequate finances. _____

38. When cost accounting and systems research techniques are applied to health care, it can be concluded that the health care needs of some citizens have not been adequately served. _____

From *Data gathering instruments for evaluating educational programs in the health sciences* by H. Stone and H. Knopke, 1978, unpublished manuscript, University of Wisconsin, Madison. Adapted by permission.

## SUBSCALES OF THE HEALTH CARE PROFESSIONAL ATTITUDE INVENTORY (AS MODIFIED BY LAWLER)

| Subscale | | |
|---|---|---|
| 1. Consumer control | 3, 11, 17, 22, 28, 34 | (6) |
| 2. Credentialing | 7, 12, 18, 23, 29, 35 | (6) |
| 3. Superordinate | 2, 8, 13, 19, 24, 30 | (6) |
| 4. Critical attitude/thinking | 4, ҃, 8, 16, 21, 27, 33 | (7) |
| 5. Impatience with need for change | 1, 14, 20, 25, 31, 37 | (7) |
| 6. Compassion for people needs | 6, 9, 15, 26, 32, 36, 38 | (7) |

### Scoring

| Agree items –<br>(reverse score) | 3, 5, 7, 9, 12 ,14, 15, 18, 19, 20, 21, 23, 24, 26, 28, 29, 30, 33, 35, 37, 38 |
|---|---|

| convert | 1 | 2 | 3 | 4 | 5 |
|---|---|---|---|---|---|
| to | 5 | 4 | 3 | 2 | 1 |

| Disagree items –<br>(score as marked) | 1, 2, 4, 6, 8, 10, 11, 13, 16, 17, 22, 25, 27, 31, 32, 34, 36 |
|---|---|

# PART II
# Measuring Clinical Performance

# 4

# Diagnostic Reasoning Protocols for Clinical Simulations in Nursing

## Jean M. Arnold

*This chapter discusses the Diagnostic Reasoning Instrument, a tool developed to clearly outline the steps used in clinical decision making in the assesment and planning stages of the nursing process.*

Diagnostic reasoning refers to the decisions made during the assessment and planning steps of the nursing process. The writer believes that critical decisions are made by the nurse as he or she collects and synthesizes data to determine client health problems. Unlike the physician, the nurse revises nursing diagnoses based on the changing health status and needs of the client at a given point in time.

Diagnostic reasoning is a process that has not been described in detail in the literature. The diagnostic reasoning model conceived by the writer includes six components, which are identified as assessment, hypothesis, objective, plan, criteric, and rationale. When a clinician encounters a situation, data are collected and an intervention plan is formulated. An assessment occurs that involves decisions about data collection for the specific client situation. The overall assessment (problem listing) is delimited, resulting in a specific hypothesis formulation. Then an intervention plan for each hypothesis (priority problem) is developed. Client objectives are specified along with expected outcomes (criteric). The actions to be taken are outlined with corresponding rationale.

## REVIEW OF LITERATURE

Literature related to the nature of the nursing process identifies diagnosis as a component of the nursing process that occurs at the completion of the assessment stage or is encompassed in this step (Marriner, 1983; Yura

& Walsh, 1978). It is implicit that the nurse is systematic when collecting data to identify client health problems (assessment and hypothesis). It is assumed that the diagnosis sets the stage for the plan of care and subsequent intervention.

Research related to diagnostic reasoning in nursing began with the examination of nurses' observations and listings of nursing actions. Kelly (1966) described the decisions made during data collection and planning of nursing care. Observation consists of three steps:

1. *Observation* is the recognition of signs and symptoms presented by the patient.
2. *Inference making* is a judgment about the state of the patient and/or the nursing needs of the patient.
3. *Decision making* is the determining of the action that should be taken that will be of optimal benefit to the patient.

Inference and decision making are critical components of nursing practice (Grier, 1981; Kelly, 1966); however, it is also important to know what observations to select (Hammond, 1966; Kelly, 1966).

Several studies related to decisions about data collection indicate that nurses do not discriminate effectively between relevant and irrelevant data. Nurses collect trivial information, that is, information that would not affect the decision-making process (Hammond, 1966; Verhonick, 1968).

Verhonick used five filmed vignettes with brief written descriptions to survey nursing observations and actions. A sample of 1,576 professional nurses was asked to list all observations seen and what action would be taken. Within the three categories of relevant, irrelevant, and inappropriate observations, 5,963 (84%) were relevant, 1,066 (15%) were irrelevant, and less than 1% were inappropriate. It is interesting to note that the greatest number of irrelevant observations were reported by doctoral respondents, and the least number were reported by those subjects who did not possess a degree (Verhonick, 1968). The two largest categories of actions were therapeutic (67%) and supportive (30%), and only two were inappropriate. A relationship was noted between observations and actions. Nurses with master's and doctoral degrees (50-53%) were more likely to relate supportive actions to observations made (26-38%).

Early literature referred to assessment and planning of care as clinical judgment. A comprehensive "lens" model, which interrelated the clinical and client situation variables by using decision theory, was applied to nursing. The lens is the clinician's past experience, knowledge, and so on, through which possible actions are filtered. Nurses were asked to infer the state of a patient by cues the patient exhibits and to determine actions and goals for a given situation. The relationships between the state of the patient and the cues and between goals and actions of nurses are probabilistic (Hammond, 1966). This model actually described diagnostic decisions for client assessment and nursing care plans.

In a research study that applied the lens model, a hospital staff of graduate nurses was asked to describe their responses to 381 clients' complaints of abdominal pain. Although 15 action categories were identified, there were no significant relationships between any one cue and selection of the action categories (Hammond 1966; Kelly, 1966). Further analysis of these data, limited to six nurses' descriptions of their responses to 100 of the 212 abdominal pain cases, confirmed the previous finding. None of the cues, either singly or grouped, conveyed more than trivial information for choosing the nursing actions, nor did the nurses discriminate between the usefulness of the various cues (Hammond, 1966; Tanner & McGuire, 1983).

Gordon (cited in Grier, 1981) provided nurses with restricted and unrestricted information and compared their data collection strategies. The nurses sought more items of information and were significantly less accurate in making a diagnosis in the unrestricted condition than in the restricted condition. This research provided evidence that nurses have difficulty deciding what data to collect.

What determines the selection process in data collection? A clinical inference, hypothesis, diagnosis, hunch, or conclusion affects the selection process (Kelly, 1966). There can be one or several conclusions reached at this time, or possibly none. Whether or not a hypothesis is reached, the field of data collection is narrowed. According to information processing theory, there is so much information available in a given situation that the limitations of short-term memory cause humans to condense it to facilitate processing. The knowledge stored in long-term memory provides the guidelines for the selection of data (Tanner & McGuire, 1983).

Do health professionals formulate hypotheses? During the initial data collection, hypotheses are formulated and then serve as guidelines for further data collection. Experienced physicians use three to five hypotheses as guides in selection patient data (Barrowa & Tambyn, 1976). Nurses tend to test multiple hypotheses simultaneously because they act as observers for physicians, they use perceptual rather than cognitive skills, they are nonselective in collecting data, and they find it time-saving (Hammond, 1966).

Tenative hypotheses are formulated at the beginning of an interaction between a client and a professional. Hypothesis formulation begins as early as the first 5 min of the encounter between a client and medical or nursing professional (Elstein, 1972). The novice differs from the expert in how this thought process is performed. The novice is taught to take a complete history before formulating a diagnosis. The expert uses a different approach in clinical practice. The expert tends to link observations with theory (Elstein, 1972; Kassirer, Kuipers, & Gorry).

Decision theory describes how one selects a course of action. Nurses make judgments about health states and choose nursing interventions (Grier, 1981). A study of 53 nurses' and 22 non-nurses' risk-taking behavior indicated that nurses with advanced education were better decision makers in situations depending on chance and nursing skill, as well as in making judgments about numbers. In situations where information had to be acquired and used in making nursing judgments, nurses did not differ according to educationsl level (Grier & Schnitzler, 1979).

Information processing theory describes problem-solving behavior as an interaction between an information processing system (the problem solver) and a task environment. The major assumption is that there are limits to the human information processing capacity, primarily in the amount of information one can attend to (Tanner, & McGuire, 1983). Fifty-four senior baccalaureate nursing students' responses to five videotapes of acute patient situations were analyzed using this theoretical approach. The major determinant of diagnostic reasoning was whether or not the correct diagnosis was included in the intitial set of hypotheses. Only a small relationship was found between diagnostic accuracy and the number of early diagnostic hypotheses (Tanner & McGuire, 1983).

## Existing Tools

Subjects' written and/or verbal responses to written and/or filmed patient situations have been used to evaluate diagnostic reasoning. In situations (simulations) the subject is presented with an opening scene, which includes the client's chief complaint. The data collection and management tasks are evaluated. They have been used to measure problem-solving behavior in medicine and nursing and have demonstrated improvement in this skill (de Tornyay, 1968; McGuire, 1967).

The writer chose simulations as a measure of diagnostic reasoning because of their advantage in approximating the clinical environment while controlling other variables typically found in this environment. A review of the literature was performed to locate suitable simulations for a research study comparing nursing students' performance.

One written patient care problem was designed to measure clinical nursing judgment in both the initial and comprehensive investigation stage of providing postoperative nursing care to a hospitalized adult. Reliability and validity data were based on 11 respondents. Agreement scores, using two methods of weighting, were described as reliability. Validity measures included an acceptable review of the simulation by practicing critical-care nurses and the faculty of an associate-degree nursing program and comparison of the 11 subjects' test performance with evaluation by their clinical instructors. There was a significant correlation coefficient (rho = .82) for the concurrent validity (Dincher & Stidler, cited in Ward & Fetler, 1979). A time requirement of 60 min and the use of only one simulation are major drawbacks of this instrument. Reliability is enhanced by using multiple client situations because it is known that a given situation affects outcomes (Grier, Tanner, & Benner, 1984; Holzemer, Schleuterman, & Miller, 1981).

A 126-item objective test of problem solving using four simulations, entitled Nursing Performance Simulation Instrument has been evaluated by its designer and other nurse researchers. The instrument was submitted for review to 42 nurse educators, 5 doctoral education students, and 3 medical educators during its development. Its reliability was assessed by the test-retest method with 50 subjects, with an $r$ of .63. Criterion-related validity measures with two different samples resulted in $r$ correlations of .30 and .35 (Gouer, cited in Ward & Fetler, 1979). The low reliability and validity coefficients and the estimated time requirement of at least 1 are major drawbacks of this instrument.

Six simulation instruments were used to measure problem-solving skills by 79 master's-degree nurses and certified practitioners. Multivariate data analysis, using correlation matrices and multiple regression statistics, provided evidence that simulations are a valid measure of clinical problem solving. The Cronbach alpha reliability coefficients ranged from a low of .71 on the multiple choice examination to a high of .98 on the colleague evaluation scale. The patient management simulation correlated significantly with the examination ($r = .54$, rho = .56)(Holzemer et al., 1981). Further investigation by this group of researchers of the construct validity of patient management problems was conducted with 46 nurse practitioners and 31 nurses. Meaningful differences were found between the nurse practitioners and nurses ($F = 16.95$, with $p < .0001$), thereby supporting the construct validity of these simulations. Mean comparisons of the subjects' performances across three simulations resulted in significant differences, suggesting that the simulation affects performance (Farrand, Holzemer, & Schleuterman, 1982).

McGuire (1967) used three techniques – Angoff Formula 12, Cronbach's coefficient alpha and principal analysis – to estimate the reliability of simulations across tests. The coefficient of reliability varied with the length of the test, with .75 to .85 for 2 to 3 problems (1 hr) and .80 to .90 for 10 to 12 problems (3-4 hr); the alpha reliability range being between .85 and .94.

The Nursing Index (Verhonick, 1968) and Nursing Process Utilization Inventory (NPUI) (Sparks, 1982) were the two instruments selected for use in the development of a diagnostic reasoning measurement tool. The five patient situations portrayed in the Nursing Index film are (1) a young housewife with a lump in her breast; (2) a middle-age photographer hospitalized with a myocardial infarction; (3) a young man who is hospitalized for hernia repair; (4) an elderly man hospitalized for medical evaluation; (5) a 5-year-old boy hospitalized for tracheobronchitis. The subjects are requested to write what they saw, actions they would perform, and reasons for their actions. A count of appropriate observations and actions ranging from 10 to 14 was established by experts for each situation. Previous researchers counted observations, actions, and reasons across situations and examined differences among types of respondents (Davis, 1972,1974; Hart, 1980; Tiffany, 1978; Verhonick, 1968). This approach did not consider each situation separately, and specific content related to factors inherent. The categories of data were defined and used to classify data. The categories of observations were relevant, irrelevant, and inappropriate; and the categories of actions were diagnostic, therapeutic, supportive, referral, and inappropriate. These categories were incorporated in the testing of the diagnostic reasoning protocols, which will be described in the Methodology section.

Content validity of the Nursing Index was established through a pilot test with 60 nurse practitioners. Reliability was established by submitting the scenarios to a panel of 10 masters-prepared faculty who viewed them three times consecutively, resulting in their recording 87% of the 55 relevant observations portrayed in the film (Verhonick, 1968).

One nurse researcher established reliability and validity measures with the Nursing Index with her sample of 112 registered nurses employed in staff nurse positions in 10 hospitals in New Jersey. Three of the five situations were used to investigate the relationship between state anxiety, creative potential, and decisions. Two medical-surgical textbooks and five doctoral students' responses were used to validate the decisions in a pilot study. Reliability of coding was determined through the use of phi coefficient for interrater reliability, with an outcome of .96, .92, and .75. No significant findings for the hypotheses were reported (Hart, 1980).

As part of a research study related to nursing organization structure, one investigator used weightings to code the responses from the Verhonick instrument, renamed it the Nursing Index, and validated the fact that it measured nursing competence, not scholastic ability. Responses of 91 first year college students without nursing education or experience were correlated with ACT scores as a measure of scholastic ability yielding a value of .16 (Tiffany, 1978).

Sparks (1982) created the Nursing Performance Simulation Instrument as a measure of problem-solving ability of 108 baccalaureate and 128 graduating associate-degree students and reported significant difference at the .01 level. The instrument uses an open-ended format for two simulations, which consist of a problem identification and a nursing care plan section. Point values were assigned to problems, objectives, criteric, and nursing actions. The responses in the present work were scored in accordance with the coding criteria developed by Sparks and used with three nurse educators, with an interrater reliability of .95 to .97. The correlations between the two situations using the Pearson product-moment correlation were .51 for total test score, .56 for the problem identification score, and .48 for the nursing care plan. Sparks explained the difference in these findings as due to the content being measured in each clinical simulation.

Further testing of the NPUI occurred with a New Jersey population of 297 nursing students with nearly equal representation from baccalaureate, associate-degree, and hospital-based educational program's (Scoloveno, 1981). The interrater reliability tests based on percentage of agreement between the two raters used in this study resulted in .97 correlation coefficient. The Cronbach alpha coefficient for the situation that refers to the Johnson Family within NPUI and another clinical simulation written by them was .85.

These research findings demonstrate that decisions involved in problem solving (nursing process) can be measured via simulations. The nursing care plan format was modified by the writer and tested using the community health situation (see Methodology section for details).

## CONCEPTUAL BASIS

A definition of the nursing process that has been used to describe problem-solving behavior by nurses has been selected for the diagnostic reasoning measurement instrument. "The nursing process is an orderly, systematic manner of determining the client's problems, making plans to solve them, initiating the plan or assigning others to implement it, and evaluating the extent to which the plan was effective in resolving the problems identified" (Yura & Walsh, 1978).

The nursing definition chosen for the measurement of diagnostic reasoning is the legal definition of nursing described in the New Jersey Practice Act. Diagnosing in the context of nursing practice means the identification of and discrimination between physical and psychosocial signs and symptoms essential to effective execution and management of the nursing regimen. Unlike the definitions of nursing by nurse theorists, this definition includes the diagnostic process and is congruent with the Diagnostic Reasoning Measurement Instrument proposed in this chapter.

The diagnostic reasoning process has been studied extensively in medicine but only recently in nursing. The diagnostic reasoning process is a complex observation/critical-thinking/data-gathering process used to identify and classify phenomena that are encountered in presenting clinical situations (Carnevali, Mitchell, Woovs, & Tanner, 1984). This classification and the knowledge associated with it in turn shape the decision or treatment regimens that can be undertaken to produce a desired outcome in patient/family response (Carnevali et al., 1984). This definition is aligned with the writer's definition because it incorporates the concepts of classification, critical thinking, and data collection, which in turn are encompassed in the writer's definition of diagnostic reasoning. The author assumed that diagnostic reasoning included a categorization of data. The manner in which the classification takes place sets the stage for the remaining steps of the nursing process. The assessment, hypothesis plan, and rationale are discrete areas that are separated and analyzed.

Carnevali and Patrick (1979) have proposed a model for nursing diagnosis and management that is interrelated with the proposed instrument. Their description of the nursing diagnostic process is as follows:

1. Collecting an adequate nursing data base and utilizing the nursing pathway of branching logic.
2. Arriving at the most accurate and precise nursing diagnosis that can be derived from the data.

3. Making a plan of nursing management that will effectively treat the defined problem area.
4. Implementing the treatment plan with the patient or family.
5. Using nursing criteria appropriate to the diagnosis to evaluate patient's family's response to nursing management.

The proposed criterion-reference measurement instrument for evaluating diagnostic reasoning in nursing simulations will focus on the areas of assessment, hypothesis formation, objectives, plan, criteric, and rationale. The assessment component evaluates the data collected; the planning component addresses the strategies for nursing intervention; the hypothesis component examines conclusions made by the subjects. The objective and criteric components are concerned with the measurable outcomes, and the rationale component focuses on cited reasons for the plan.

## DEFINITIONS

*Diagnostic reasoning.* Analysis of data organized for determination of client's nursing diagnosis at a particular time; includes assessment, hypothesis (diagnosis) objective, plan, criteric, and rationale.

*Assessment.* The collection of data about a given client situation. It may include history, patient observations, laboratory test results, information about the family. There are three classifications, as described below.

*Assessment with validity.* Assessment is classified as valid because relevant substantiating data are included. No inappropriate data are included.

*Assessment with some validity.* Data collection consists of a mixture of relevant substantiating data and some inappropriate data.

*Assessment without validity.* Data collection primarily consists of data that are inappropriate to a client situation.

*Data.* Sightings and notations comprising observations about a given client situation.

*Relevant data.* Observations of items or conditions that fit the client situation and could influence nursing intervention, these include subjective and objective data and provide substantiating data for a hypothesis, or significant signs and symptoms.

*Irrelevant data.* Observations of items or conditions that occur but are insignificant to a hypothesis and do not fit the client situation; not significant for the given situation.

*Hypothesis.* Conclusion(s) or inference(s) about a client situation; generally an unsophisticated diagnosis because it describes the problem component but not the etiology.

*Appropriate hypothesis.* A conclusion that is relevant to a given client situation and can be supported by relevant data.

*Mixed hypothesis.* Two or more hypotheses are made for a given client situation with a mixture of appropriate and inappropriate.

*Inappropriate hypothesis.* An interpretation of data that is unreasonable, cannot be supported by relevant data not related to client situation, may be based on assumption, and includes inappropriate data.

*No hypothesis.* No hypothesis is given for the client situation.

*Objective.* A measurable behavior expected in client to guide the nursing plan; classified as correct or incorrect.

*Plan.* Strategies for intervention designed by a nurse for providing care to a client. Interventions are further classified as described below.

*Correct intervention.* Nursing actions cited in the literature and/or by experts as relevant for a specific client problem; may or may not be based on relevant data or hypothesis.

*Intervention with some validity.* Nursing actions that are not cited in the literature or by experts as being appropriate for the given situation.

*Rationale.* Reason given by a nurse for nursing intervention.

*Relevant rationale.* Reason is related to intervention specified for a given situation.

*Incorrect rationale.* Information cited is not a reason or is not related to nursing intervention. Rationale is incomplete because a partial reason is given for an intervention, or a rationale is provided for some intervention, but not all.

*Mixed rationale.* Two or more rationales are given for a nursing intervention, with a mixture of correct and incorrect rationales.

## PURPOSE

The purpose of the study was to examine critically the diagnostic reasoning processes performed during the assessment and planning steps of the nursing process, using clinical simulations.

## OBJECTIVES

The study objectives were as follows:

1. To develop an instrument that measures diagnostic reasoning processes occurring during assessment and planning steps of the nursing process, using clinical simulations (situations).
2. To develop a critique procedure for analyzing nursing decisions made during the assessment and planning phases of the nursing process, using clinical simulations.
3. To use diagnostic reasoning protocols with a variety of clinical simulations.

## INSTRUMENT DEVELOPMENT

The initial development of diagnostic reasoning protocols emerged from coding of open-ended responses to the Nursing Index. The purpose of that study was to compare undergraduate and graduate students' decisions (Arnold, 1985). The writer's analysis of 79 nursing students' written responses to the five situations within the Nursing Index produced an unexpected outcome. Although the undergraduate and graduate students were directed to list their observations, actions, and rationales for their actions, a majority of them stated a conclusion or hypothesis. The respondents wrote their hypotheses within any of the three categories, indicating that the sequence of hypothesis formulation varied. Thus, a fourth classification of data occurred and was labeled hypothesis.

The research review substantiated the use of simulations as a measure of problem-solving behavior that is also equated with the nursing process. The assumption that decisions occur at each step of the nursing process provided the foundation for the diagnostic reasoning instrument. It was recognized that written simulations limit examination of diagnostic reasoning to the confines of situation and respondent and do not include the variables found in the clinical environment.

The diagnostic reasoning protocols include assessment, hypothesis, objective, plan, criteric, and rationale as illustrated in the flow diagram in Figure 4.1. The assessment label refers to the observation section of Nursing Index and the problem-listing section of NPUI. The hypothesis was an

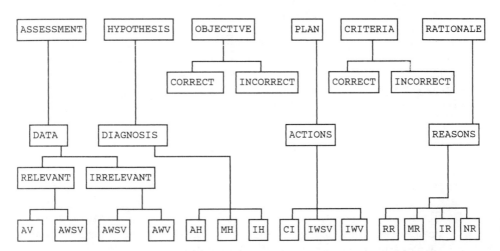

**FIGURE 4.1** Flow diagram of Diagnostic Reasoning Instrument. AV, assessment with validity; AWSV, assessment with some validity; AWV, assessment without validity; AH, appropriate hypothesis; MH, mixed hypothesis; IH, inappropriate hypothesis; CI, correct intervention; IWSV, intervention with some validity; IWV, intervention without validity; RR, relevant rationale; MR, mixed rationale; IR, irrevelant rationale; NR, no rationale.

added coding category of the Nursing Index and the priority problem listing of the NPUI. The objective and criteria component were equivalent to those used in the NPUI but were not tested in this study because of limited data. So few subjects submitted responses for these categories that statistical analysis was not possible. "Plan" referred to the listing of actions in the six simulations, and "rationale" referred to reasons for these actions. The subcategories of assessment, hypothesis plan, and rationale were conceived by the writer.

## ADMINISTRATION AND SCORING

The writer superimposed the diagnostic reasoning protocols on the coding criteric developed for the Nursing Index and the NPUI. The subclassifications of the diagnostic reasoning protocols were based on scoring procedures developed by the writer for each instrument (see Definitions).

The diagnostic reasoning protocols of assessment, intervention, hypothesis, and rationale were tested with the Nursing Index. The coding system developed by previous researchers for observations and actions was used (Davis, 1974; Tiffany, 1978; Verhonick, 1968). The coding guidelines for hypothesis and rationale were developed by Arnold (1985), using experts, since no such guidelines were available. The rater made judgment's regarding the classification of assessment, hypothesis, intervention, and rationale using the coding system developed by author.

The more appropriate the category, the higher the weighting. The subject's score and weighting was calculated by averaging the three raters' results. The subject's rating for each diagnostic reasoning protocol was based on a weighting of 3 for appropriate subclassification, 2 for mixed subclassification, and 1 for inappropriate subclassification.

### Nursing Index

*Assessment* was a weighted score (1-9) determined by adding the assigned weighting in each subcategory of observations written by the subject. The number of observations in each subcategory was determined by a decimal point. The resulting figures were divided by the number of subcategories used, ranging from 1 to 3. Note that observations were classified as appropriate, inappropriate, or irrelevant by Verhonick (1968). The assigned weighting for assessment was as follows: Assessment without validity, 1 to 3; assessment with some validity, 4 to 6; assessment with validity, 7 to 8; irrelevant and/or inappropriate observations were added.

### Intervention

First the action was classified as diagnostic, supportive, therapeutic, referral, or inappropriate. Then the judge placed these responses in the category of intervention with validity, intervention with some validity, or intervention without validity. A weighted score (1-14) was calculated by adding the assigned weighting in each subcategory of intervention written by the subject. The number of actions was determined by a decimal point. The resulting figures were determined by dividing by the number of action categories used: intervention without validity, 1 to 5; intervention with some validity, 7 to 10; intervention with validity, 11 to 14.

## Hypothesis and Rationale

The rationale and hypothesis were weighted 1 to 3 in accordance with the three subclassifications: appropriate hypothesis, 1; mixed hypothesis, 2; irrelevant hypothesis, 1; no hypothesis, 0; relevant rationale, 3; mixed rationale, 2; irrelevant rationale, 1; no rationale, 0.

# NPUI
## Assessment

This instrument required the subject to make a problem list for the Johnson Family Simulation that was supported by substantiating data. The problem identification section of the instrument was equated with the assessment and data diagnostic protocols. The assessment score was based on number of correct problems according to (Sparks, 1982). The maximum number of points was 24, based on 3-point values for six major problems and 1-point value's for six minor problems. The rating ranged from 1 to 3 appropriate assessment, 3; inappropriate assessment, 1. A score of 1 point was given for inappropriate responses due to emphasis on process, rather than on the correct response when making ratings for any subcomponent within diagnostic reasoning protocols.

## Hypothesis

The priority problems were labeled as hypothesis by the writer. The hypothesis score was based on six major problems identified by Sparks (1982). Since only three hypotheses were required, the maximum score was 9, with a range of 3 to 9. The hypothesis rating, ranging from 1 to 3 points, was the same as that used for the assessment protocol.

## Intervention and Rationale

The scoring system for the intervention plan and rationale subcomponents deviated slightly from the Sparks system. A score of 1 point was given for each nursing intervention and related rationale cited by the subject. Sparks (1982) recommended a score of 1 point for each action only if it was provided by an appropriate rationale. The assigning of separate scores facilitated testing of these diaagnostic reasoning protocols. The intervention score was calculated by multiplying correct action, according to Sparks's criteria, by the weighting assigned to the subcategory of intervention. The maximum number of actions and rationale for each problem was five. The rationale score was determined by multiplying correct rationale, according to Spark's criteria, by the weighting assigned to the subcategory of intervention. The rating system used for the assessment and hypothesis protocols was also used for the plan and rationale components.

The scoring systems described were used by three judges to analyze responses from 141 undergraduate and graduate students. Criteria for the coders include master's preparation in a clinical specialty and current employment in nursing. Two of the judges were master's prepared, and one was doctorally prepared.

A schedule of instrument administration was established by the researcher and circulated to subjects who agreed to participate in the research. The required for completion of six simulations was 2 hr. Data collection occurred during a 3-month period.

## Reliability

A combination of measurement frameworks was used to establish the reliability and validity of the Diagnostic Reasoning Instrument. First, a subject's performance was assessed on a clinical simulation, using explicit criteria developed by previous researchers, and its validity established through the use of expert panels. Next, the subject's responses were analyzed using a norm-referenced approach. The mean score for each simulation was calculated to determine the patterns of behavior by all respondents on each situation. For example, when the diagnostic reasoning protocols were used with the Nursing Index, the mean score for assessment of each simulation was determined. Using a range of 1 to 8 points, the mean score was 3.7, indicating that the assessment pattern for this situation was assessment with some validity as opposed to the extremes of the continuum. A mean score of 6 to 8 was classified as an appropriate assessment with maximum validity pattern, whereas a score of 1 to 3 points was classified as an assessment without validity. These findings confirm the construct of the three subcategories of assessment. Similar calculations were performed with the intervention, hypothesis, and rationale categories.

Interrater reliability was chosen, due to the use of open-ended clinical simulations. Interrater reliability was established by using the following procedure: Three experts employing predetermined criteria were used to judge responses from 141 subjects. Each rater was required to judge all of the subjects' responses. Separate coding sheets were used by each rater, and scoring was performed independently by each expert at a different time and place. The response sheets were rotated to each coder. Training sessions were scheduled as needed to discuss problems associated with using the coding criteria. The Pearson product-moment correlation procedure was used to determine the interrater reliability for each of the six simulations used for the following diagnostic reasoning protocols: assessment, intervention, rationale, and hypothesis. The data were not rescored by the same rater because of time commitments for coding the subjective criteria.

## Validity

*Construct* validity was assumed by determining if the demographic (independent) variables affected the subject's responses. The independent variables included age, rank in college, licensure status, years of experience, level of education, and employment. Construct validity involved the use of two contrasted groups: baccalaureate and graduate nursing students. First, the Nursing Index only was used with nursing students at sophomore, senior, and graduate levels as a pilot test. A one-way analysis of variance statistic was used to determine differences among student groups for each subcategory of the Diagnostic Reasoning Instrument.

Interrater reliability was calculated for each simulation using the Pearson product-moment correlation procedure. Intercorrelations were performed among the scores and ratings on each simulation. There were 20 by 20 correlations for the five simulations with the Nursing Index and four diagnostic reasoning protocols.

*Content* validity involved the use of three experts to act as raters. These raters used the coding criteria established by a panel of content experts in previous research when the clinical simulations were developed. The raters possessed a variety of clinical expertise. Two raters had experiences in pediatric and adult acute care nursing and master's preparation in their clinical speciality. Another had master's preparation and clinical experience in adult and psychiatric nursing. The experts' clinical expertise corresponded with the clinical content of the simulations.

*Face* validity was established through the use of experts who agreed that the simulations represented realistic clinical situations. In addition, the developers of the simulations had established the content validity of the answer key through the use of a panel of nursing experts. A 90% affirmative response was obtained for each item included in the NPUI (Sparks, 1982).

*Criterion-related* validity assumed that the students' performance on simulations would predict behavior in actual clinical setting.

The Diagnostic Reasoning Measurement Instrument evolved through the writer's previous research of decisions made by nursing students using two instruments: the Nursing Index and the NPUI. The scoring guidelines developed by authors of these instruments were enhanced through the addition of the diagnostic reasoning protocols. Subcomponents of these four diagnostic reasoning protocols were developed through previous research by this author (Arnold, 1985). Thus, the rating for each diagnostic protocol was based on the subject's performance within that protocol.

## MAJOR FINDINGS AND RESULTS

### Demographic Data

Intercorrelations among the demographic data of college rank, nursing experience, age, and licensure status of 141 undergraduate and graduate students was examined. Moderately high and moderately positive correlations were observed between college rank (.70) and age (.45). Licensure status reflected high to moderate negative correlations with the following variables: college rank (−.75), experience (−.54), and age (−.36). Age was positively correlated with experience (.41). Correlations between these demographic variables and components of diagnostic reasoning protocols using the six simulations did not produce any statistically significant relationships that were above .50. Thus, college rank, age, and experience are variables to consider when examining diagnostic reasoning by nursing students.

### Nursing Index

Interrater agreement among three judges on 141 subjects' responses on the five simulations within the Nursing Index were computed (see Table 4.1). The results of the Pearson product-moment correlation coefficients do not illustrate a significant pattern by simulation or among raters. The simulations appeared to influence interrater agreement. This instrument had a less structured scoring guideline than the NPUI. Highest agreement among raters occurred for the plan-of-actions protocol within the Diagnostic Reasoning Instrument.

Ideally, interrater reliability figures should have been calculated, but neither the funding nor the time was available. On one occasion, one judge repeated ratings on 20 subjects' performance on this instrument and noted the lack of consistency in ratings. The other two judges voiced concern about their ability to be consistent in their scoring of the data. Approximately 25 subjects' responses were evaluated by a judge during one time period. Thus, six evaluation periods occurred for each judge and required 3 months for completion.

The Pearson product-moment correlation procedure was also used to examine interrater reliability among three judges for diagnostic reasoning protocols using the NPUI. The results of the assessment protocol within the NPUI are presented in Table 4.2. The findings indicate that these outcomes are affected by rater and by client problem identified for the situation that refers to the Johnson Family Situation. The highest correlations were observed for Problem 1 because most respondents name the same problem. Another high correlation was the assessment score (.75-.86), which was based on summary points for problem listing.

**TABLE 4.1** Interrater Reliability for Nursing Index

| Outcome/situation | Pearson | P | N | Pearson | P | N |
|---|---|---|---|---|---|---|
| Assessment | Simulation 1 | | | Simulation 2 | | |
| Rater 1 with Rater 2 | .771 | .000 | 141 | .217 | .005 | 141 |
| Rater 1 with Rater 3 | .5871 | .000 | 141 | .175 | .019 | 141 |
| Rater 2 with Rater 3 | .5755 | .000 | 141 | .270 | .001 | 141 |
| Intervention | | | | | | |
| Rater 1 with Rater 2 | .800 | .000 | 141 | .760 | .000 | 141 |
| Rater 1 with Rater 3 | .642 | .000 | 141 | .767 | .000 | 141 |
| Rater 2 with Rater 3 | .608 | .000 | 141 | .696 | .000 | 141 |
| Rationale | | | | | | |
| Rater 1 with Rater 2 | .376 | .000 | 141 | .417 | .000 | 140 |
| Rater 1 with Rater 3 | .407 | .000 | 141 | .119 | .081 | 140 |
| Rater 1 with Rater 3 | .272 | .001 | 141 | .252 | .001 | 140 |
| Hypothesis | | | | | | |
| Rater 1 with Rater 2 | .523 | .000 | 101 | .515 | .000 | 127 |
| Rater 1 with Rater 3 | .326 | .000 | 109 | .333 | .000 | 124 |
| Rater 1 with Rater 3 | .397 | .000 | 105 | .485 | .000 | 125 |
| Assessment | Simulation 3 | | | Simulation 4 | | |
| Rater 1 with Rater 2 | .716 | .000 | 141 | .694 | .000 | 141 |
| Rater 1 with Rater 3 | .669 | .000 | 141 | .644 | .000 | 141 |
| Rater 2 with Rater 3 | .630 | .000 | 141 | .693 | .000 | 141 |
| Intervention | | | | | | |
| Rater 1 with Rater 2 | .601 | .000 | 140 | .201 | .008 | 141 |
| Rater 1 with Rater 3 | .613 | .000 | 140 | .325 | .000 | 141 |
| Rater 2 with Rater 3 | .609 | .000 | 140 | .196 | .010 | 141 |
| Rationale | | | | | | |
| Rater 1 with Rater 2 | .358 | .000 | 139 | .561 | .000 | 141 |
| Rater 1 with Rater 3 | .340 | .000 | 139 | .398 | .000 | 141 |
| Rater 2 with Rater 3 | .434 | .000 | 139 | .512 | .000 | 141 |
| Hypothesis | | | | | | |
| Rater 1 with Rater 2 | .607 | .000 | 102 | .522 | .000 | 122 |
| Rater 1 with Rater 3 | .596 | .000 | 114 | .315 | .000 | 127 |
| Rater 2 with Rater 3 | .720 | .000 | 101 | .535 | .000 | 115 |
| Assessment | Simulation 5 | | | | | |
| Rater 1 with Rater 2 | .337 | .000 | 141 | | | |
| Rater 1 with Rater 3 | .276 | .000 | 141 | | | |
| Rater 2 with Rater 3 | .367 | .000 | 141 | | | |
| Intervention | | | | | | |
| Rater 1 with Rater 2 | .449 | .000 | 141 | | | |
| Rater 1 with Rater 3 | .573 | .000 | 141 | | | |
| Rater 2 with Rater 3 | .501 | .000 | 141 | | | |
| Rationale | | | | | | |
| Rater 1 with Rater 2 | .470 | .000 | 137 | | | |
| Rater 1 with Rater 3 | .396 | .000 | 138 | | | |
| Rater 2 with Rater 3 | .245 | .000 | 137 | | | |
| Hypothesis | | | | | | |
| Rater 1 with Rater 2 | .461 | .000 | 109 | | | |
| Rater 1 with Rater 3 | .490 | .000 | 135 | | | |
| Rater 2 with Rater 3 | .298 | .001 | 109 | | | |

**TABLE 4.2** Interrater Reliability for NPUI Assessment (Six Major Problems)

| Outcome/problem | Person | P | N[a] | Pearson | P | N[a] |
|---|---|---|---|---|---|---|
| | Problem 1 | | | Problem 2 | | |
| Rater 1 with Rater 2 | .772 | .000 | 73 | .586 | .000 | 66 |
| Rater 1 with Rater 3 | .780 | .000 | 79 | .750 | .000 | 71 |
| Rater 2 with Rater 3 | .701 | .000 | 74 | .452 | .000 | 64 |
| | Problem 3 | | | Problem 4 | | |
| Rater 1 with Rater 2 | .425 | .009 | 30 | .640 | .012 | 12 |
| Rater 1 with Rater 3 | .375 | .016 | 33 | .666 | .003 | 15 |
| Rater 2 with Rater 3 | .468 | .009 | 25 | .866 | .000 | 12 |
| | Problem 5 | | | Problem 6 | | |
| Rater 1 with Rater 2 | .354 | .194 | 8 | .657 | .000 | 33 |
| Rater 1 with Rater 3 | .667 | .017 | 10 | .486 | .002 | 35 |
| Rater 2 with Rater 3 | .354 | .194 | 8 | .361 | .032 | 27 |
| Total Assessment score and rating | | | | | | |
| Rater 1 with Rater 2 | .817 | .000 | 133 | .715 | .000 | 134 |
| Rater 2 with Rater 3 | .866 | .000 | 133 | .604 | .000 | 134 |
| Rater 2 with Rater 3 | .745 | .000 | 133 | .441 | .000 | 134 |

[a]The N value varies due to choice of problem by subjects.

The range (.60-.99) for the hypotheses across the three priority problems for the Johnson Family indicated high rates or agreement among the three judges. Other correlations to note are those for the intervention scores on priority problems (hypotheses 1 and 2, .79-.84) and rationale score on all three hypotheses (.63-.77). The agreements among the raters on the ratings for hypothesis, intervention, and rationale diagnostic reasoning protocols were generally lower than on the scores for these protocols (see Table 4.3). These results affected the writer's decision to modify the scoring system for ratings in the computerized version that was developed at a later date.

The findings of interrater reliability for diagnostic reasoning protocols with both the Nursing Index and NPUI illustrate the difficulty of raters interpreting open-ended responses consistently. The use of a computer problem to rate responses to clinical simulations may be a more suitable methodology due to its objectivity.

The Pearson product-moment correlation procedure was also used to examine relationships between components within the diagnostic reasoning instrument. The responses of 141 students' scores and ratings on the six simulations used provide the data base for these statistical results.

Intercorrelations among the assessment, hypothesis, rationale, and intervention components were calculated using the five simulations within the Nursing Index. Intercorrelations of the assessment component of clinical Simulation 1 in relation to the other three diagnostic reasoning protocols

**TABLE 4.3** Interrater Reliability for NPUI (Three Priority Problems)

| Outcome/situation | Person | P | N[a] | Pearson | P | N[a] |
|---|---|---|---|---|---|---|
| | Assessment Score | | | Assessment Rating | | |
| Rater 1 with Rater 2 | .817 | .000 | 133 | .715 | .000 | 134 |
| Rater 1 with Rater 3 | .866 | .000 | 133 | .604 | .000 | 134 |
| Rater 2 with Rater 3 | .745 | .000 | 133 | .441 | .000 | 134 |
| | Priority Problem 1 | | | Priority Problem 2 | | |
| Hypothesis | | | | | | |
| Rater 1 with Rater 2 | .819 | .000 | 128 | .887 | .000 | 126 |
| Rater 1 with Rater 3 | .604 | .000 | 130 | .743 | .000 | 128 |
| Rater 2 with Rater 3 | .710 | .000 | 129 | .810 | .000 | 127 |
| Nursing intervention score | | | | | | |
| Rater 1 with Rater 2 | .822 | .000 | 127 | .845 | .000 | 113 |
| Rater 1 with Rater 3 | .822 | .000 | 128 | .821 | .000 | 112 |
| Rater 2 with Rater 3 | .819 | .000 | 127 | .792 | .000 | 112 |
| Nursing intervention rating | | | | | | |
| Rater 1 with Rater 2 | .567 | .000 | 126 | .468 | .000 | 113 |
| Rater 1 with Rater 3 | .637 | .000 | 128 | .610 | .000 | 112 |
| Rater 2 with Rater 3 | .512 | .000 | 126 | .545 | .000 | 112 |
| Nursing rationale score | | | | | | |
| Rater 1 with Rater 2 | .778 | .000 | 118 | .767 | .000 | 97 |
| Rater 1 with Rater 3 | .746 | .000 | 119 | .745 | .000 | 97 |
| Rater 2 with Rater 3 | .678 | .000 | 118 | .638 | .000 | 97 |
| Nursing rationale rating | | | | | | |
| Rater 1 with Rater 2 | .544 | .000 | 117 | .458 | .000 | 97 |
| Rater 1 with Rater 3 | .547 | .000 | 119 | .461 | .000 | 96 |
| Rater 2 with Rater 3 | .340 | .000 | 117 | .383 | .000 | 97 |
| | Priority Problem 3 | | | | | |
| Hypothesis | | | | | | |
| Rater 1 with Rater 2 | .848 | .000 | 118 | | | |
| Rater 1 with Rater 3 | .778 | .000 | 118 | | | |
| Rater 2 with Rater 3 | .768 | .000 | 119 | | | |
| Nursing intervention score | | | | | | |
| Rater 1 with Rater 2 | .777 | .000 | 103 | | | |
| Rater 1 with Rater 3 | −.047 | .324 | 97 | | | |
| Rater 2 with Rater 3 | −0.21 | .420 | 95 | | | |
| Nursing intervention rating | | | | | | |
| Rater 1 with Rater 2 | .449 | .000 | 104 | | | |
| Rater 1 with Rater 3 | .390 | .000 | 104 | | | |
| Rater 2 with Rater 3 | .440 | .000 | 103 | | | |
| Nursing rationale score | | | | | | |
| Rater 1 with Rater 2 | .757 | .000 | 95 | | | |
| Rater 1 with Rater 3 | .770 | .000 | 95 | | | |
| Rater 2 with Rater 3 | .658 | .000 | 93 | | | |
| Nursing rationale rating | | | | | | |
| Rater 1 with Rater 2 | .301 | .001 | 96 | | | |
| Rater 1 with Rater 3 | .578 | .000 | 95 | | | |
| Rater 2 with Rater 3 | .291 | .002 | 94 | | | |

within that situation resulted in the following: Assessment 1 with Intervention 1, .16; Assessment 1 with Rationale 1, 19; Assessment 1 with Hypothesis 1, .55. This latter finding is logical, since a hypothesis is based on the data collected. Other calculations performed among the five assessment components of the Nursing Index (.11-.25) indicate that each assessment is unique to a given situation. The highest correlation expected was between assessment and hypothesis.

When the assessment component for the Simulation 1 on the Nursing Index was compared with the hypothesis component within the same situation and among the other four simulations of the Nursing Index, there was hardly any correlation (.08-.23). The findings of a positive correlation of .16 between the assessment of Simulation 1 with the intervention of Simulation 1 and negative correlations between Assessment 1 and the intervention components of simulations 2, 3, 4, and 5 (−.04-.07) are to be expected. Also, there was no correlation among the assessment component of simulation 1 with the rationale component of this same situation and the other simulations (.0006-.18).

The expectation that there would be some degree of correlation between assessment and hypothesis component was realized with testing of the Nursing Index (.16-.59). However, the simulation affected the outcome of these calculations (see Table 4.4). The degree of correlation between intervention and rationale categories was low, with the exception of simulation 3, which was .59.

Further testing of the diagnostic reasoning measurement instrument was conducted for the situation that refers to the Johnson Family simulation from the NPUI. Only a small portion of the subjects wrote objectives and criteria, making statistical analysis impossible. The four diagnostic reasoning protocols of assessment, hypothesis, intervention, and rationale were tested through use of the Pearson product-moment correlations procedure.

The problem listing for the situation that refers to Johnson Family constituted the assessment component, and the listing of the three priority problems constituted the hypothesis component. There was no correlation among these items, which may be due to the fact that the data base for these components could vary in number and content as a result of the open-ended nature of the NPUI.

The correlations within the intervention and rationale scores were based on the nursing care section for the three priority problems identified for the Johnson Family. The findings for their scores and ratings are reported in Table 4.4. Note the high correlations that occurred within the intervention and rationale scores across all three priority problems (hypotheses) identified for the Johnson Family. Further correlations were computed between intervention scores and rating and the rationale scores and rating. These findings demonstrated a range of outcomes. The highest correlation was between intervention and rationale scores (.80-.84). There was also a moderate relationship between

**TABLE 4.4** Correlations among Components of Diagnostic Reasoning
Protocols

| Nursing Index, Assessment and Hypothesis | | Nursing Index, Intervention and Rationale | |
|---|---|---|---|
| Simulation | Pearson corr. | Simulation | Pearson corr. |
| 1 | .554 | 1 | .161 |
| 2 | .164 | 2 | .351 |
| 3 | .191 | 3 | .591 |
| 4 | .598 | 4 | .331 |
| 5 | .423 | 5 | .381 |

*Nursing Process Utilization Inventory, Assessment Score and Rating*

| | |
|---|---|
| Assessment core and Hypothesis 1 | −.103 |
| Assessment score and Hypothesis 2 | .098 |
| Assessment score and Hypothesis 3 | .087 |
| Assessment rating and Hypothesis 1 | −.006 |
| Assessment rating and Hypothesis 2 | .129 |
| Assessment rating and Hypothesis 3 | .184 |
| Hypothesis 1 with Intervention 1 score | .092 |
| Hypothesis 1 with Intervention 1 rating | .229 |
| Hypothesis 2 with Intervention 2 score | .413 |
| Hypothesis 2 with Intervention 2 rating | .470 |
| Hypothesis 3 with Intervention 3 score | .390 |
| Hypothesis 3 with Intervention 3 rating | .524 |

| Intracorrelations between Intevention and Rationale Scores | | Intracorrelations between Intervention and Rationale Ratings | |
|---|---|---|---|
| Problem | Pearson corr. | Problem | Pearson corr. |
| 1 | .865 | 1 | .448 |
| 2 | .851 | 2 | .801 |
| 3 | .838 | 3 | .708 |

| Intracorrelations between Intevention Scores and Ratings | | Intracorrelations betwween Rationale Scores and Ratings | |
|---|---|---|---|
| Problem | Pearson corr. | Problem | Pearson corr. |
| 1 | .394 | 1 | .577 |
| 2 | .532 | 2 | .585 |
| 3 | .451 | 3 | .450 |

| Intercorrelations among Intervention Scores | | | | Intercorrelations among Intervention Ratings | | | |
|---|---|---|---|---|---|---|---|
| Problem | Corr. | N | P | Problem | Corr. | N | P |
| 1 & 2 | .48 | 113 | .000 | 1 & 2 | .230 | 113 | .007 |
| 1 & 2 | .42 | 105 | .000 | 1 & 3 | .064 | 113 | .005 |
| 2 & 3 | .38 | 113 | .000 | 2 & 3 | .208 | 113 | .001 |

| Intercorrelations among Intervention Scores and Rationale Scores | | | | Intercorrelation among Rationale Scores | | | |
|---|---|---|---|---|---|---|---|
| Problem | Corr. | N | P | Problem | Corr. | N | P |
| 1 & 1 | .82 | 118 | .000 | 1 & 2 | .50 | 97 | .000 |
| 2 & 2 | .80 | 99 | .000 | 1 & 3 | .33 | 95 | .001 |
| 3 & 3 | .84 | 96 | .000 | 2 & 3 | .34 | 88 | .001 |

*Intercorrelations among Rationale Scores and Ratings*

| Problem | Corr. | N | P |
| --- | --- | --- | --- |
| 1 & 1 | .38 | 119 | .000 |
| 2 & 2 | .51 | 98 | .000 |
| 3 & 3 | .41 | 97 | .000 |

intervention and rationale ratings. Intercorrelations between the intervention scores and ratings and rationale scores and ratings were generally moderately positive. These findings support the fact that nursing students do identify rationales for their nursing actions via this written simulation.

The results of the analysis of variance statistical testing indicated some differences among the three groups of students tested. Due to space limitation, the data are not presented here. There was no difference on hypothesis formation amont 59 sophomores, 20 seniors, and 62 graduate students with any of the six clinical simulations within NPUI and Nursing Index. Some differences occurred with the assessment component on two of five simulations during pilot testing of the Nursing Index and the NPUI. Also, there were significant differences among these students on intervention and rationale scored on some of the simulations within the Nursing Index and all of those within the NPUI.

## CONCLUSIONS, RECOMMENDATIONS, AND IMPLICATIONS

These conclusions are based on the testing of the Diagnostic Reasoning Instrument with six simulations: (1) the construct of four diagnostic reasoning protocols – assessment, hypothesis formation, plan of action, and rationale-were realized through their testing with six clinical simulations; (2) testing with the Nursing Index yielded correlations between assessment and hypothesis protocols but generally not between intervention and rationale components; (3) testing with NPUI yielded correlations between intervention and rationale components but not between assessment and hypothesis components; (4) the clinical simulation affected the measurement of diagnostic reasoning; (5) the demographic variables of college rank and experience affected diagnostic reasoning.

Recommendations for further study include (1) the devlopment of computer software programs that can be used to rate responses on clinical simulations, instead of human judges; (2) the use of this instrument as a teaching tool to analyze an individual's diagnostic reasoning process for a given clinical simulation; (3) testing this instrument with a variety of clinical simulations; (4) further development and testing of the diagnostic reasoning processes that occur within all steps of the nursing process.

Implications for nursing include the following: (1) nursing and nursing education should examine diagnostic reasoning processes in greater detail through the use of clinical simulations, and (2) nursing education should include teaching the diagnostic reasoning process within its curriculum.

## FUTURE DIRECTIONS FOR MEASUREMENT OF DIAGNOSTIC REASONING

The need to make the rating process more objective and to perform individualized analysis led to the development of a computer software program that automates the evaluation process. The diagnostic reasoning protocols as outlined in Figure 4.1 served as specifications for the program. The software, which consists of two disks, a test disk and an answer disk, is used only to analyze each individual's responses to a given situation. The subject is still required to complete the diagnostic reasoning process by responding to the written situation without benefit of the computer. The choices are restricted by the use of a closed, rather than an open-ended, format. A listing of choices for the assessment, hypothesis, objective, criteric, intervention, and rationale components are provided and coded by number. The answer code for the situation that refers to the Johnson simulation limited responses as follows: 12 problems for assessment, 3 priority problems (hypotheses), 1 objective for each hypothesis, 3 criteria for each hypothesis, 5 nursing actions and rationales for each hypothesis. The answer key is entered on the answer disk of the computer software.

The simulation was submitted to three content experts for further face validity and delimitation of five nursing actions and corresponding rationale for the major problems. The answer disk was then used to correct each subject's responses. The computer printout of the individual's diagnostic reasoning pattern refelcts the scoring system. The numerical scoring is identical to that originally recommended by Sparks, yielding a separate score for assessment and plan. The embellishments are within the derivation of a rating label for a given subject's response for each diagnostic protocol, as follows:

*Assessment* (maximum,12). If the correct-answer range is 9 to 12, rating is assessment with validity. If the correct-answer range is 6 to 8, rating is assessment with some validity. If the correct-answer range is 0 to 4, rating is assessment without validity.

*Hypothesis* (maximum, 3). If the correct-answer range is 3, appropriate rating is given. If the correct-answer range is 2, mixed hypothesis rating is given. If the correct-answer range is 1, rating given is inappropriate hypothesis.

*Intervention and rationale*. If the correct-answer range is 5, rating is assessed with validity. If the correct-answer range is 3 to 4, rating is assessed with some validity. If two or fewer correct answers are given, rating is assessed without validity.

The rating is now a descriptive statement that yields an individual's pattern. Only the three numerical scores – assessment, plan, and total score – can be subjected to statistical analysis using grouped data.

The advantage of computerizing the diagnostic reasoning protocols is the capability to analyze a variety of simulations using this single format. Plans are to use this instrument with practicing nurses as well as with students. The content of the situation used will determine the type of nursing population tested (i.e., the community health situation with community health nurses). Another advantage is versatility in that this Diagnostic Reasoning Instrument can be applied in other fields, using situations analogous to a particular discipline. The speed of the computer provides immediate feedback and analysis, offering direction for individualized instruction. A program of this design provides a window on human thought processes. It is anticipated that patterns of diagnostic reasoning will be identified and thereby provide models for teaching the diagnostic reasoning process.

## REFERENCES

Arnold, J. (1985, January). *Decision making by nursing students.* Paper presented at society for Research in Nursing Education, San Francisco.

Barrows, H. S., & Tamblyn, R. M. (1976). An evaluation of problem-based learning in small groups utilizing a simulated patient. *Journal of Medical Education, 51,* 52-54.

Carnevali, D., Mitchel, P. H., Woods, N. F., & Tanner, C. A. (1984). *Diagnostic reasoning in nursing.* Philadelphia: J. B. Lippincott.

Davis, B. G. (1972). Clinical expertise as a function of educational preparation. *Nursing Research, 21*(5), 531-534.

Davis, B. (1974). Effect of levels of nursing education on patient care: A replication. *Nursing Research, 23*(2), 150-155.

de Tornyay, R. (1968). Measuring problem-solving skills by means of the simulated clinical nursing problem test. *Journal of Nursing Education, (7),* 3-8, 34-35.

Elstein, A. S. (1972). Methods and theory in the study of medical inquiry. *Journal of Medical Education, 47,* 85-92.

Farrand, L., Holzemer, W. L., & Schleutermann, J. A. (1982). A study of construct validity. Simulations as a measure of nurse practitioners' problem solving skills. *Nursing Research, 31*(1), 37-42.

Grier, M. R. (1981). The need for data in making nursing decisions. In H. H. Werley & M. R. Grier (Eds.), *Nursing information systems* (pp. 15-31). New York: Springer Publishing Co.

Grier, M. R., & Schnitzler, C. P. (1979). Nurses' propensity to risk. *Nursing Research, 28*(3), 186-190.

Grier, M., Tanner, C., & Benner, P. (1984, January). Symposium on clinical knowledge: Controversies and countercurrents. Audio-tape of paper presented at meeting of Society for Research in Nursing Education, San Francisco.

Hammond, K. R. (1966). Clinical inference in nursing. *Nursing Research, 15*(1), 27-38.

Hart, J. (1980). *The relationship between state anxiety, creative potential and decisions reported in stimulated decisions.* Unpublished doctoral dissertation, New York University, New York.

Holzemer, W. L., Schleutermann, J. L., & Miller, A. G. A. (1981). Validation study: Simulations as a measure of nurse practitioners' problem-solving skills. *Nursing Research, 30*(3), 139-44.

Kassirer, J. P., Kuipers, B. J., & Gorry, A. G. (1982). Toward a theory of clinical expertise. *American Journal of Nursing, 73,* 251-259.

Kelly, K. (1966). Clinical inference in nursing. *Nursing Research, 15*(1), 23-26.

Marriner, A. (1983). *The nursing process: A scientific approach to nursing care.* St. Louis: C. V. Mosby.

McGuire, C. H. (1967). Simulation technique in the measurement of problem solving skills. *Journal of Educational Measurement, 4*(1), 1-10.

Scoloveno, M. A. (1981). *Problem-solving ability of senior nursing students in three program types.* Unpublished doctoral dissertation, Rutgers-The State University, New Brunswick, NJ.

Sparks, R. K. (1982). Problem solving ability of graduates from associate and baccalaureate degree nursing program, *Journal of Nursing Education, 21*(8), 68-69.

Tanner, C. A., & McGuire, C. (1983). Research on clinical judgement. *In Review of Research in Nursing Education* (pp. 2-32). Thorofare, NJ: Slack Incorporated.

Tiffany, C. (1978). *Nursing organizational structure and the real goals of hospitals: A correlational study.* Unpublished doctoral dissertation, Indiana University, Bloomington, IN.

Verhonick, P. (1968). I came, I saw, I responded: Nursing observation and action survey. *Nursing Research, 17*(1), 38-44.

Ward, M. J., & Fetler, M. E. (1979). *Instruments for use in nursing education.* Boulder, CO: Western Interstate Commission for Higher Education.

Yura, H., & Walsh, M. B. (1978). *The nursing proces: Assessing, planning, implementing, evaluating* (3rd). New York: Appleton-Century-Crofts.

# 5

# The Reliability and Validity of a Nurse Performance Evaluation Tool

## Margaret R. Kostopoulos

*This chapter discusses the Performance Evaluation Tool (Registered Nurse, Medical/Surgical Unit), a measure of nursing job performance.*

## BACKGROUND OF STUDY

Prior to the 1980 Standards of the Joint Commission on Accreditation of Hospitals (JCAH), the employee performance evaluation tool in use in nearly all hospitals used global traits as the criteria for measurement. These highly subjective categories of "dependability, initiative, cooperation, appearance," and so on were used for all employees whether in maintenance, dietary, medical records, or nursing. Although there were some who were advocating objective criterion-based evaluation (Brief, 1979; del Bueno, 1977; Dracup, 1979; Krumme, 1975), it was the impetus from JCAH that resulted in the transition to criterion-referenced measurement.

Employee performance evaluation is an essential tool of management. It can serve as a determiner for promotion and salary increases, a motivator toward professional growth, and an indicator of quality of patient care (Burns, Chubinski, & Freiburger, 1983; Davis, Greig, Burkholder, & Keating, 1984; Lerch, 1982). In order to do so, the performance evaluation must define the standard of care expected of an employee in a particular position so that the actual performance can be measured against those standards and staff are motivated to excel as their areas for professional growth are clarified (Deckers, Oldenburg, Pattison, & Swartz, 1984). Areas for attention by the staff development department can be identified if there is consistent inadequacy among employees. "Measurement of performance against realistic and attainable standards of nursing will enable nurses to know they are being held accountable and responsible for their nursing performance" (O'Loughlin & Kaulbach, 1981).

## REVIEW OF THE LITERATURE

Although nursing literature has included much on performance evaluation, the emphasis has been on evaluation of students. There has also been much written on the evaluation of nursing care from both the process and outcome viewpoints that is, quality assurance. But there is comparatively little written about the comprehensive evaluation of employee performance and about methods of evaluation that have been tested for reliability and validity (Waltz, Strickland, & Lenz, 1984). Concurrent investigation and reporting of reliability and validity has been absent in the majority of cases, and content validity has been relied heavily. The technical and manual tasks involved in nursing are not difficult to measure and have been handled through a skill inventory of some sort in most hospitals. But the quantifying of intellectual and interpersonal activities has been more difficult to define and measure.

Performance can be evaluated if the content of the evaluation is based on specific expectations stated in behavioral terms (Dracup, 1979; del Bueno, 1979; Goodykoontz, 1981; Smith, 1982; West, Sudbury, & Ayers, 1979). These expectations must be consistent with the job description and specific to the job (Burns et al., 1983; del Bueno, 1979; Krumme, 1975).

Criterion-referenced evaluation is advocated if there is to be validity of the tool and if the tool is to address its intended purpose because in criterion-referenced measurement one's performance is evaluated on the basis of criteria or standards rather than compared to the performance of others (del Bueno, 1979; Krumme, 1975). Validity can be viewed from two aspects: (1) Does the evaluation tool actually measure the true performance of the employee, and (2) do the supervisors and staff believe the system has credibility (Brief, 1979)? Del Bueno (1979) states that "validity is insured by basing the content on the performance expectations." By explicitly stating the expectation, the employee and supervisor are clear on the level of performance to be achieved (Smith, 1982). But in addition to knowledge of the level of performance, the employee must consider the defined criteria to be important to the optimum performance of the job (Cook, 1979). There must be congruence between the employee's appraised performance and his/her actual performance if there is to be validity (Brief, 1979). And the appraisal system will have no credibility if unacceptable performance is tolerated at any level (del Bueno, 1979).

The validity of the evaluation tool is first dependent on a high reliability. However, reliability does not insure validity (Waltz et al., 1984). To be reliable, an evaluation tool must have clearly defined criteria that are measurable and not subject to interpretation. Clearly defined criteria are necessary because interpretations of quality differ (O'Loughlin & Kaulbach, 1981). "Although it is impossible for an evaluator to be completely objective, by limiting judgments to measurable behaviors, a greater degree of objectivity can be achieved. Evaluation of attitudes are unreliable and subjective" (del Bueno, 1977, p.23). Therefore, self-rating scales cannot be effectively used for evaluation when used alone.

Del Bueno (1977) advocates a yes/no rating scale to increase reliability. She contends that an employee either does or does not meet the criterion. Using a rating scale invites unreliability because the evaluator must rely on his/her own interpretations of the rating. To recognize and reward excellence, she suggests using a weighting technique. "A specified group of standards represent an acceptable minimum. An excellent performance means meeting standards beyond the minimum for a particular level" (del Bueno, 1977, p.51).

Cook (1979) states that using a percentage of the time is not completely descriptive or objective, but it does give a clearer idea of how the employee is performing and what performance goals need to be met. Further differentiating a yes response serves to encourage professional growth and stimulate motivation.

If a system of performance evaluation is to be both reliable and valid, "a standard of behavior that cannot be put into measurable terms should not be formally evaluated" (del Bueno, 1979, p.51).

## PURPOSE

The purpose of this study was to determine whether the Performance Evaluation (Registered Nurse, Medical/Surgical Unit) that was developed for Doctors' Hospital of Prince George's County is both valid and reliable.

## CONCEPTUAL FRAMEWORK

The concepts important in Dorothea Orem's (1980) self-care framework serve as the basis for determining the components of the content domains for the performance evaluation of the registered nurse on the medical/surgical unit.

Section 1 includes those nursing activities that demonstrate the utilization of the nursing process, such as an initial and ongoing assessment, an initial plan of care with revisions as necessary, the implementation of that plan, and evaluation of the effectiveness of the interventions.

The second section is designed to enable an evaluation of the supportive-educative role of the professional nurse, a role defined by Orem (1980) as a valid way of assisting the patient and/or family to achieve self-care. It includes the assessment of learning needs, the use of appropriate teaching methods and resources, and the evaluation of learning that has taken place.

The ability to meet patient needs in an organized manner is the focus of the third section of the evaluation tool. Included are those activities and characteristics of the professional nurse that fulfill the other roles defined by Orem (1980) – doing for another or providing a helping environment.

The fourth section of the evaluation tool addresses the professional nurse's responsibility for self-development. If the nurse is truly to assist the patient in the maintenance or resumption of self-care activities, he/she must grow professionally and increase his/her effectiveness as a resource for the patient.

The last section is directed toward the professional nurse's responsibility and accountability for quality care and includes his/her contributions to increasing the effectiveness of nursing practice.

Throughout the evaluation tool the focus is on those activities of the nurse that facilitate the meeting of identified holistic self-care needs that the patient cannot meet independently.

## TOOL DEVELOPMENT

Several objectives guided the development of the evaluation tool for the registered nurse on a medical/surgical unit.

- The tool should be criterion-referenced.
- The criteria should reflect major concepts of Orem's (1980) self-care framework.
- The tool should reflect the standards of performance established by the Department of Nursing Services, Doctor's Hospital of Prince George's County.
- The criteria should reflect the role of the registered nurse as defined in the Maryland Nurse Practice Act.

Initial work on the tool was done by a task force that was developing a career ladder program. This task force included both nursing managers and nursing staff. Building on this work, the criteria were further developed, reviewed, and accepted by the nursing managers. In retrospect, it is acknowledged that nursing staff should have had an opportunity to participate at this level of development also. This tool is used for both the probationary and annual evaluation of the medical/surgical registered nurse.

## ADMINISTRATION AND SCORING

The nurse is rated by an individual familiar with her performance in the work setting, such as a supervisor or head nurse. The items are rated on a Likert scale from 1 (representing below standard performance) to 4 (representing outstanding performance). Each item is scored according to the ranking guidelines listed at the beginning of the tool, and the numbers are totaled and divided by the number of items scored for an average overall rating. Although each criterion has equal weight at present, the effectiveness of the tool could be increased by using a weight factor to indicate critical behaviors.

# METHODOLOGY

A descriptive study was conducted that focused on two methods to measure content validity and one method to measure reliability of the performance evaluation tool that is utilized for the medical/surgical registered nurse. The position description on which the performance evaluation tool was based and copy of the tool can be found at the end of the chapter.

## Content Validity

Four registered nurses who are considered content specialists examined the performance evaluation to see whether the criteria statements within each domain measured the domain. Two were educators teaching in a graduate program in nursing, and two were clinical specialists familiar with self-care theory. Each content specialist rated the congruence of each item against the following questions:

- Is the criterion measurable?
- Does the criterion reflect the expectation of performance by a registered nurse on a medical/surgical unit?
- Is the criterion relevant to the domain statement?
- Does the criterion fit the rating scale?
- Does the criterion represent the performance expectation for the domain?

A +1 was used to indicate if the item was judged to be congruent, 0 if undecided and −1 if incongruent.

A questionnaire was distributed to all of the registered nurses employed at Doctors' Hospital of Prince George's County who worked on a medical/sugical unit and who had been evaluated using the study tool. The questionnaire was designed to measure employee acceptance of the evaluation tool as applicable for evaluating their performance. Using a 4-point rating scale measuring acceptance from Strongly Agree to Strongly Disagree (see Table 5.1), the registered nurses responded to these items:

**TABLE 5.1 Registered Nurses' Assessment of the Registered Nurse Performance Evaluation Tool**

| | Strongly agree | Agree | Disagree | Strongly disagree | % Agree |
|---|---|---|---|---|---|
| 1. Generally, the performance evaluation describes the expectation for an RN. | | | | | |
| (With A) | 7 | 30 | 10 | 11 | 63.8 |
| (Without A) | 7 | 29 | 10 | 3 | 73.5 |
| 2. I know what is expected of me based on the statements of the performance evaluation. | | | | | |
| (With A) | 8 | 29 | 11 | 10 | 63.8 |
| (Without A) | 8 | 28 | 11 | 2 | 73.5 |
| 3. The statements in Section A relate to the objective A. | | | | | |
| (With A) | 6 | 38 | 7 | 7 | 75.9 |
| (Without A) | 6 | 36 | 7 | 0 | 85.7 |
| 4. The statements in Section B relate to the objective B. | | | | | |
| (With A) | 8 | 40 | 3 | 7 | 82.8 |
| (Without A) | 8 | 38 | 3 | 0 | 93.9 |
| 5. The statements in Section C relate to the objective C. | | | | | |
| (With A) | 13 | 35 | 3 | 7 | 82.8 |
| (Without A) | 13 | 33 | 3 | 0 | 93.9 |
| 6. The statements in Section D relate to the objective D. | | | | | |
| (With A) | 10 | 35 | 6 | 7 | 77.6 |
| (Without A) | 10 | 33 | 6 | 0 | 87.8 |
| 7. The statements in Section E relate to the objective E. | | | | | |
| (With A) | 7 | 39 | 5 | 7 | 79.3 |
| (Without A) | 7 | 37 | 5 | 0 | 89.8 |
| 8. I would rather be rated on a rating scale (1-2-3-4) than a yes/no scale. | | | | | |
| (With A) | 22 | 24 | 7 | 4 | 80.7 |
| (Without A) | 15 | 24 | 7 | 2 | 81.3 |
| 9. This performance evaluation form has helped me to identify areas in which I excel. | | | | | |
| (With A) | 7 | 21 | 17 | 13 | 48.3 |
| (Without A) | 7 | 21 | 16 | 5 | 57.1 |
| 10. This performance evaluation form has heped me to identify areas for professional growth. | | | | | |
| (With A) | 4 | 26 | 16 | 12 | 51.7 |
| WIthout A) | 4 | 26 | 14 | 4 | 62.5 |

*N* with Unit A, 58; *N* without Unit A, 49.

- Generally, the performance evaluation describes the expectation for an RN.
- I know what is expected of me based on the statements of the performance evaluation.
- The statements in section A relate to the objective A.
- The statements in section B relate to the objective B.
- The statements in section C relate to the objective C.
- The statements in section D relate to the objective D.
- The statements in section E relate to the objective E.
- I would rather be rated on a rating scale (1-2-3-4) than on a yes/no scale.
- This performance evaluation form has helped me to identify areas in which I excel.
- This performance evaluation form has helped me to identify areas for professional growth.

## Reliability

The clinical supervisor and three assistant clinical supervisors of a medical/surgical unit discussed together the performance of 10 registered nurses who worked on that unit. Independently, they then completed the annual evaluation form for each of the 10 and the results were compared for interrater reliability using percentage of agreement. The evaluations for study were the first 10 received from the personnel department beginning with a specified data.

## MAJOR FINDINGS

### Content Validity

In nearly all instances, the content specialists agreed on the validity of the evaluation tool. Calculating the percentage of agreement among them, in 28 of the 42 total criteria there was 100% agreement with validity. Of the remaining 14, there were only 4 criteria (9.5%) in which there was less than 75% agreement with one or more of the 5 congruency questions. These criteria and the corresponding questions in which there was less than 75% agreement are as follows:

*Objective*: C. Synchronizes the nursing activities toward achievement of patient and nurse goals safely, efficiently, and effectively.
    Criterion: 3. Establishes priorities appropriately.
              d. Identifies stress-producing situations.
        50% agreement with congruency to the following questions:
              Is the criterion measurable?
              Does the criterion fit in a rating scale?
    Criterion: 6. Is accessible and approachable.
        50% agreement with congruency to the following questions:

Does the criterion reflect the expectation of performance by a registerd nurse on a medical/surgical unit?
Is the criterion relevant to the domain statement?
25% agreement with congruency to the following question:
Does the criterion represent the performance expectations for the domain?

Criterion: 7. Participates in group process and facilitates communication.

50% agreement with congruency to the following question:
Is the criterion measurable?

*Objective:* E. Participates in programs designed to increase the effectiveness of nursing practice.

Criterion: 5. Demonstrates responsibility for maintaining certification in CPR and for reviews in isolation and fire safety as designated in nursing policy.

50% agreement with congruency to the following question:
Does the criterion fit in a rating scale?

The registered nurses viewed the evaluation tool favorably in judging its content to be applicable to the content domains. Over 75% agreed that the statements on the tool related to their respective objective, and 63.8% felt that the performance evaluation describes the expectation for a registered nurse and that the tool helped them to know what is expected of them. They were less in agreement with its usefulness in helping them identify areas of strength (48.3%) and the need for professional growth (51.7).

Of the 58 respondents, 7 of 9 from one unit were extremely negative in their responses. This was inconsistent with the range of responses from all other respondents and is felt to be significant of a unit problem that will require further investigation. When this unit was excluded, the results indicated that more than 82% agreed with the compatibility of the rating tool with the objectives, and 73.5% believed that the evaluation tool describes the expectation for a registered nurse and that it helped them to know what was expected of them. The percentage of agreement was determined by combining the number of responses of Strongly Agree and Agree, dividing them by the number of responses to each statement, and multiplying by 100.

With a possible range of scores from 10 to 40 (10 being the highest agreement), distribution of individual scores for the survey is as follows:

| | |
|---|---|
| 10-15 | 6 |
| 16-20 | 18 |
| 21-25 | 20 |
| 26-30 | 7 |
| 31-35 | 1 |
| 36-40 | 7 |

It should be noted that all seven of the surveys showing the least agreement were from Unit A.

The mean score, including all respondents, was 22.33. Without Unit A, the mean score was 20.59. In either case the mode was 21.

## Reliability

In the evaluation of the 10 registered nurses, 75% agreement by the four nursing managers was considered acceptable. The reliability was examined in two ways: (1) by the percentage of agreement about each registered nurse, and (2) by the percentage of agreement about each item for all registered nurses. The average percentage of items for which there was at least 75% agreement between raters for a specific nurse was 59.0%, with a range of 42.9% to 81.0% (see Table 5.2).

An item was considered reliable if 7 of the 10 responses had 75% or greater agreement by the four raters. These items are indicated in Table 5.3 by an asterisk. Nineteen of the 42 items were found to be reliable. Table 5.3 presents the level of agreement between raters for each item.

It is interesting to note that the items in Section C of the performance evaluation indicate reliability in 9 of the 12 items, but it is these items that showed the least congruency in validity. Interrater reliability for the entire tool ranges from .10 to 1.00 for the evaluations of the registered nurses.

## CONCLUSION

Although the results of this study indicated a basically useful tool for the performance evaluation of the medical/surgical registered nurse, the study gives concrete direction for improvement of the tool. Based on the findings of this study, each criterion for which there was less than 75% agreement by either the content specialists or nursing managers should be critically examined. Repetition of the study after revision will allow measurement of the revised criteria until a valid and reliable tool is developed. However, it is possible that interrater reliability could be improved if raters are trained in the interpretation of items and use of this tool. Therefore, training of raters and provision of clear explanations of the item meanings and related behaviors are needed.

A structured continuing education program for managers on the process of employee performance evaluations may increase the importance placed on identification of areas of strength and areas for professional growth for the employee. If these are emphasized during the evaluation conference, the employee may be better able to relate future goals for practice based on previous practice and the usefulness of the tool will be increased.

**TABLE 5.2** Number of Items with 75%
Interrater Agreement between Raters per RN

| RN | Number of items with 75% | % Total items in which 75% agree |
|----|----|----|
| A | 34 | 81.0 |
| B | 30 | 71.4 |
| C | 28 | 66.7 |
| D | 28 | 66.7 |
| E | 27 | 64.2 |
| F | 23 | 54.8 |
| G | 21 | 50.0 |
| H | 20 | 47.6 |
| I | 19 | 45.0 |
| J | 18 | 42.9 |

**TABLE 5.3** Agreement between Raters for Each Item

| Item | No. with 75% agreement | Item | No. with 75% agreement |
|----|----|----|----|
| A-1 | 10* | C-1 | 10* |
| A-2 | 8* | C-2 | 8* |
| A-3a | 6 | C-3a | 8* |
| A-3b | 4 | C-3b | 9* |
| A-3c | 3 | C-3c | 7* |
| A-3d | 4 | C-3d | 5 |
| A-3e | 2 | C-4 | 7* |
| A-4 | 8* | C-5 | 5 |
| A-5 | 7* | C-6 | 7* |
| A-6 | 5 | C-7 | 4 |
| A-7 | 4 | C-8 | 9* |
| A-8 | 7* | C-9 | 8* |
| A-9 | 6 | D-1 | 8* |
| A-10 | 3 | D-2 | 5 |
| B-1 | 4 | D-3 | 5 |
| B-2 | 9* | D-4 | 3 |
| B-3 | 2 | E-1 | 5 |
| B-4 | 7* | E-2 | 6 |
| B-5 | 7* | E-3 | 1 |
| B-6 | 6 | E-4 | 3 |
| B-7 | 6 | E-5 | 8* |

* Level of agreement was at least 75%.

The benefits of a valid and reliable performance evaluation will be felt by both employee and employer as direction for professional growth, recognition for performance, and an assurance of a standard of quality care can be demonstrated.

## REFERENCES

Brief, A. P. (1979). Developing a usable performance appraisal system. *Journal of Nursing Administration, 10*, 7-10.

Burns, C., Chubinski, S., & Freiburger, O. (1983). A criteria-based performance appraisal for the critical care nurse. *Nursing Administration Quarterly, 3*, 46-58.

Cook, P. A. (1979). Painless performance evaluations-that work. *RN, 10*, 75-85.

Davis, D. S., Greig, A. E., Burkholder, J., & Keating, T. (1984). Evaluating advanced practice nurses. *Nursing Management, 3*, 44-47.

Deckert, B., Oldenburg, C., Pattison, K. A., & Swartz, S. L. (1984). Clinical ladders. *Nursing Management, 3*, 54-62.

del Bueno, D. J. (1977). Performance evaluation: When all is said and done, more is said than done. *Journal of Nursing Administration, 12*, 21-23.

del Bueno, D. (1979). Implementing a performance evalution system. *Supervisor Nurse, 2*, 48-52.

Dracup, K. (1979). Improving clinical evaluation. *Supervisor Nurse, 6*, 24-27.

Goodykoontz, L. (1981). Performance evaluation of staff nurses. *Supervisor Nurse, 8*, 39-43.

Joint Commission on Accreditation of Hospitals (1980). *Accreditation manual for hospitals.* Chicago: JCAH.

Krumme, U. S. (1975). The case for criterion-referenced measurement. *Nursing Outlook, 12*, 764-770.

Lerch, E. M. (1982). Criteria-based performance appraisals. *Nursing Management, 7*, 28-31.

O'Loughlin, E. L., & Kaulbach, D. (1981). Peer review: A perspective for performance appraisal. *Journal of Nursing Administration, 9*, 22-27.

Orem, D. E. (1980). *Nursing: Concepts of practice.* New York: McGraw-Hill.

Smith, J. (1982). Managing employee performance. *Nursing Management, 8*, 14-16.

Waltz, F., Strickland, O. L., & Lenz, E. R. (1984). *Measurement in nursing research,* Philadelphia: F. A. Davis.

West, N., Sudbury, J., & Ayers, M. (1979). An objective appraisal instrument for registered nurses. *Supervisor Nurse, 3*, 32-38.

# Performance Evaluation Tool
# (Registered Nurse, Medical/Surgical Unit)

## POSITION DESCRIPTION

The following is a description of the position for which the following Performance Evaluation Tool was developed.

Title: Registered Nurse
Supervisor: Clinical Supervisor

I.  Summary of Responsibilities:
    The Registered Nurse is responsible for assessing the self-care needs of each patient in his/her care and for planning with the patient/family the actions of both nurse and patient necessary to meet those self-care needs which may be physiological, psychological, social or spiritual. Once planned, the Registered Nurse is responsible for implementing the plan of care directly and/or through leadership of unit personnel. The Registered Nurse utilizes principles of teaching and learning to assist patients, staff, and self in the identification of the need for new knowledge and skills.

II. Qualifications:
    A.  Graduate from an accredited School of Nursing.
    B.  Current registration as a professional nurse in the State of Maryland.
    C.  One year's previous experience in medical/surgical nursing within the past five years.
    D.  Ability to assess, plan, direct and/or implement, and evaluate the activities necessary to meet the self-care needs of the patients in his/her care.
    E.  Ability to communicate effectively.

III. Job relationships:
    A.  Responsible to:
        1.  The patient for whom care is provided.
        2.  Self and peers as professional nurses.
        3.  Clinical Supervisor or Assistant Clinical Supervisor.
        4.  Evening Assistant Clinical Supervisor or Administrative Nursing Supervisor when working the evening shift.
        5.  Charge Nurse or Administrative Nursing Supervisor when working the night shift.
    B.  Employees supervised:
        1.  Licensed Practical Nurses and unlicensed patient care givers.
        2.  As preceptor, orientees and nursing graduates.

C. Interdisciplinary relationships:
  1. Works effectively toward collaborative relationships with the Medical Staff, other members of the health team and administrative personnel.
  2. Maintains a cooperative working relationship with ancillary departments.

IV. Responsibilities:
  A. Adheres to the Purpose and Objectives of Nursing Practice of the Department of Nursing Services, utilizing the Nursing Process to assist patients in meeting their self-care needs.
    1. Assesses the patient on admission and documents appropriate data.
    2. Initiates and maintains an individualized Patient Care Plan which includes nursing diagnosis, patient and nurse goals, nursing system to be utilized, patient and nurse actions, and evaluation of plan using outcomes.
    3. Implements the medical and nursing plan of care and revises plan according to ongoing evaluation.
    4. Identifies, documents, and reports appropriately changes in patient's status.
    5. Coordinates the plan of care in preparation for discharge.
  B. Organizes and carries out a plan for teaching the self-care required to patient and/or family.
    1. Utilizes principles of teaching and learning.
    2. Identifies barriers to learning.
    3. Displays the attitudes, knowledge and skills necessary to stimulate motivation in patients to achieve results appropriate to the patient's condition and circumstances.
    4. Evaluates learning and modifies teaching plan as necessary.
    5. Contacts other hospital departments/services and community resources to assist with self-care.
  C. Synchronizes the nursing activities toward achievement of patient and nurse goals safely, efficiently and effectively.
    1. Formulates a plan of care based on priority self-care needs.
    2. Utilizes resources and other nursing personnel commensurate with their educational preparation and experience.
    3. Instructs, supervises, and evaluates activities of other members of the nursing team.
    4. Contributes to the promotion of a climate that fosters supportive communication and problem solving.
  D. Identifies and pursues his/her professional self-development plan.
    1. Utilizes the current literature and pertinent workshops in nursing and related fields to enhance his/her professional development.
    2. Continually evaluates own practice and outcome of care in light of emerging knowledge.
  E. Participates in programs designed to increase the effectiveness of nursing practice.
    1. Demonstrates awareness of the value and relevance of research in nursing.
    2. Suggests need for and participates in quality assurance measures.

## PERFORMANCE EVALUATION TOOL
## (REGISTERED NURSE, MEDICAL/SURGICAL UNIT)

| _____ | _____ |
| (Employee Name) | (Department – Unit) |

_____      FROM _____ TO _____
(Reason for Review)

Ranking Guidelines:

Below Standard (1) – Fulfills defined expectation inconsistently, requiring repeated assistance and follow-up.

Meets Standard (2) – Fulfills defined expectation consistently (90% of the time) in routine situations, requiring assistance initially and/or with difficult or unusual situations.

Above Standard (3) – Fulfills defined expectation consistently (90% of the time) in routine situations, requiring assistance some of the time with difficult or unusual situations.

Outstanding (4) – Fulfills defined expectation independently and consistently in almost all situations.

A. Adheres to the "Purpose and Objectives of Nursing Practice" of the Department of Nursing Services, utilizing the nursing process to assist patients in meeting their self-care needs.

1. Identifies in the admission nursing assessment progress note the relationship between data collected from the nursing history, systems assessment, and self-care needs within 24 hours of admission.      1   2   3   4

_____

_____

2. Documents nursing diagnoses in the nursing progress notes and on the master problem list within 24 hours of admission. 1   2   3   4

_____

_____

3. Initiates a written plan of care within 24 hours of admission collaborating with the physician, patient, and family, utilizing:
   a. Nursing diagnosis      1   2   3   4

_____

   b. Long- and short-term goals      1   2   3   4

_____

_____

    c.   Nursing systems        1  2  3  4

_____

_____

    d.   Specific patient/nurse actions        1  2  3  4

_____

_____

    e.   Measurable outcome criteria        1  2  3  4

_____

_____

4.   Documents implementation of the medical/nursing plan of care in the nursing progress notes.     1  2  3  4

_____

_____

5.   Documents an evaluation of the patient's compliance and response to the therapeutic regimen.     1  2  3  4

_____

_____

6.   Reviews/revises and updates patient care plan at least every 48 hours to reflect resolution of problems, new nursing diagnoses, and/or revisions in patient/nurse actions.     1  2  3  4

_____

_____

7.   Documents the reason for changes in patient care plan in nursing progress note.     1  2  3  4

_____

_____

8.   Revises master problem list as status of active and inactive problems change.     1  2  3  4

_____

_____

9.   Identifies need for and includes preparation for discharge on the patient care plan as appropriate.     1  2  3  4

_____

_____

10. Documents progress of patient/family in preparation for discharge in nursing progress note.     1  2  3  4

_____

_____

B.  Organizes and carries out a plan for teaching the self-care
    required to patient and/or family.
    1.  Documents learning needs, readiness to learn and motiva-
        tion of patient and family in the nursing progress notes.     1   2   3   4

    _____

    2.  Includes patient and family while developing goals for the
        teaching/learning plans.                                      1   2   3   4

    _____

    3.  Documents the teaching/learning plans on the patient care
        plan.                                                         1   2   3   4

    _____

    4.  Selects teaching tools consistent with the patient's ability
        to learn.                                                     1   2   3   4

    _____

    5.  Documents use of community resources in teaching more
        complex self-care activities.                                 1   2   3   4

    _____

    6.  Documents patient's behavioral response to teaching.          1   2   3   4

    _____

    7.  Revises teaching/learning plans in response to patient
        need.                                                         1   2   3   4

    _____

C.  Synchronizes the nursing activities toward achievement of
    patient and nurse goals safely, efficiently, and effectively.
    1.  Completes nursing activities within established time frame
        and with consideration of patient desires.                    1   2   3   4

    _____

    2.  Collaborates with other members of the health team
        to establish priorities of patient care.                      1   2   3   4

    _____

3. Establishes priorities appropriately.
   a. Gives immediate priority to emergency situations.  1 2 3 4

   _____

   _____

   b. Identifies time sequences for completion of
      procedures.  1 2 3 4

   _____

   _____

   c. Seeks assistance, if necessary, in order to accomplish
      immediate priorities without loss of control.  1 2 3 4

   _____

   _____

   d. Identifies stress-producing situations.  1 2 3 4

   _____

   _____

4. Assigns nursing activities to those qualified to perform
   them.  1 2 3 4

   _____

   _____

5. Assesses learning needs of nursing personnel and makes
   recommendations for and/or provides instruction.  1 2 3 4

   _____

   _____

6. Is accessible and approachable.  1 2 3 4

   _____

   _____

7. Participates in group process and facilitates
   communication.  1 2 3 4

   _____

   _____

8. Organizes nursing activities and uses equipment and
   supplies as intended, resulting in cost containment.  1 2 3 4

   _____

   _____

9. Demonstrates knowledge and skill while performing
   technical skills indicated on skill inventory checklist.  1 2 3 4

   _____

   _____

D.  Identifies and pursues his/her professional self-development plan.
    1.  Incorporates new concepts, procedures, and skills obtained
        from continuing education into clinical practice.              1   2   3   4

    _____

    _____

    2.  With assistance of unit supervisor, identifies areas of strength
        and those needing further development at appropriate
        intervals.                                                    1   2   3   4

    _____

    _____

    3.  Formulates goals for professional growth as part of
        probationary and yearly evaluations.                          1   2   3   4

    _____

    _____

    4.  Meets previous goals or demonstrates pursuit of alternatives
        within clearly defined time frames.                           1   2   3   4

    _____

    _____

E.  Participates in programs designed to increase the effectiveness
    of nursing practice.
    1.  Communicates nursing research reported in the literature
        in formal and/or informal settings, as appropriate to specific
        patient and/or unit needs.                                    1   2   3   4

    _____

    _____

    2.  Participates in unit and staff meetings.                      1   2   3   4

    _____

    _____

    3.  Conducts patient care conferences.                            1   2   3   4

    _____

    _____

    4.  Makes suggestions for topics for investigation to unit
        representatives of appropriate nursing/hospital
        committees.                                                   1   2   3   4

    _____

    _____

    5.  Demonstrates responsibility for maintaining certification
        in CPR and for reviews in isolation and fire/safety as
        designated in nursing policy.                                 1   2   3   4

    _____

    _____

SIGNATURES OF REPORTING OFFICERS:
This report is based on my observation and/or knowledge. It represents my best judgment of the employee's performance.

RATED BY _____DATE _____

REVIEWED BY _____DATE _____

APPROVED BY _____        DATE _____

Report discussed with and copy given to employee

BY _____DATE _____

This report has been discussed with me

Employee's signature _____DATE _____
Received in Personnel Office for Review

BY _____ DIRECTOR        Date _____

# 6

# Development of a Clinical Performance Examination for Critical Care Nurses

## Barbara Clark Mims

*This chapter discusses the Clinical Performance Examination for Critical-Care Nurses, a measure of nurses' clinical performance in the critical-care setting.*

### PURPOSE

Evaluation of clinical performance is a pervasive problem encountered by nursing faculty, educators in practice settings, and nursing service administrators, who all share responsibility for ensuring the quality of nursing care delivered to the health care consumer. Unfortunately, however, the measurement of clinical performance is indeed problematical. While paper-and-pencil tests can reliably measure theoretical knowledge, knowledge does not guarantee one's ability to perform patient care in the clinical setting (Cantor, 1975). In fact, a study performed by O'Donohue and Wegin (cited in Ramsberg, 1983) showed no relationship between scores on written examinations and assessment of clinical performance. It follows, therefore, that attending staff development programs may increase a nurse's knowledge base, yet not after her clinical performance. "Evaluation of the learner's ability to transfer classroom theory to behavioral performance is a critical concern" (Uphold, 1983, p. 397). During this era of cost containment and intense administrative scrutiny of educational expenditures, it is essential that methods be developed to evaluate objectively the impact staff development programs have on clinical performance. Therefore, the purpose of this study was to develop an instrument to measure clinical performance of nurses employed in critical-care settings. This criterion-referenced instrument can be utilized to evaluate the impact that educational programs have on nurses' clinical performance.

# CONCEPTUAL BASIS

The review of literature indicated evidence of interest in evaluating clinical performance dating back to 1900. However, the first competency-based clinical performance examination that was widely accepted in nursing was developed between 1972 and 1975 as part of the New York Regents' External Degree Nursing Program. During the last decade, movement toward competency-based education has heightened interest in performance testing using a criterion-referenced approach. This type of performance evaluation focuses on how well an examinee is able to meet specified performance standards. The examinee's competence level is then judged on how well standards are met. The New York Regent's External Degree Nursing Program differs from conventional program in that it is noninstructional and is based on assessment of learning. How, where, and when learning takes place is the responsibility of the learner. To obtain the degree, candidates must demonstrate clinical competence. During the program's initial development, the faculty agreed that paper-and-pencil tests are insufficient to measure nursing competence. Therefore, the development of the Clinical Performance Examination was an absolute necessity (Morgan & Irby, 1978). This is a "comprehensive, hospital-based, patient-oriented, objective clinical performance examination" (Lenburg, 1979, p.xiii). It serves as a model for others interested in developing competency-based clinical examinations.

## Competency-Based Education

Competency-based education has gained increasing popularity among nurse educators in practice settings. Spady (cited in Scott, 1982), has defined competency-based education as "a data-based, adaptive, performance-oriented set of integrated processes that facilitate, measure, record, and certify within the context of flexible time parameters the demonstration of known, explicitly stated, and agreed upon learning outcomes that reflect successful functioning in life roles" (p. 119). These definitions support the idea that professional education should assist the learner in acquiring the ability to function successfully in the designated role. The Minnesota State Board of Nursing supports this concept and "has considered rules to include demonstration of skill in approved programs to meet mandatory continuing education offerings" (Sonnen, 1983, p. 28). One of the most difficult tasks in implementing a competency-based learning program is the evaluation of competence. This is due to the existing measurement tools, which Spady has described as "inadequate, weak in validity, and questionable in reliability" (cited in Scott, 1982, p. 122). Therefore, Houston and Warner (cited in Scott, 1982, p. 123), have stated, "The future of competency-based training may well be linked to its development in three areas – new bases for specifying competencies, linking training procedures with outcome specifications and competency assessment". The notion of competence as the goal of staff development programs is attractive, as it indicates that learners will be able to function as a result of their participation. Significantly, documentation of competent performance achieved through staff development programs is consistent with JCAH standards (del Bueno & Altano, 1984).

## DEVELOPMENT OF INSTRUMENT

The concept of clinical performance includes the actual observable behaviors expected of a practicing clinical nurse; that is, the way in which a nurse carries out the tasks or duties expected of her reflects her clinical performance. For the purpose of this study, clinical performance was operationalized into five categories: assessment, clinical/technical skill, communication, documentation, and general employment policies.

These categories were derived through interviews with practicing critical-care nurses, including both staff nurses and nurse managers. Discussions with critical-care nurse educators and a review of widely accepted critical-care nursing texts confirmed that the five categories encompass the major aspects of job performance required of nurses functioning in a critical-care setting. When linked together, these five categories give a complete description of the clinical duties and responsibilities of a critical-care nurse.

## CONSTRUCTION OF TOOL

The five categories identified above were divided into subcategories, each of which had one test objective. The categories and objectives were refined during reliability and validity testing. The final tool has the following 24 test objectives.

*Category I (assessment).* When caring for a critically ill adult, the nurse performs a head-to-toe assessment within 1 hr of arriving at the bedside.

Performs complete neurological system assessment.
Performs complete cardiovascular system assessment.
Performs complete pulmonary system assessment.
Performs complete gastrointestinal system assessment.
Performs complete renal/metabolic system assessment.
Performs complete musculoskeletal system assessment.

*Category II (clinical/technical skills).* When caring for a critically ill adult patient, the nurse performs the clinical/technical skills that are common in critical-care nursing practice.
Adheres to safety procedures.
Performs general physical care.
Administers medications.

Administers intravenous therapy.
Performs hemodynamic monitoring.
Manages the patient-ventilator system.
Administers tube feedings.
Administers hyperalimentation.
Changes peripheral IV/arterial line dressings.
Changes central line dressings.
Changes dressings of open wounds every shift or as ordered by
   physician.

*Category III (communication).* The nurse interacts and communicates with others in a courteous and professional manner.

Participates in unit activities and interacts effectively with co-workers.
Communicates effectively with patients.
Communicates with and provides support for family members.

*Category IV (documentation).* The nurse completes all aspects of documentation.

Documents all nursing interventions, including patient's response when
   appropriate.
Maintains complete and current care plan for each patient.

*Category V (general employment policies).* The nurse follows hospital policy regarding dress and punctuality.
Adheres to uniform regulations.
Adheres to policies regarding punctuality.

Competency statements were developed for each of the test objectives. Since initial utilization of the tool was to be within the Critical Care and Trauma Nurse Internship at Parkland Memorial Hospital, the internship faculty participated in formulating the competency statements. Documents utilized in constructing the tool included the internship evaluation tool, the quality assurance audit tools, and the staff nurse job description developed at Parkland Memorial Hospital, and the American Association of Critical-Care Nurses' *Standards for Nursing Care of the Critically Ill* (American Association of Critical-Care Nurses, 1981).

## ADMINISTRATION OF THE EXAM

The final tool actually consists of 24 individual tests. Since each test is scored separately, each can be administered separately. Ideally, the tests will be treated as an aggregate, and the entire exam will be administered at one time.
   Testing must take place in a critical-care unit. Subjects should be given

a copy of the test ahead of time and given ample notice of when the testing will take place. If all of the 24 tests are to be administered, the patient must have the following equipment in use: Ventilator, Swan-Ganz catheter, ECG monitor, IV, and Foley catheter.

The person administering the test will observe the nurse for a minimum of 4 hr during an 8-hr shift. Periods of observation may vary from 5 min to 1 hr. The observer will not participate in the patient's care unless an emergency arises or the patient's safety is jeopardized.

## PROCEDURES FOR SCORING

### Rating Items

Each individual test (capital letters) within each major category (Roman numerals) is scored separately. There are four possible ratings for each item on this criterion-referenced tool. If the item was performed as stated, it is rated Done. If the nurse does not perform the item as stated or if she omits the item, it is rated Not Done. If the item does not apply during this particular patient care situation, it is rated Not Applicable. If the item is appropriate to the patient care situation but the opportunity to observe the behavior does not arise, it is rated Not Observed.

### Raw Score and Maximum Possible Raw Score

The raw score for each test is calculated by summing the number of items rated Done. The maximum possible raw score is calculated by subtracting the number of items rated Not Applicable and Not Observed from the total number of items on the test.

### Cut Score

In order to establish the criteria for categorizing subjects as masters or nonmasters, it was necessary to establish a cut score for each test. The panel of experts was asked to rate each test item on a scale from 1 to 10 as to its importance relative to the test objective. Each expert's ratings across all items on the test were then averaged. Finally, the mean of averages from all four experts was calculated, then converted into a proportion that became the cut score (Waltz, Strickland, & Lenz, 1984). The cut scores and maximum obtainable raw scores are shown in Table 6.1.

### Master/Nonmaster

Before comparing the subject's raw score to the cut score, the number of items rated Not Observed and Not Applicable is subtracted from the expert's cut score. In order for the subject to be labeled as master on the test, the raw score must equal or exceed the cut score obtained in this manner.

**TABLE 6.1** Cut Scores for Classifying Subjects as Master/Nonmaster

| Objective (test) | Maximum possible raw score | Cut score |
|---|---|---|
| Category I | | |
| A | 5 | 5 |
| B | 10 | 10 |
| C | 4 | 4 |
| D | 5 | 5 |
| E | 4 | 4 |
| F | 3 | 3 |
| Category II | | |
| A | 15 | 13 |
| B | 6 | 5 |
| C | 5 | 5 |
| D | 7 | 6 |
| E | 9 | 9 |
| F | 5 | 5 |
| G | 5 | 4 |
| H | 6 | 5 |
| I | 8 | 3 |
| J | 7 | 7 |
| K | 9 | 9 |
| Category III | | |
| A | 4 | 3 |
| B | 7 | 7 |
| C | 2 | 2 |
| Category IV | | |
| A | 12 | 9 |
| B | 3 | 3 |
| Category V | | |
| A | 3 | 3 |
| B | 4 | 4 |

## Percentage Score

A percentage score is then calculated for each test (capital letters), using the following formula:

$$\text{Percentage Score} = \frac{\text{Subject's Raw Score}}{\text{Maximum Possible Raw Score}} \times 100$$

If the 24 tests are administered as an aggregate, the percentage scores for all tests (capital letters) are averaged to arrive at a score for the category (Roman numerals). Although the percentage score is not used to classify subjects as master/nonmaster, it provides useful information and enables the subject to follow his/her progress when taking the same test multiple times.

# RELIABILITY ASSESSMENT

The tool was field-tested in the critical-care units at Parkland Memorial Hospital. Interrater reliability was established by having two trained observers simultaneously rate subjects in performing the behaviors identified in the test items. The number of subjects observed for each test ranged from 16 to 24. The subjects were critical-care nurses with 1 to 5 years experience. Most of the subjects were employed in the surgical intensive care unit. The majority were female, and most were graduates of baccalaureate nursing programs.

The statistics utilized were $P_0$ and K. $P_0$ represented the proportion of subjects classified the same (master/nonmaster) by both observers. K represented the proportion of persons classified the same beyond that expected by chance. The minimum acceptable K value was 0.50. If K was less than 0.50, the test items were revised or deleted. The results of interrater reliability testing are shown in Table 6.2. Out of 24 tests that were assessed for interrater reliability, six had K values less than 0.5. Substantial revisions were made, and the final tool appears at the end of the chapter.

## Item Analysis

Item analysis was performed to ensure that the items on the tool represent the specified content domain. The most commonly employed criterion-referenced item analysis procedures involve either pretest/posttest measurements with one group or two independent measurements with two different groups. Neither of these approaches was appropriate with the tool under study. The tool is used to measure actual clinical practice, and it is not feasible to test a group of nurses on clinical practice before they have been taught to function in a critical-care unit. Therefore, only the adjunct item discrimination index was used (Waltz et al., 1984).

The discrimination index was computed to measure the effectiveness of an item in relation to the total test in classifying subjects as masters/nonmasters. This was done by checking the proportion of subjects who were classified as masters and nonmasters on the overall test against the proportion of masters and nonmasters on the item (Waltz et al., 1984).

$P_0$, K, $K_{max}$, and $K/K_{max}$ ratio are the statistics that were utilized. $K_{max}$ indicates an upper limit value for K with a particular distribution of test results. $K/K_{max}$ ratio provides a value that can be interpreted on a standard scale. The upper limit of this ratio is 1.00 (Waltz et al., 1984). During this study, the minimum acceptable value for the $K/K_{max}$ ratio was 0.50. If an item had an index of less than 0.50, the item was discarded or revised. Although there were a few items that required revision based on the adjunct item discrimination index, the mean of $K/K_{max}$ for the 24 tests ranged from 0.542 to 1.000. The results are shown in Table 6.3.

**TABLE 6.2** Results of Interrater Reliability Testing

| Objective | $P_0$ | K |
|---|---|---|
| Category I | | |
| A | 0.894 | 0.777 |
| B | 0.895 | −0.006 |
| C | 0.895 | 0.441 |
| D | 0.875 | 0.733 |
| E | 0.941 | 0.821 |
| F | 0.944 | 0.770 |
| Category II | | |
| A | 1.000 | 1.000 |
| B | 0.931 | 0.848 |
| C | 0.952 | 0.904 |
| D | 0.895 | 0.784 |
| E | 0.875 | 0.449 |
| F | 0.875 | −0.059 |
| G | 1.000 | 1.000 |
| H | 1.000 | 1.000 |
| I | 0.944 | 0.870 |
| J | 0.850 | 0.659 |
| K | 1.000 | 1.000 |
| Category III | | |
| A | 0.000 | 0.000 |
| B | 0.739 | 0.405 |
| C | 1.000 | 1.000 |
| Category IV | | |
| A | 0.958 | 0.000 |
| B | 1.000 | 1.000 |
| Category V | | |
| A | 1.000 | 1.000 |
| B | 1.000 | 1.000 |

## VALIDITY ASSESSMENTS

### Panel of Experts

Content validity was considered at the item and test levels. A panel of experts was utilized to assess the relevance of items and the extent to which they measure the content domain. Since there are 24 objectives on this tool, the items that are measures of each objective were treated as separate tests. The panel of experts was composed of four nurses. One was an assistant nurse coordinator for the medical intensive care unit/coronary care unit. She had a B.S.N. and 4 years of critical-care experience. She was a certified Critical Care Registered Nurse and a Clinical Nurse I. The second expert was a master's-prepared nurse who has

**TABLE 6.3** Adjunct Item Discrimination Index

| Objective | $P_0$ range | Mean of $P_0$ | K range | Mean of K | $K_{max}$ range | Mean of $K_{max}$ | $K/K_{max}$ range | Mean of $K/K_{max}$ |
|---|---|---|---|---|---|---|---|---|
| Category I | | | | | | | | |
| A | 0.421-0.800 | 0.594 | 0.063-0.569 | 0.294 | 0.128-0.569 | 0.294 | 1.000-1.000 | 1.000 |
| B | 0.080-0.875 | 0.354 | 0.003-0.440 | 0.106 | 0.003-0.537 | 0.138 | 0.424-1.000 | 0.942 |
| C | 0.211-1.000 | 0.579 | 0.021-0.769 | 0.395 | 0.021-1.000 | 0.511 | 0.769-1.000 | 0.923 |
| D | 0.529-0.793 | 0.666 | 0.172-0.600 | 0.408 | 0.172-0.600 | 0.408 | 1.000-1.000 | 1.000 |
| E | 0.235-0.971 | 0.802 | 0.016-1.000 | 0.733 | 0.016-1.000 | 0.733 | 1.000-1.000 | 1.000 |
| F | 0.697-0.862 | 0.784 | 0.315-0.582 | 0.459 | 0.315-0.791 | 0.529 | 0.736-1.000 | 0.912 |
| Category II | | | | | | | | |
| A | 0.296-1.000 | 0.637 | 0.000-1.000 | 0.366 | 0.000-1.000 | 0.427 | 0.125-1.000 | 0.542 |
| B | 0.408-1.000 | 0.728 | 0.123-0.550 | 0.511 | 0.123-0.767 | 0.450 | 0.401-1.000 | 0.962 |
| C | 0.525-0.900 | 0.704 | 0.009-0.796 | 0.431 | 0.183-0.796 | 0.474 | 0.474-1.000 | 0.869 |
| D | 0.400-0.706 | 0.538 | 0.105-0.452 | 0.216 | 0.114-0.452 | 0.233 | 0.467-1.000 | 0.924 |
| E | 0.156-0.834 | 0.365 | 0.009-0.469 | 0.122 | 0.009-0.469 | 0.122 | 1.000-1.000 | 1.000 |
| F | 0.182-0.935 | 0.376 | 0.000-0.537 | 0.119 | 0.000-0.846 | 0.163 | 0.121-1.000 | 0.822 |
| G | 0.334-0.818 | 0.720 | 0.000-0.645 | 0.379 | 0.000-0.645 | 0.379 | 1.000-1.000 | 1.000 |
| H | 0.500-0.750 | 0.639 | 0.182-0.500 | 0.361 | 0.182-0.500 | 0.361 | 1.000-1.000 | 1.000 |
| I | 0.289-0.680 | 0.546 | 0.000-0.350 | 0.170 | 0.000-0.350 | 0.170 | 1.000-1.000 | 1.000 |
| J | 0.625-0.923 | 0.744 | 0.000-0.806 | 0.335 | 0.000-0.806 | 0.335 | 1.000-1.000 | 1.000 |
| K | 0.125-1.000 | 0.525 | 0.000-1.000 | 0.339 | 0.000-0.876 | 9.339 | 1.000-1.000 | 1.000 |
| Category III | | | | | | | | |
| A | 0.666-1.000 | 0.053 | 1.000-1.000 | 0.500 | 0.000-1.000 | 0.500 | 1.000-1.000 | 1.000 |
| B | 0.591-0.865 | 0.728 | 0.000-0.732 | 0.511 | 0.000-0.732 | 0.450 | 0.774-1.000 | 0.962 |
| C | 1.000-1.000 | 1.000 | 1.000-1.000 | 1.000 | 1.000-1.000 | 1.000 | 1.000-1.000 | 1.000 |
| Category IV | | | | | | | | |
| A | 0.216-1.000 | 0.704 | 0.044-0.483 | 0.151 | 0.013-0.483 | 0.151 | 1.560-1.000 | 1.000 |
| B | 0.167-0.942 | 0.613 | 0.000-0.000 | 0.000 | 0.000-0.000 | 0.000 | Indeterminate | 1.000 |
| Category V | | | | | | | | |
| A | 0.172-0.769 | 0.470 | 0.000-0.451 | 0.226 | 0.000-0.451 | 0.226 | 1.000-1.000 | 1.000 |
| B | 0.417-0.417 | 0.417 | 0.125-0.125 | 0.125 | 0.125-0.125 | 0.125 | 1.000-1.000 | 1.000 |

worked as a clinical specialist and nurse educator in critical care. She was also a Critical Care Registered Nurse and at the time of this study, worked part-time in the surgical intensive care unit and the burn intensive care unit. The third expert had a B.S.N. and 4 years of critical-care experience and was a Critical Care Registered Nurse. She was the staff development coordinator for the medical intensive care unit. The fourth expert had a B.S.N. and 4 years of critical care experience and was a certified Critical

Care Registered Nurse. She was the staff development coordinator for the surgical intensive care unit.

## Item-Objective Congruence

Item-objective congruence was determined using the method described by Rovinelli and Hambleton (cited in Waltz et al., 1984). Content specialists assigned a value of +1, 0, or −1 for each item, depending upon the item's congruence with the test objective. A value of +1 indicated that the item was a definite measure of the objective, a value of 0 meant that the judge was undecided, and a rating of −1 indicated that the item was not a measure of the objective. These data were then used to compute the index of item-objective congruence. The limits of this index range from minus 1.00 to +1.00, with +1.00 indicating perfect positive item-objective congruence. After the index was computed for each item, only those items with an index of +0.80 or greater were retained.

The range of coefficients for item-objective congruence appears in Table 6.4. Of a total of 149 items, there were 13 with an index of item-objective congruence less than 0.80. Such items were refined, moved to a different section on the test, or deleted.

## Interrater Agreement

The content specialists were asked to rate the relevance of each item to the content domain. Interrater agreement was then determined. $P_0$ was calculated and reflects the items given a rating of Not/Somewhat Relevant and Quite/Very Relevant by two content specialists. Therefore, $P_0$ represents the "consistency of judges' ratings of the relevance of the group of items within the test to the specified content domain" (Waltz et al., 1984, p. 198). K represents $P_0$ corrected for chance agreements. $P_0$ was calculated to be 0.97; K was calculated to be 0.40.

## Average Congruency Percentage

The average congruency percentage was calculated as a further estimation of content validity. This involved calculating the proportion of items rated congruent by each judge and converting this to a percentage (Waltz et al., 1984). The average congruency percentage was then calculated by figuring the mean percentage for all four judges (Table 6.5).

Only three objectives had average congruencies of less than 90%. Items for each of these objectives were carefully scrutinized, and possible reasons for the low ratings were considered. Some of the items were then changed, some moved to a different section on the test, and some were discarded. The tool appearing at the end of this chapter includes the revisions made after validity and reliability testing was done.

**TABLE 6.4** Index of Item Objective Congruence

| Objective | Index (range) | No. of items with index of item-objective congruence 0.800 |
|---|---|---|
| Category I | | |
| A | 0.938-0.981 | |
| B | 0.875-0.969 | |
| C | 0.644-0.963 | 2 |
| D | 0.944-0.981 | |
| E | 0.956-0.981 | |
| F | 0.912-0.969 | |
| Category II | | |
| A | 0.731-1.000 | 1 |
| B | 0.600-0.988 | 4 |
| C | 0.938-0.944 | 1 |
| D | 0.938-0.981 | |
| E | 0.694-0.994 | 1 |
| F | 0.731-0.988 | 1 |
| G | 0.950-0.956 | |
| H | 0.950-0.975 | |
| Category III | | |
| A | 0.625-1.000 | 1 |
| B | 0.981-1.000 | |
| C | 1.000-1.000 | |
| Category IV | | |
| A | 0.863-1.000 | |
| B | 0.994-1.000 | |
| Category V | | |
| A | 0.875-1.000 | |
| B | 0.750-1.000 | 2 |

## IMPLICATIONS FOR NURSING

This study resulted in the development of a criterion-referenced tool for the objective evaluation of clinical performance of critical-care nurses. The tool may be used by nurse managers, educators in practice settings, or nursing school faculty to document competence in critical-care nursing. Since it provides a mechanism for competency assessment, the tool may prove useful in documenting the impact of staff development programs on clinical performance of critical-care nurses.

The results of reliability testing showed that 18 of the 24 tests had evidence of interrater reliability. Substantial revisions were made in the remaining six tests.

Validity exercises indicated that the tool is valuable for assessing clinical performance of critical-care nurses. When the index of item-objective congruence was computed for each of the 149 items, only 13 were found to have values less than 0.80. Appropriate revisions were made in these items. Interrater agreement was assessed to evaluate the relevance of items to the content domain of the test. Strong evidence of relevance was demonstrated by a $P_0$ of 0.97 and a K of 0.40. Further evidence of content validity was demonstrated when the average congruency percentage was calculated. Of 24 objectives, only three were found to have values less than 90%. Appropriate revisions were made.

Information obtained during item analysis further supported the relevance of test items to the content domain of the test. The adjunct item discrimination index was computed, and 0.50 for $K/K_{max}$ was used as a cutoff for retaining items. Although this value is fairly lenient, it was appropriate for this initial validity testing.

## FUTURE DIRECTIONS

Further testing of established cut scores, reliability, and validity should be done now that revisions based on initial testing have been made. Additional work should include development of a guide to be used by examiners, specifying precisely the behaviors that must be demonstrated in order for an item to be rated Done.

**TABLE 6.5** Average Congruency Percentages

| Objective | Average congruency percentages |
|---|---|
| Category I | |
| A | 100 |
| B | 100 |
| C | 100 |
| D | 100 |
| E | 100 |
| F | 100 |
| Category II | |
| A | 96 |
| B | 83 |
| C | 100 |
| D | 100 |
| E | 98 |
| F | 94 |
| G | 100 |
| H | 100 |
| Category III | |
| A | 87 |
| B | 100 |
| C | 100 |
| Category IV | |
| A | 94 |
| B | 100 |
| Category V | |
| A | 94 |
| B | 88 |

Priority setting is the one aspect of clinical performance that is not addressed in this tool. A mechanism for evaluating priority setting in clinical practice needs to be incorporated as evolution of the tool continues.

## REFERENCES

American Association of Critical-Care Nurses. (1981). *Standards for Nursing Care of the Critically Ill*. Reston, VA: Reston Publishing.

Cantor, M. L. (1975). Certifying competencies of personnel. *Journal of Nursing Administration, 5*(6), 8.

del Bueno, D., & Altano, R. (1984). Competency-based education: No magic feather. *Nursing Management, 15,* 52.

Lenburg, C. B. (1979). *The clinical performance examination*. New York: Appleton-Century-Crofts.

Morgan, M. K., & Irby, D. W. (1978). *Evaluating clinical competence in the health professions*. St. Louis: C. V. Mosby.

Ramsberg, G. C. (1983). Evaluation of clinical performance: part I. *Journal of the American Association of Nurse Anesthetists, 51*(2), 59.

Scott, B. (1982). Competency-based learning: A literature review. *International Journal of Nursing Studies, 19*(3), 119-124.

Sonnen, B. E. (1983). Clinical practice in continuing education offerings: Practical considerations. *Journal of Continuing Education in Nursing, 14*(3),28.

Uphold, C. R. (1983). Using an individualized clinical evaluation strategy to motivate the R.N. student. *Journal of Nursing Education, 22,* 397.

Waltz, C. F., Strickland, O. L., & Lenz, E. R. (1984). *Measurement in nursing research*. Philadelphia: F. A. Davis.

# Clinical Performance Examination for Critical-Care Nurses

| | |
|---|---|
| Name | Employee number |

| | |
|---|---|
| Examination date | Unit |

## I. ASSESSMENT

Score ___

When caring for a critically ill adult patient, the nurse performs a head-to-toe assessment within one hour of arriving at the bedside

| | Done | Not done | Not observed | Not applicable |
|---|---|---|---|---|
| Raw Score ___  Maximum Possible Raw Score ___  Percentage Score ___  Cut Score 5-___  Master ___  Nonmaster ___ | | | | |
| A. Performs complete neurological system assessment | | | | |
| 1. Assesses level of consciousness | ___ | ___ | ___ | ___ |
| 2. Assesses orientation | ___ | ___ | ___ | ___ |
| a. person | ___ | ___ | ___ | ___ |
| b. place | ___ | ___ | ___ | ___ |
| c. time | ___ | ___ | ___ | ___ |
| 3. Checks pupils | | | | |
| a. size | ___ | ___ | ___ | ___ |
| b. reaction to light | ___ | ___ | ___ | ___ |
| 4. Evaluates ability to move extremities, purposeful or not | ___ | ___ | ___ | ___ |
| 5. Checks grasps | ___ | ___ | ___ | ___ |
| a. strength | ___ | ___ | ___ | ___ |
| b. equality | ___ | ___ | ___ | ___ |

Raw Score __          B. Performs complete cardio-
Maximum Possible         vascular system
  Raw Score __           assessment
Percentage
  Score __                  1. Obtains cardiac moni-
Cut Score 10–                  tor strip                    __    __    __    __
  Master __
  Nonmaster __              2. Interprets cardiac
                               monitor strip                __    __    __    __

                            3. Checks blood pressure    __    __    __    __

                            4. Checks heart rate        __    __    __    __

                            5. Assesses skin            __    __    __    __

                               a. warm or cool          __    __    __    __
                               b. moist or dry          __    __    __    __

                            6. Auscultates heart
                               sounds                        __    __    __    __

                            7. Palpates peripheral
                               pulses                        __    __    __    __

                            8. Checks IV                 __    __    __    __

                               a. patency               __    __    __    __
                               b. type of fluid as
                                  ordered                    __    __    __    __
                               c. rate                       __    __    __    __

                            9. Checks Swan-Ganz
                               catheter                      __    __    __    __

                               a. system intact         __    __    __    __
                               b. PA waveform visible   __    __    __    __
                               c. line free of air
                                  bubbles                    __    __    __    __

                           10. Checks arterial line     __    __    __    __

                               a. evaluates circulation
                                  in extremity distal to
                                  insertion site             __    __    __    __
                               b. line free of air
                                  bubbles                    __    __    __    __

Raw Score __          C. Performs complete pulmo-
Maximum Possible         nary system assessment
  Raw Score __              1. Checks oxygen admin-
Percentage                     istration device             __    __    __    __
  Score __
Cut Score 4–                2. Evaluates respirations   __    __    __    __
  Master __
  Nonmaster __              3. Auscultates breath
                               sounds                        __    __    __    __

                            4. Checks chest tubes       __    __    __    __

                               a. system intact         __    __    __    __

       b. underwater seal
intact    ___ ___ ___ ___

       c. suction set as
ordered    ___ ___ ___ ___

       d. fluctuating?    ___ ___ ___ ___

       e. bubbling?    ___ ___ ___ ___

       f. subcutaneous
crepitus    ___ ___ ___ ___

Raw Score ___  
Maximum Possible  
  Raw Score ___  
Percentage  
  Score ___  
Cut Score 5–___  
  Master ___  
  Nonmaster ___

D. Performs complete gastro-intestinal system assessment

   1. Checks for abdominal distention (girth if applicable)    ___ ___ ___ ___

   2. Checks for tenderness on palpation    ___ ___ ___ ___

   3. Auscultates bowel sounds    ___ ___ ___ ___

   4. Checks NG tube    ___ ___ ___ ___

      a. color of aspirate    ___ ___ ___ ___  
      b. PH if appropriate    ___ ___ ___ ___  
      c. suction (if ordered)    ___ ___ ___ ___

   5. Checks abdominal drains    ___ ___ ___ ___

      a. checks functioning of drain    ___ ___ ___ ___  
      b. describes drainage    ___ ___ ___ ___

Raw Score ___  
Maximum Possible  
  Raw Score ___  
Percentage  
  Score ___  
Cut Score 4–___  
  Master ___  
  Nonmaster ___

E. Performs complete renal/-metabolic system assessment

   1. Checks urinary drainage system    ___ ___ ___ ___

   2. Checks results of last SAD (within 1 hour of arrival at bedside)    ___ ___ ___ ___

   3. Takes temperature    ___ ___ ___ ___

   4. Checks hypothermia unit (when present)    ___ ___ ___ ___

Raw Score ___  
Maximum Possible  
  Raw Score ___  
Percentage  
  Score ___  
Cut Score 3–___  
  Master ___  
  Nonmaster ___

F. Performs complete musculoskeletal system assessment

   1. Checks restraints    ___ ___ ___ ___

      a. safely applied    ___ ___ ___ ___  
      b. explanation given to patient    ___ ___ ___ ___

2. Checks integrity of skin   ____   ____   ____   ____

3. Notes measures uti-
   lized to prevent
   decubiti                   ____   ____   ____   ____

   a. pillo pump              ____   ____   ____   ____
   b. heel protectors         ____   ____   ____   ____

# II. CLINICAL/TECHNICAL SKILLS

Score ____

When caring for a critically ill adult patient, the nurse intern performs the clinical/technical skills that are common in critical care nursing practice.

Raw Score ____
Maximum Possible
  Raw Score ____
Percentage
  Score ____
Cut Score 13–____
  Master ____
  Nonmaster ____

A. Adheres to Safety Procedures

1. Checks emergency
   equipment within 30
   minutes of arriving at
   bedside                    ____   ____   ____   ____

   a. Ambu bag                ____   ____   ____   ____
   b. flow meter              ____   ____   ____   ____
   c. $O_2$ tubing            ____   ____   ____   ____
   d. nipple                  ____   ____   ____   ____
   e. suction                 ____   ____   ____   ____

2. Replaces missing items
   of emergency
   equipment                  ____   ____   ____   ____

3. Keeps side rails up
   when not at bedside        ____   ____   ____   ____

4. Restrains wrists of
   intubated patients
   when not at bedside        ____   ____   ____   ____

5. Checks cardiac moni-
   tor alarms for proper
   functioning within 30
   minutes of arriving at
   bedside                    ____   ____   ____   ____

6. Sets cardiac monitor
   limits at 25% +/–
   heart rate                 ____   ____   ____   ____

7. Checks to be sure disconnect alarm (low pressure or low volume) on ventilator is on and functioning within 30 minutes of arriving at bedside ___ ___ ___ ___

8. Maintains secure position of endotracheal/tracheostomy tube ___ ___ ___ ___

9. Tapes eyelids closed if patient is Pavulonized ___ ___ ___ ___

10. Verifies NG tube placement prior to instilling fluids/medications ___ ___ ___ ___

11. Covers stopcock ports with injection caps ___ ___ ___ ___

12. Ensures that patient is wearing a legible arm band ___ ___ ___ ___

13. Washes hands prior to performing "clean" procedures ___ ___ ___ ___

14. Washes hands after performing "dirty" procedures ___ ___ ___ ___

15. Ensures that special electrical equipment has current certification label ___ ___ ___ ___

Raw Score ___
Maximum Possible Raw Score ___
Percentage Score ___
Cut Score 5–___
Master ___
Nonmaster ___

B. Performs general physical care

1. Turns immobilized patients at least every 2 hours (unless contraindicated by patient's condition) ___ ___ ___ ___

2. Provides for privacy when giving bath, bedpan, etc. ___ ___ ___ ___

3. Applies heel protectors if indicated ___ ___ ___ ___

4. Gives passive ROM to immobilized patients 1 × per shift (unless contraindicated) ___ ___ ___ ___

5. Performs Foley care
   1 × per shift                      ___    ___    ___    ___

6. Correctly measures
   and records I & O:                 ___    ___    ___    ___

   a. Measures and
      records urine output
      +/− 10 minutes of
      the hour                        ___    ___    ___    ___
   b. Records all IV fluids
      infused during shift            ___    ___    ___    ___
   c. Measures amounts
      in all drainage bags/
      bottles and records
      at end of shift (or as
      indicated) (NG, CT,
      axioms, etc.)                   ___    ___    ___    ___
   d. Totals I's and O's
      correctly                       ___    ___    ___    ___
   e. Leaves IV credits
      for next shift                  ___    ___    ___    ___

Raw Score ___          C. Administers medications
Maximum Possible
   Raw Score ___          1. Looks up medications
Percentage                  prior to administering
   Score ___                if unfamiliar with nor-
Cut Score 5−___             mal dose, action, side
Master ___                  effects and route         ___    ___    ___    ___
Nonmaster ___
                         2. Checks appropriate
                            parameters prior to
                            giving medications
                            (blood pressure with
                            antihypertensives,
                            SAD/dextrostik with
                            insulin, PCWP, UOP,
                            K+ with Lasix, HR
                            and K+ with dig, BP
                            with MS, Valium, etc.)    ___    ___    ___    ___

                         3. Administers all medi-
                            cations within 30 min-
                            utes before or after
                            time due                  ___    ___    ___    ___

                         4. Clamps NG tube for
                            30 minutes after
                            instilling medications
                            (not including antacids)  ___    ___    ___    ___

                         5. Signs out controlled
                            substances and follows
                            correct wastage
                            procedure                 ___    ___    ___    ___

Raw Score ___
Maximum Possible
Raw Score ___
Percentage
Score ___
Cut Score 6-___
Master ___
Nonmaster ___

D. Administers intravenous
therapy

   1. Maintains flow rate
within 10% +/−
ordered rate

   2. Time tapes IV bag
(unless KO rate)   ___   ___        ___

   3. Changes IV tubing
according to unit
routine   ___   ___   ___   ___

   4. Calculates mcg/kg/
min of cardiovascular
infusions within 15
minutes of changing
infusion rate   ___   ___   ___   ___

   5. Calculates mcg/kg/
min of cardiovascular
infusion within 1 hour
of arrival at bedside   ___   ___   ___   ___

   6. Identifies line for
emergency drug infu-
sion within 1 hour of
arrival at bedside   ___   ___   ___   ___

   7. Checks reference
source to determine
amount of fluid and
infusion rate of PB
medications   ___   ___   ___   ___

Raw Score ___
Maximum Possible
Raw Score ___
Percentage
Score ___
Cut Score 9-___
Master ___
Nonmaster ___

E. Performs hemodynamic
monitoring

   1. Levels air fluid interface with right atrium
(4th ICS, midaxillary
line)   ___   ___   ___   ___

   2. Calibrates monitor
prior to obtaining first
readings each shift   ___   ___   ___   ___

   3. Assures that pressure
gauge on blood pump
is set at 300 mmHg   ___   ___   ___   ___

   4. Changes flush bag and
tubing according to
unit policy   ___   ___   ___   ___

5. Obtains PA systolic, diastolic, mean, and PCWP correctly and records every 2 hours (or as ordered)        ___   ___   ___   ___

6. Displays Swan-Ganz wave form on oscilloscope to monitor for wedging of Swan        ___   ___   ___   ___

7. Checks cuff BP and compares to arterial line BP within 1 hour of arrival at bedside        ___   ___   ___   ___

8. Draws blood specimens correctly from arterial line        ___   ___   ___   ___

9. Obtains cardiac output values correctly        ___   ___   ___   ___

Raw Score ___        F. Manages patient-ventilator
Maximum Possible         system
   Raw Score ___
Percentage            1. Keeps ventilator tub-
   Score ___             ing free of water
Cut Score 5–               (empties into recepta-
Master ___                 cle, not into cascade)        ___   ___   ___   ___
Nonmaster ___
                      2. Suctions patient PRN        ___   ___   ___   ___

                         a. Recognizes when patient needs to be suctioned        ___   ___   ___   ___

                         b. Sets suction regulator at −80 to −120 mmHg        ___   ___   ___   ___

                         c. Maintains sterile technique during entire suctioning process; discards catheter if contaminated and begins again if task is not completed

                         d. Places finger over hole and withdraws catheter using a rotating motion        ___   ___   ___   ___

                         e. Uses continuous suction and limits suction time to a maximum of 10 seconds        ___   ___   ___   ___

f. Observes the cardiac monitor for dysrhythmias and patient for signs of distress ___ ___ ___ ___

g. Disposes of contaminated catheter ___ ___ ___ ___

3. Calculates SEC (per unit routine or if asked to do so) ___ ___ ___ ___

4. Takes appropriate action when alarms sound or can describe these actions when asked ___ ___ ___ ___

5. Administers sedatives PRN for patients receiving Pavulon ___ ___ ___ ___

Raw Score ___  
Maximum Possible Raw Score ___  
Percentage Score ___  
Cut Score 4–___  
Master ___  
Nonmaster ___

G. Administers tube feedings ___ ___ ___ ___

1. Rinses administration bag and tubing with tap water when adding new formula ___ ___ ___ ___

2. Delivers correct formula ___ ___ ___ ___

3. Maintains correct flow rate ___ ___ ___ ___

4. Hangs new formula every 8 hours ___ ___ ___ ___

5. Irrigates feeding tube every 4 hours with 10 cc saline ___ ___ ___ ___

Raw Score ___  
Maximum Possible Raw Score ___  
Percentage Score ___  
Cut Score 5–___  
Master ___  
Nonmaster ___

H. Administers hyperalimentation

1. Checks label on bottle with physician's order sheet ___ ___ ___ ___

2. Checks patient's latest SMA results (K+, glucose) and notifies physician of abnormalities ___ ___ ___ ___

3. Hangs bottle using aseptic technique ___ ___ ___ ___

4. Checks fluid level with time tape every 2 hours ___ ___ ___ ___

5. Checks SADs every 6
   hours                          ___    ___    ___    ___

6. Changes IV dressing
   and tubing to hub
   acording to unit policy        ___    ___    ___    ___

Raw Score ___        I. Changes peripheral
Maximum Possible        IV/arterial line dressings
   Raw Score ___
Percentage              1. If needed, changes IV
   Score ___               tubing to catheter hub
Cut Score 8-___            prior to cleansing IV
   Master ___              site                    ___    ___    ___    ___
   Nonmaster ___        2. Dons sterile glove      ___    ___    ___    ___

                        3. Cleanses IV site with
                           Betadine solution        ___    ___    ___    ___

                        4. Applies Betadine
                           ointment                 ___    ___    ___    ___

                        5. Covers IV site with
                           sterile dressing         ___    ___    ___    ___

                        6. Documents appear-
                           ance of IV site          ___    ___    ___    ___

                        7. Writes date, time, and
                           initials on new dressing ___    ___    ___    ___

                        8. Maintains sterile tech-
                           nique throughout
                           dressing change          ___    ___    ___    ___

Raw Score ___        J. Changes central line
Maximum Possible        dressing
   Raw Score ___
Percentage              1. Dons sterile gloves      ___    ___    ___    ___
   Score ___
Cut Score 7-___         2. Cleanses insertion site
   Master ___              with acetone if soiled   ___    ___    ___    ___
   Nonmaster ___
                        3. Cleanses with
                           Betadine solution        ___    ___    ___    ___

                        4. Applies Betadine oint-
                           ment and Benzoin (if
                           needed)                  ___    ___    ___    ___

                        5. Applies tape             ___    ___    ___    ___

                        6. Writes date, time,
                           and initals on new
                           dressing                 ___    ___    ___    ___

                        7. Maintains sterile tech-
                           nique throughout
                           dressing change          ___    ___    ___    ___

Raw Score ___
Maximum Possible
   Raw Score ___
Percentage
   Score ___
Cut Score 9-__
   Master ___
   Nonmaster ___

K. Changes dressings of open wound every shift or as ordered by physician

   1. Dons mask, cap, and nonsterile gloves ___ ___ ___ ___

   2. Removes and deposits old dressing in plastic bag. If unable to remove entire dressing, dons sterile gloves to remove inner layers ___ ___ ___ ___

   3. Changes sterile gloves ___ ___ ___ ___

   4. Cleanses wound with 4×4 soaked with solution ordered ___ ___ ___ ___

   5. Dresses wound according to physician's order ___ ___ ___ ___

   6. Secures dressing correctly ___ ___ ___ ___

   7. Notifies MD of any deteriorating change in wound appearance (dusky appearance, necrotic areas) ___ ___ ___ ___

   8. Closes bag containing old dressing and deposits in trash ___ ___ ___ ___

   9. Maintains sterile technique throughout dressing change ___ ___ ___ ___

# III. COMMUNICATION

Score ___

The nurse intern interacts and comunicates with others in a courteous and professional manner.

Raw Score ___
Maximum Possible
   Raw Score ___
Percentage
   Score ___
Cut Score 3-__
   Master ___
   Nonmaster ___

A. Participates in unit activities and interacts effectively with co-workers

   1. Readily assists other nurses when indicated ___ ___ ___ ___

   2. Gives thorough, concise, verbal reports using systems approach ___ ___ ___ ___

3. States name of unit
and own name when
answering telephone     ____   ____   ____   ____

4. Refrains from inappro-
priate conversation at
the bedside     ____   ____   ____   ____

Raw Score ____      B. Communicates effectively
Maximum Possible       with patients
  Raw Score ____
Percentage          1. Introduces self to
  Score ____          patient at beginning of
Cut Score 7–           shift     ____   ____   ____   ____
Master ____
Nonmaster ____      2. Orients patient to time
and place if necessary   ____   ____   ____   ____

3. Provides means of
communication for
patients who are
intubated     ____   ____   ____   ____

4. Informs patient prior
to drawing blood, giv-
ing injections, etc.     ____   ____   ____   ____

5. Provides verbal sup-
port and comfort dur-
ing painful procedures
(Swan-Ganz, CVP,
arterial line, CT
insertion)     ____   ____   ____   ____

6. Refrains from discuss-
ing patient at the
bedside     ____   ____   ____   ____

7. Ensures that call light
is within reach when
not present at the
bedside     ____   ____   ____   ____

Raw Score ____      C. Communicates with and
Maximum Possible       provides support for fam-
  Raw Score ____       ily members
Percentage
  Score ____          1. If family is available,
Cut Score 2–           makes contact with
Master ____            them at least once per
Nonmaster ____         shift     ____   ____   ____   ____

2. Stays with family dur-
ing visits at bedside to
provide support and
answer questions     ____   ____   ____   ____

# IV. DOCUMENTATION

Score ___

Raw Score ___
Maximum Possible
  Raw Score ___
Percentage
  Score ___
Cut Score 9–___
Master ___
Nonmaster ___

The nurse intern completes
all aspects of documentation.

A. Documents all nursing
   interventions, including
   patient's response when
   appropriate

   1. Charts complete phys-
      ical assessment within
      3 hours of arriving at
      bedside                    ___  ___  ___  ___

   2. Records within 10
      minutes of taking vital
      signs                      ___  ___  ___  ___

   3. Documents all medica-
      tions within 10 min-
      utes of administering      ___  ___  ___  ___

   4. Documents effects of
      PRN medication             ___  ___  ___  ___

   5. Documents lab results
      within 30 minutes of
      receiving                  ___  ___  ___  ___

   6. Documents support of
      family or significant
      others                     ___  ___  ___  ___

   7. Documents
      explanations/patient
      teaching performed         ___  ___  ___  ___

   8. Documents patient's
      anxiety and appropri-
      ate nursing
      interventions              ___  ___  ___  ___

   9. Completes patient
      classification units
      each shift                 ___  ___  ___  ___

  10. Uses no unauthorized
      abbreviations              ___  ___  ___  ___

  11. Signs name using first
      name, last name, R.N.      ___  ___  ___  ___

  12. Documents verbal
      orders on physician's
      order sheet                ___  ___  ___  ___

Raw Score ___      B. Maintains complete and
Maximum Possible       current care plan for each
  Raw Score ___        patient
Percentage                 1. Ensures that care plan
  Score ___                   incudes one problem
Cut Score 3-___              in each of the follow-
  Master ___                 ing areas:                    ___   ___   ___   ___
  Nonmaster ___
                              a. physical                  ___   ___   ___   ___
                              b. psychosocial              ___   ___   ___   ___
                              c. teaching                  ___   ___   ___   ___

                           2. Includes long-term or
                              discharge goals on
                              care plan                    ___   ___   ___   ___

                           3. Updates Kardex on a
                              daily basis                  ___   ___   ___   ___

## V. GENERAL EMPLOYMENT POLICIES

Score ___              Follows hospital policy
                       regarding dress and
                       punctuality

Raw Score ___      A. Adheres to uniform
Maximum Possible       regulations
  Raw Score ___            1. Wears white uniform,
Percentage                    light-colored top over
  Score ___                   white uniform pants,
Cut Score 3-___               or scrub clothes            ___   ___   ___   ___
  Master ___
  Nonmaster ___            2. Wears I.D. card or
                              name badge                   ___   ___   ___   ___

                           3. If hair is longer than
                              shoulder length, wears
                              it pulled back or
                              pinned off the neck          ___   ___   ___   ___

# 7

# Measuring Clinical Performance

## Kathryn S. Hegedus, Eloise M. Balasco, and Anne S. Black

*This chapter discusses a tool developed to measure the clinical performance of advanced-level nurses at Children's Hospital in Boston. The entire tool is not included (see end of chapter for where to obtain).*

As a practice, nursing has sought methods to evaluate the performance of its practitioners. A variety of contemporary issues contribute to an intensified focus on evaluation of the performance of nurses involved in the direct care of patients. Some of these issues relate to the economics of care and professional worth, diverse career avenues open to women, and changing consumer demands. Most compelling are needs to identify clinical nursing practice as the central professional endeavor and to recognize the progression of that practice to the expert level.

### PURPOSE

The purpose of this study was to devise a tool to measure the clinical performance of the Staff Nurse III at The Children's Hospital, Boston. It was part of a larger effort to define three levels of practice and develop measures for each. Incumbents in the Staff Nurse III role were designated as expert practitioners of nursing.

The measurement tool flows from a body of work of the Professional Advancement and Evaluation Committee Members: Pat Kraepelian-Bartels, R.N.C., M.S., head nurse; Jill Stanely-Brown, R.N., B.S.N., B.A., staff nurse; Ann Colangelo, R.N., B.S.N., staff nurse; Ruth Fisk, R.N.C., M.S., clinical specialist; Roberta Harding, R.N., M.S.N., head nurse; Ann Jenks, R.N., B.S.N., head nurse; Susan Shaw, R.N., head nurse.

## CONCEPTUAL BASIS

Professional nursing practice incorporates the elements of competency, accountability, scientific inquiry, leadership, and humanistic orientation to individuals and the community. Attempts to measure these variables have been elusive, and the elements in existing tools most frequently address processes nurses use to provide care. While it is important to know what the nurse does, the behaviors that identify the qualitative dimensions inherent in progressive practice and identify them in ways that can be reasonably measured have not been adequately described.

Delineating behaviors that describe the complex knowledge and competencies that nurses are expected to exhibit is central to principles of autonomy and accountability. McClure (1978) notes that the concept of accountability has been given considerable importance in the literature but elaborates on the difficulty experienced in operationalizing the concept. She cites, for example, the reluctance on the part of both individual nurses and the profession to differentiate among practitioners on the basis of their knowledge and ability.

Passos (1973) has a similar view. She questions how, if we cannot find solutions for the problems of how accountability is to be manifested, monitored, regulated, and controlled, will we know that a nurse behaving in a particular way in a given situation is performing with the professionalism for which she is accountable?

Gortner (1974) lists several hospitals in different parts of the country that attract practitioners to their settings. She speculates that accountability for nursing practice figures prominently in drawing nurses to these institutions. Fagen (1971) sees the essence of the concept to be one of holding service professions accountable for the success or failure of their methods and performance.

## Measurement and Recognition of Practice

In the past, the traditional system of organizing nursing service often rewarded clinical competence by moving the expert nurse away from direct care activities into a management position. The assumption that good clinicians were automatically good administrators was incorrect and frequently led to the appointment of nurse managers who were ill-prepared to provide management expertise to the profession. In any event, managerial or teaching tracks were, for many years, the only ways in which expert practice was tangibly rewarded.

Currently, trends are directed toward the recognition and reward of progressive and increasingly effective practice within the framework of horizontal promotion models. Historically, however, hospitals have tended to adapt existing models and have designed advancement systems to meet their own needs. Zimmer (1972) described one of the first ladders for clinical advancement in nursing practice and was an early advocate of recognizing expertise through a promotional system. The clinical ladder concept, developed by the nursing services of the University of California health care facilities, has also been extensively described in the literature (Colavecchio, Tescher, & Scalzi, 1974; Mullins, Colavecchio, & Tescher, 1979; Tescher & Colavecchio, 1977).

As hospitals design models for career advancement, several interfacing patterns emerge. A number of levels of practice are identified (Colavecchio et al., 1974; Weeks & Vestal, 1983), and the components of practice are delineated. Several of these authors comment on their attempts to measure performance levels, eligibility criteria, and entry processes.

## Existing Instruments

A review of the literature indicates that several instruments are available to measure quality of nursing care and to examine the performance of individual practitioners. They provide background information and are useful for directing new tool development.

Three measures are pertinent here: (a) The Rush-Medicus Nursing Process Methodology (Jelinek, Haussman, Hegyvary, & Neuman, 1974); (b) Quality Patient Care Scale (Qual Pacs) (Wandelt & Ager, 1974); (c) Criterion Measures of Nursing Care (Horn & Swain, 1979). Numerous investigators have utilized these instruments in gathering data for evaluating care (Hegedus, 1980; Ventura, Hagerman, Slater, & Fox, 1982). Ventura and associates (1982) found that the Rush-Medicus instrument and Qual Pacs examine similar variables and both underscore the complex, multidimensional factors involved in patient care delivery. In a more recent publication, Fox and Ventura (1984) elaborated on the ability of Qual Pacs to measure specific domains of care that are reflective of quality of nursing care.

One of the earliest tools available for measuring individual performance was the Slater Nursing Competencies Scale (Slater, 1967). A second type of methodology was demonstrated by examinations devised as part of the New York State Regents Degree Program (Lenburg, 1979): (a) Clinical Performance in Nursing, (b) Health Assessment Performance Examination, (c) Professional Performance Examination. In the above examples, Slater and Lenburg both address the competencies of beginning practitioners. Wolley (1977) provided a concise historical perspective of the various approaches used to evaluate the clinical performance of a nursing student.

Benner (1982b; 1984) categorizes five incremental levels of practice found in nursing. She identifies (a) novice, (b) advanced beginner, (c) competent, (d) proficient, and (e) expert. Benner uses data obtained from interviews and observations to illustrate the differences in skill performance between a competent nurse and proficient nurse. The difficulty in measuring levels of performance is also commented on (Benner, 1982a), and the observation is made that testing strategies effective in measuring the beginning level of practice are less well suited to identifying the expert's range of capabilities.

## SETTING

The Children's Hospital is a 339-bed inpatient facility that is the primary pediatric teaching hospital of the Harvard Medical School. The major portion of the staff (98%) is professionally prepared, with more than 70% having the minimum of a baccalaureate degree. Primary nursing is the system of nursing care delivery.

### Professional Advancement Program

The purpose of the Professional Advancement Program at the Children's Hospital is to define nursing practice behaviors descriptive of movement toward expert practice and to recognize and reward that practice (Black, 1984). The program now recognizes three levels of practice, which are described in performance criteria. A formal process for advancement is in place.

The system is built on the premise that the Staff Nurse I role is the first level of nursing practice that is a fully acceptable level of practice. Certain nurses, within varying time frames, will choose to seek advancement beyond the Staff Nurse I role. Progression beyond this first designation requires high levels of competency in professional practice, combined with distinctive integration of leadership, educational, and research competencies and activities. The characteristics ascribed to a Staff Nurse III are the ability to reason intuitively, reduce artifacts, and quickly grasp the whole. They rely less on deliberative analysis of the clinical situation; thus, their performance is more holistic. This is in contrast to the staff nurse's I and II, who perform in a more incremental manner and rely to a higher degree on procedure and process.

Responsibilities for seeking promotion to advanced practice levels reside primarily with each individual nurse. A board of review of the Professional Advancement Program has been established to provide a strong component of peer review for all candidates seeking promotion to Staff Nurse III. The board affirms attainment of Staff Nurse III role requirements, recommends for or against appointment, assures standardization of expectations and processes, monitors system equity, and compiles system data relevant to Staff Nurse III profiles.

## METHODOLOGY

### Criterion-Referenced Measurement

A criterion refers to a set standard of behavior. Criterion-referenced measurement is used to determine an individual's performance against specific behavioral criteria. The measurement tool devised to examine the clinical performance of the Staff Nurse III utilizes a criterion-referenced approach to measurement.

Criterion-referenced testing is most useful at the mastery level of learning because the outcomes are relatively simple, behavior domain is limited, and learning is sequential in nature (Kneedler, 1976). Krumme (1975) stresses the advantages of criterion-referenced testing over norm-referenced or other modes of measurement reported in the literature for clinical evaluation, and also notes that these measures have not yet had full impact on the development of clinical nursing performance tools.

Gronlund (1973) provides principles for constructing criterion-referenced tests. These principles necessitate a succinctly defined and delimited domain of learning tasks, clearly specified standards of performance, test items that clearly reflect specified behavior, a scoring mechanism, and a reporting system.

## Description of Instrument

Within the frame of the Professional Advancement Program, the following four practice domains have been identified for the Staff Nurse III level: (a) clinical practice, (b) clinical leadership, (c) professional growth/ continuing education, and (d) nursing research. Stem statements that operationalize the domain in a qualitative way were generated. In addition, for each stem, critical elements were developed that describe specific behaviors for each domain. The final tool has a total of seven stems and 27 critical elements. Table 7.1 provides an example of a stem and the critical elements.

## Administration and Scoring

This tool is a rating scale that allows the supervisor or head nurse to rate the nurse's performance, or the nurse may do a self-rating.

The instrument has two columns or possible choices for determining

**TABLE 7.1 Sample Items: Stem and Critical Elements Showing Domain of Nursing Research**

| Demonstrates competency in nursing research | Consistently | Intermittently |
|---|---|---|
| 1. Critically analyzes research studies to justify the inclusion/exclusion of findings in the rationale for nursing decisions | | |
| 2. Collaborates in the research activities of colleagues as appropriate | | |
| 3. Identifies researchable problems and communicates these in a spirit of inquiry | | |
| 4. Designs and implements research studies and reports these findings at professional meetings or in professional publications | | |

performance as being present either "consistently" or "intermittently." Data that follow provide findings using this model, but it is recognized that this portion of the tool requires further evaluation. Acceptable performance levels specifying the percentage of items or specific items in each practice domain that must receive a rating of "consistently" have not yet been determined by the tool's developers. The concluding portion of this chapter addresses future measurement concerns related to scoring.

## Pilot Testing

Members of the Professional Advancement and Evaluation Committee were responsible for devising the tool utilizing content from a long progression of developmental work and, most recently, incorporating the work of Benner (1984). The committee membership includes directors of nursing, clinical nurse specialists, head nurses, and staff nurses, all of whom serve as content specialists in the establishment of the criteria.

A pilot test of the instrument was conducted to assess the congruence between the self-ratings of nurses in the Staff Nurse III role and that of their supervisors. Each nurse in the Staff Nurse III role utilized the tool independently to evaluate the performance of the nurse or nurses reporting to her. It is important to note that for purposes of the piloting phase, persons were asked to utilize the tool at the time of entry into the role, although the tool is designed to be used both as a pre-entry guide and as an assessment tool for the nurse designated as a staff nurse.

The pilot sample of staff nurses consisted of five women, four of whom held a bachelor's degree and one of whom held a master's degree. They ranged in age from 30 to 32, having practiced in nursing between 6 and 10 years, with 5 to 7 of those years at the Children's Hospital.

## Reliability

Because of the small sample size and limited variability in scores, a measure of internal consistency has not been obtained. As sample size increases, the Kuder-Richardson 20 will be used to obtain a reliability measure.

## Validity

Content validity (Waltz, Strickland, & Lenz, 1984) was established by using a panel of qualified experts (three staff nurses and three head nurses who were not members of the committee). They determined, independently of one another, the adequacy of each critical element for representing the domain of practice. The range for percentage of agreement was from 74 to 100% (Table 7.2). This tool was determined to be valid and was used for the pilot test.

**TABLE 7.2** Percentage of Agreement for the Stems and Critical Elements

| Stem | No. of items | % Agreement |
|---|---|---|
| Clinical practice | | |
| I | 5 | 100 |
| II | 4 | 74 |
| Clinical leadership | | |
| III | 3 | 100 |
| IV | 3 | 96 |
| Professional growth/continuing education | | |
| V | 4 | 88 |
| VI | 4 | 96 |
| Nursing research | | |
| VII | 4 | 96 |

Each Staff Nurse III and her respective manager received a package containing the tool and directions for completion of the tool. The directions for completion of the instrument required placing a check mark for each of the 27 items in the column (either consistently or intermittently) that best described their current practice in relation to each of the items, and working independently of others.

The staff nurses rated their performance by marking the critical elements "consistent" 80% of the time, in comparison to the head nurses, who marked the items as "consistent" 89% of the time. The staff nurses chose "intermittent" 20% of the time in contrast to the head nurses, who made this choice 11% of the time. The 9% discrepancy between staff nurses and head nurses occurred predominantly in the areas of professional growth/continuing education and nursing research. The domains of clinical practice and clinical leadership were congruent.

When the scores for the Staff Nurse III self-ratings and ratings by the head nurses were correlated for the five subjects, the Pearson product-moment correlation coefficient was $r = .85$. This provides a validity index that reflects a fairly high level of congruence between the self-ratings and the head nurse rating.

## Approaches for Further Development of Tool

Clearly, the issues of scoring need further assessment and continuing development. One possible new approach is the assignment of a combined score from the subject's assessment of his/her own performance and that of a peer evaluator. Another strategy that might be applied to the tool is factor analysis by subscale. This second strategy would give a measure of internal consistency providing an additional reliability estimate, (i.e.,theta coefficient) (Armor, 1974).

Additional work is needed for establishing pass or cut scores. It is recognized that the final tool will allow for differences in proficiency level and that some domains will have higher standards than others. For example, clinical practice and clinical leadership would require high levels of competency, whereas professional growth/continuing education and research could have lower passing points.

# CONCLUSIONS

This study demonstrates the value of research directed toward measurement of behaviors associated with advancing clinical practice. The valuable involvement of staff nurses in the research process has also been described. By design, qualitative research methodology has been utilized. Qualitative research, by its very essence, is applicable and appropriate to nursing studies in practice settings (Leininger, 1985; Swanson & Chenitz, 1982).

Members of the Professional Advancement and Evaluation Committee of the Children's Hospital have utilized the four domains described in the Staff Nurse III criteria and devised critical elements to examine the performance of staff nurses I and II. A panel of experts has established content validity, and these tools are now ready for further testing. These tools all allow for assessment of nursing competencies and move in the direction of examining behaviors, not processes. The comparison of the three instruments now indicates the need to revise the tool for Staff Nurse III.

## Implications for Nursing

Implications for nursing are seen from the perspective of both the individual and the discipline. The interface between the two is based on the assumption that nursing is a practice discipline; thus, its theory base can best be described and tested in the arena of care.

The ability to establish measures that would identify practice behaviors along a continuum from novice to expert allows for the portrayal of nursing with all its complex scientific and artistic dimensions. The tool permits examination of individual performance, and from this description, patterns of practice emerge that signify a body of knowledge inductively built. In turn, hypotheses are formulated and tested with implications for strengthening and building a science of practice.

This tool may be obtained from:
  Kathryn S. Hegedus, R.N., D.N.Sc.
  Director, Staff Development and Research
  The Children's Hospital
  300 Longwood Avenue
  Boston, MA 02115

# REFERENCES

Armor, D. F. (1974). Theta reliability and factor scaling. In H.L. Costner (Ed.), *Sociological methodology* (pp.17-50). San Francisco: Jossey-Bass.

Benner, P. (1982a). Issues in competency-based testing. *Nursing Outlook, 30*, 303-309.

Benner, P. (1982b). From novice to expert. *American Journal of Nursing, 82*, 402-407.

Benner, P. (1984). *From novice to expert: Excellence and power in clinical nursing practice*. Menlo Park; CA: Addison-Wesley.

Black, A. (1984). Clinical advancement program for registered nurses. *Memorandum*, Boston: The Children's Hospital.

Colavecchio, R., Tescher, B., & Scalzi, C. (1974). A clinical ladder for nursing practice. *Journal of Nursing Administration, 4*, 54-58.

Fagen, C. (1971). Accountability. *Nursing Outlook, 19*, 249-251.

Fox, R. N., & Ventura, M. R. (1984). Internal psychometric characteristics of the Quality Patient Care Scale. *Nursing Research, 33*, 112-117.

Gortner, S. R. (1974). Scientific accountability in nursing. *Nursing Outlook, 22*, 764-768.

Gronlund, N. E. (1973). *Preparing criterion-referenced tests for classroom instruction*. New York: Macmillan.

Hegedus, K. S. (1980). Primary nursing: Evaluation of professional nursing practice. In K. G. Ciske, & G. A. Mayer (Eds.) (Special Issue), *Nursing Dimensions, 7*, 85-89.

Horn, B., & Swain, M. (1979). *Development of criterion measures of nursing care* (NHS No. PB 267-004 and 267-005). Ann Arbor, MI: University of Michigan, School of Public Health.

Jelinek, R., Haussman, R. K. D., Hegyvary, S. T., & Newman, J. E. (1974). *A methodology for monitoring quality of nursing care* (DHEW Publication No.HRA 76-25). Washington, DC: Department of Health, Education and Welfare.

Kneedler, J. (1976). Criterion-referenced measurement for one continuing education offering: Pre and post operative visits by operating room nurses. *The Journal of Continuing Education, 7*, 26-36.

Krumme, U. S. (1975). The case for criterion-referenced measurement. *Nursing Outlook, 23*, 764-770.

Leininger, M. M. (1985). *Qualitative research methods in nursing*. New York: Grune and Stratton.

Lenburg, C. B. (1979). *The Clinical Performance Examination*. New York: Appleton-Century-Crofts.

McClure, M. L. (1978). The long road to accountability. *Nursing Outlook, 26*, 47-50.

Mullins, A. C., Colavecchio, R. E., & Tescher, B. E. (1979). Peer review: A model for professional accountability. *Journal of Nursing Administration, 9*, 25-29.

Passos, J. Y. (1973). Accountability: Myth or mandate. *Journal of Nursing Administration, 3*, 17-22.

Slater, D. (1967). *The Slater Nursing Competencies Rating Scale*. Detroit: Wayne State University.

Swanson, J. M., & Chenitz, W. C. (1982). Why qualitative research in nursing? *Nursing Outlook, 30*, 241-245.

Tescher, B. E., & Colavecchio, R. (1977). Definition of a standard for clinical nursing practice. *Journal of Nursing Administration, 7*, 32-44.

Waltz, C. F., Strickland, O. L.,& Lenz, E. R. (1984). *Measurement in nursing research*, Philadelphia: F. A. Davis.

Wandelt, M., & Ager, J. (1974). *Quality Patient Care Scale*, New York: Appleton-Century-Crofts.

Weeks, L. C., & Vestal, K. W. (1983). PACE: A unique career development program. *Journal of Nursing Administration, 13*, 29-32.

Woolley, A. S. (1977). The long and tortured history of clinical evaluation. *Nursing Outlook, 25*, 308-315.

Ventura, M. R., Hageman, P. T.,Slakter, M. J., & Fox, R. N. (1982). Correlation of two quality of nursing care measures. *Research in Nursing and Health, 5*, 37-43.

Zimmer, M. J. (1972). Rationale for a ladder for clinical advancement in nursing practice. *Journal of Nursing Administration, 2*, 18-24.

# 8

# Measurement of Helping Outcomes in Nursing

## Doris E. Nicholas

*This chapter discusses the Helping Outcomes Rating Scale, a measure of nurses' helping skills.*

Nurse educators recognize that nursing as a profession must devote its greatest effort over the next decades to the construction of a knowledge base for its professional practice. This knowledge base will consist of a body of theoretical formulations derived from the generation and repeated testing of hypotheses and application of findings from these tests to practice (Chaska, 1983, p. 33). However, the lack of a clear definition of what comprises nursing practice inhibits the formulation of a conceptual model with stages of helping that are easily understood by students of nursing, educators, and nurses in clinical settings.

Nursing theorists have long recognized that helping is a main concern of nursing practice. However, helping has not been systematically acknowledged as a major theme in nursing theory and conceptual models during the past decade. Specifically, the concepts named as central to nursing – man (person), environment, health, and nursing – have been described by Cronewett (1983, p. 342) as complex and multidimensional and are therefore almost useless in terms of guiding research and practice. Similarly, the nursing process assists the nurse to think reflectively. However, this process does not direct attention to the behavioral changes that occur as the nurse helps the client.

Interestingly, current nursing literature shows an increasing focus on the importance of clearly telling what helping skills are and how they are acquired (Long & Phrophet, 1981). These authors used components from Carl Rogers's theories in addition to Carkhuff's helping frameworks in the construction of a communication manual for nurses. Similarly, Smitherson (1981) emphasized the importance of helping in nursing practice. Although Smitherson's titles of the helping phases differ from those of Long and Phrophet, both works document the collaborative activity of the nurse and the client in specific phases of the helping process.

Carkhuff (1971) felt that health professionals and laypersons can use the same model of facilitative interpersonal process. The framework that is proposed by Carkhuff and Bernesen (1977) allows the cooperative movement of the client and the nurse through three phases of helping. It would seem that this systematic collaborative process would improve the efficacy of the nurse. Furthermore, changes in health care delivery and health care financing – for example, Diagnostic Related Groups – encourage the adoption of a facilitative model that promotes clients' collaboration and self-responsibility.

## THE PURPOSE

In spite of health professionals' efforts to be helpful, many people in the United States believe that health care is too impersonal (Gazda, Walters, & Childers, 1975, p. 1). The expertise of the nurse has moved along with great advances in technology and medical science. However, it is clear that a deficit in human relations development continues. Therefore, a practical model of helping that clearly outlines the steps in the helping process is indicated. In addition, the helper must be able to determine whether helping has worked (Egan, 1982b, p. 7). Carkhuff and Berensen (1977) suggest that the outcomes of helping must be measured in terms of holistic growth (physical, emotional, and intellectual) or lack of growth in these domains. Furthermore, client learning is the major factor in determining when helping is successful.

The purpose of this project was to test a theory-guided instrument that measures helping outcomes in nursing. Specifically, the instrument measures the extent of the nurse's facilitative action as the client (1) explores the problem, (2) understands him/herself better, and (3) acts more effectively. To achieve the goals of this project, raters were trained to observe directly each nurse participating in this investigation as the nurse and the client collaboratively experienced each of the aforementioned phases of the helping process. Reliability and validity data were collected and analyzed.

## THEORETICAL PERSPECTIVE

Carkhuff (1971) and Egan (1982a, b) have constructed helping models that can be used by a wide variety of health professionals in addition to laypersons. The models clearly outlined the following three steps in the helping process: (1) exploring, (2) understanding, and (3) acting. Carl Rogers's client-centered approach (Rogers, Gendin, & Traux, 1967) provided the central theme for Carkhuff's helping model. However, Carkhuff expanded the model to include behavioral learning theory. The model presented by Egan also reflects core dimensions of helping: for example, empathy, respect, and concreteness, as proposed by Carl Rogers. Egan's facilitative model emphasized problem-solving management. In addition, Egan directed attention to social influence as an important element in the helping process. Egan proposed that if both the person needing help and the person helping believe in the power of each other, a more effective interpersonal process can be established. It is clear that the humanistic focus of the helping models previously mentioned cuts across nursing theoretical boundaries.

The literature documents the measurement of coping and helping behaviors focused on ill and non-ill persons. Specifically, the Jalowiec Coping Scale (JCS) (1979) has long been used in nursing practice and research. The JCS measures a person's reaction to stress and tension, focusing on what a person does when stressful situations are encountered. Examples of Jalowiec's coping behaviors follow: (1) worry, (2) cry, (3) work off tension with physical activity or exercise. The JCS defines the client's adaptation as the environment changes. Similarly, other instruments have been designed by nurses that focus on the adaptation potentials of adults and children. Roy's model (1980) emphasized the client's adaptation in a changing environment. Therefore, Roy provides a theoretical frame of reference for the nurse as clients are helped in the process of adapting. Cronewett's (1983) analysis of helping in nursing models suggests that nursing approaches developed by Hall (1963) and Kinlein (1977) identify how the nurse helps the client to manage problems better. However, the literature does not reveal an instrument that clearly and systematically identifies the nurse's objective with respective client behaviors in specified phases of helping. Therefore, a model that reflected the main concern of nursing (helping) was investigated. In addition, a model of helping that has experienced extensive empirical testing was selected and modified to show how nursing processing skills articulate with the client's processing skills in defining the client's problem, achieving accurate perception of self and health problems, and, finally, implementing an action program.

## APPLICATION OF HELPING MODELS TO NURSING

Historically, nurses have been cast in the role of helper, although different personal philosophies, theoretical frameworks, and technical expertise have been experienced. In spite of the differences in the academic and clinical preparation of health professionals, Carkhuff (1971), Gazda and associates (1975), and Egan (1982b) propose that under appropriate conditions some people are successful in helping others. Furthermore, the same facilitative model may be used by all health professionals and laypersons.

The client-centered, problem-solving emphasis of the aforementioned three-phase helping models is not new to nursing. Carkhuff and Berensen (1977) suggest that all helpers are client-centered in the sense that they serve for the benefit of their client's (p. 59). Furthermore, nurses have participated in behavioral programs for many years, particularly in psychiatric nursing. In addition, nurses are familiar with sequential processes as illustrated by the nursing process. Course offerings, licensure, and certification examinations are central for the safe practice of nursing.

It would seem that since the helping models documented in the literature are supported by extensive research, nurse educators and nurses in clinical settings could direct efforts to determining how these existing frameworks can be incorporated into nursing. The helping models that have been mentioned are open to development or change. Therefore, a model of helping could be adapted that would be congruent with the nurse's personal philosophy and conceptual frame of reference.

In addition to the suitability of helping models for varied clinical areas (for example, medical-surgical, psychiatric, and pediatric nursing), helping models may be used at varied points along the health/illness continuum, preparing clients to live or to die. Both ends of the continuum require systematic sequential helping skills.

## IMPLICATIONS FOR THE MEASUREMENT OF HELPING OUTCOMES IN NURSING

The literature indicates that an instrument that measures helping outcomes is needed in clinical nursing. Specifically, the instrument must show that the nurse has systematically helped the client (Long & Phrophet, 1981). If this instrument documents the magnitude of three phases of helping as measured by the client's behavior, the nurse can be evaluated in this clinical domain. Nurse educators and practicing nurses have attempted to delineate the capacity of the nurse to function appropriately in clinical settings. Terminal objectives have been constructed. However, difficulty has been encountered in formulating clear outcomes that can be measured. The literature documents a lack of agreement among faculty, students, nursing service managers, and staff nurses in the identification of nursing clinical behaviors. Therefore, it would seem that in the formative period of behavioral identification, guidelines from established helping models may be necessary in the development of defensible nursing outcomes.

Increasingly, nurses are held accountable for their own behavior. Increased consumer awareness, increased health care costs, changes in health care delivery, particularly the prospective payment plan with earlier discharge of the client, demand that there must be congruence among nurses in what helping behaviors are and how these behaviors lead to the expected outcome of moving the client toward a more productive life.

Similar to the lack of agreement between practicing nurses in determining defensible clinical behaviors is the fact that nurse educators do not present a unified theory of nursing. Chaska (1983) states that there is no

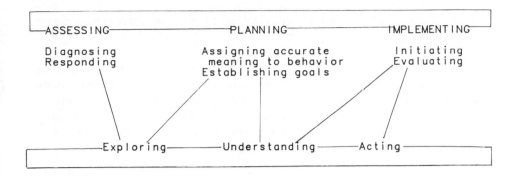

**FIGURE 8.1** Articulation of the nursing and helping processes. Source: from *The Art of Helping* by Dr. R. R. Carkhuff, 1983, Amherst, MA: Human Resources Press. © 1982. Adapted by permission.

shared body of knowledge that is the same for all nursing. Each nursing theory will build its own body of knowledge even though diverse theories may examine the same raw data (p. 711). The main concern of the project was to develop an instrument that measured helping outcomes in nursing. In addition, the outcome measure was designed to unite varied theoretical frameworks. It would seem that the nursing outcomes contained in the Helping Outcomes Rating Scale (HORS) could be used for a group of research studies using a single theory of helping that has experienced intensive empirical testing. In addition to cutting across theoretical boundaries, the HORS encourages collaboration with other health professionals. The articulation of Carkhuff's helping model with the nursing process, the problem-management model of nursing, is shown in Figure 8.1.

The helping model, despite its rather complex appearance, can be readily articulated with the nursing process. Subsequently, it can be aligned with the theoretical frameworks for nursing. The nurse is aware that complete availability (attending) is necessary for the successful establishment of an interaction, in addition to promoting client involvement. Therefore, attending as a prehelping strategy can be easily understood. Assessment is the first step in the nursing process, but it occurs in each of the phases of helping. Similarly, Carl Rogers's (Rogers et al., 1967) conditions for helping are essential elements throughout the helping process. Examples of these conditions for helping are empathy, respect, and concreteness. Carkhuff (1983a, b) suggests that recycling the feedback from the client's action stimulates more intensive action.

The primary level of the aforementioned conditions appears in the first phase and step of helping. The advanced level of the conditions is experienced in the second and third phases of helping. Examples of primary level accurate empathy follow:

You *feel* lonely *because* your husband did not come to the hospital
tonight. (an experience)
You feel guilty because you told him not to leave the children alone. (a
behavior).

A working relationship has been established and exploration of the client's
problem has been achieved in the first step of helping. Advanced-level helping strategies offer the client a new, deeper, more objective way to express
feelings. Egan (1982b) described advanced accurate empathy as sharing
hunches about the client's overt and covert experiences and feelings.
Examples of advanced accurate empathy follow:

I think I might also be hearing you say that you are more than anxious,
    perhaps frightened of your forthcoming mastectomy. (client's indi-
    rect or implied expression)
From all that you have told me about the surgery, it seems that you are
    wondering about the effects that your mastectomy will have on your
    marriage. (drawing logical conclusions from the client's implied or
    indirect expression)

In addition to advanced accurate empathy, probing and confrontation
are other helping strategies that may be employed in the second and third
steps of the helping process.

## DEVELOPMENT OF THE INSTRUMENT

The HORS was constructed to measure the outcomes of nurse/client
interpersonal processes. The specific goals of the instrument have been
to determine the extent of helping in three phases of nurse/client interaction. The initial scale contained 28 items derived from the literature that
focused on Carkhuff's (1971) model of helping. In addition, Egan's
(1982a, b) problem-management helping model contributed to the construction of the HORS. In contrast to Carkhuff's model, which addresses
the helper's interpersonal and information processing skills, the present
model directs attention to nursing processing skills. The literature indicates that nurses perceive the problem-solving process performed by
nurses (the nursing process) as the central method of helping (Cronewett,
1983). The nursing process addresses models and nursing approaches that
are congruent with the central theme of Carkhuff's and Egan's models.
For example, Peplau (cited in Fitzpatrick & Whall, 1983) defines nursing
as a significant therapeutic interpersonal process functioning comparatively with other human processes that make health possible for individuals (p. 27). Similar to the conditions for helping that are embodied in
Carkhuff's and Egan's models, Orem (cited in Fitzpatrick & Whall, 1983)
suggests that shared respect, belief, trust, recognition, and fostering

developmental potential are essential to helping. Furthermore, Orem proposes that each person strives to earn respect and trust as he/she assumes or attempts to assume responsibility for personal development (p. 139).

Both the psychological and nursing models and approaches contributed to the construction of items for the norm-referenced HORS. The literature focused on helping was searched for statements that represented behaviors in each of the three phases of helping. Then a set of salient client behaviors was entered on the scale. Items had to be constructed so that they could be easily understood and accepted by nurses using the scale. Items for each of the three categories of the scale were presented to several nurses, who provided preliminary evaluation of content and format. Subsequently, eight items were deleted with revision of some of the remaining items. In addition, intermediate points were deleted to form a 5-point scale: (1) Very Unsuccessful, (2) Unsuccessful, (3) Minimally Successful, (4) Successful, (5) Very Successful. Scores for each helping phase are summed to comprise a total score that represents the helping outcomes. The final 20-item instrument was submitted to two experts, who judged the content validity of the scale. The investigator believed that a short scale would increase its suitability for nurses in clinical settings.

## Administration and Scoring

The HORS was constructed to measure the outcomes of nurse/client interpersonal processes. The specific goal of the instrument has been to determine the extent of helping in three phases of nurse/client interaction. Many other assessment tools designed to measure nursing outcomes have been self-inventories that did not clearly tell what the client is doing as the nurse systematically engages in the helping process.

The present endeavor is intended primarily for use with a wide variety of clinical specialties, for example, medical-surgical nursing, pediatrics, community health, and mental health. This scale is designed principally for problem solving. Therefore, if clients in psychiatric clinical settings can problem-solve, this instrument may be useful. However, psychiatrically disturbed persons or intensely confused medical-surgical clients may not be suitable subjects for the application of this rating scale. The instrument is intended mainly for socially functioning persons. The instrument contains 20 items and yields a total score, although subscores are available for each of the three phases of helping.

The HORS includes the phases listed below, which are designed to address important steps in the helping process and emphasize the behavioral clustering that exists among them.

Phase I: Exploring
1. Experiences
2. Feels

3. Clarifies
4. Involves
5. Specifies
6. Defines

Phase II: Understanding

1. Informs
2. Needs
3. Changes
4. Repeats
5. Perceives
6. Shares
7. Constructs

Phase III: Acting

1. Operationalizes
2. Problem-solves
3. Reflects
4. Analyzes
5. Grows
6. Evaluates

## Administration

The HORS may be used by a rater who directly observes the client/nurse interaction. Observations are usually achieved within 20 to 30 min. However, less or additional time may be experienced.

No strict conditions are necessary to achieve valid and useful observation results. The scale has been tried with nurses and clients in varied environments and circumstances. For example, the nurse may be engaged in bedside activities or in a conference room. Ideal interacting conditions are preferred. However, modification is expected to ensure the instrument's suitability for varied populations.

Raters are encouraged to use their own judgment. If an item seems especially difficult to an observer, he/she may leave the item blank.

## Scoring

Scoring of the scale is easily accomplished. The rater is required to circle one of the following points on the continuum that represents the magnitude of the nurse's helping: Very Unsuccessful (1), Unsuccessful (2), Minimally Successful (3), Successful (4), Very Successful (5). The scores for each phase of helping are summed to comprise a single score.

## The Individual Phases

The names of the phases were selected to reflect the behavior that the client is expected to manifest. The nurse's objective for each phase precedes specific client behaviors. The nurse's success in stimulating the expected behaviors are expressed on the following continuum: Very Unsuccessful, which carries a value of 1, to Very Successful, with a value of 5. For example, in phase I the nurse receives a rating of successful (5) if it is clear that the client discusses his/her feelings and experiences. The ultimate expected client behavior in the exploring phase is problem identification. Each phase of helping contains approximately the same number of items and extent of difficulty.

## Interaction Among Phases

Although the nurse's magnitude of helping can be rated for each of the three phases, the instrument is constructed to focus on patterns and combinations of high and low scores across the scale. Until further research is accomplished, the discussion of patterns of interaction is tentative. Some nurses may present consistently low scores or a combination of high and low scores among the three phases.

The paradigm shown in Table 8.1 describes behavior that may be seen in high and low scores.

### TABLE 8.1 Guide to Assigning Low and High Scores

| High scores – client's behaviors | Phases and nurse's objectives | Low scores – client's behaviors |
|---|---|---|
| Explores specifically the feelings, experiences, and behaviors relevant to the problem | 1. Exploring to help the client explore his/her problems | Avoids discussion of issues, lacks self-confidence, passive, distrustful, cannot clarify the problem |
| Sees the problem situation in new ways, identifies alternatives, formulates goals, recognizes the need for action | 2. Understanding to help the client understand himself/herself better | Confused, blames others for his/her resources, defensive, constricted in selecting alternatives, uncertain of plans that would correct the problem, inflexible, goals are not defined |
| Explores the best alternative for achieving goals, seeks supportive resources with self and environment, implements action programs, evaluates the helping process | 3. Acting to help the client take actions to correct the problem | Awkward, cautious, unambitious, retiring, dependent, cannot operationalize goals, cannot determine if the interaction has been helpful |

# METHODOLOGY FOR TESTING

## Reliability

The reliability of the HORS was assessed by an internal consistency procedure. This strategy is usually employed to estimate the reliability of norm-referenced measures. Furthermore, internal consistency reliability addressed the concern for consistency of performance of a psychiatric nursing group and a medical-surgical nursing group across the items on the HORS. The alpha coefficient was calculated as the estimate of reliability. This index of internal consistency was selected because it has a single value for any given set of data. In addition, internal consistency reliability measured the extent to which performance on any one item on the HORS is a good indicator of performance on any other item on the HORS (Waltz, Strickland, & Lenz, 1984, p. 136).

Interrater reliability determines the degree of agreement among the two raters (judges) in assigning scores to the same observation. Administrators of clinical centers that participated in the project assisted in the selection of the raters. Outstanding evaluation of the raters' interpersonal processes was a criterion for selecting. A baccalaureate or higher degree for the registered nurses who served as raters were additional criteria. A 2-hr training session was provided to familiarize both the interraters and intraraters with the following: (1) purpose of the project, (2) helping model, (3) HORS, and (4) sampling procedures, in addition to a 2-hr practice session.

Raters served as nonparticipant observers for a 30-min client/nurse interaction. The Pearson product-moment correlation coefficient was employed for the two raters who directly observed each event. The coefficient reflected the degree of agreement between the different raters in assigning scores. Interrater reliability has been documented to be especially important when observational and subjective measures are employed (Waltz et al., 1984).

The consistency with which one rater assigned scores to each scale level of client behaviors on two occasions (intrarater reliability) was difficult to achieve for both the medical-surgical and psychiatric groups. Inhibiting factors for collecting intrarater reliability data follow: (1) time required for an additional observation; (2) frequent changes in clients' behaviors, particularly for the psychiatric group; and (3) changes in the client setting. Therefore, intrarater data were not employed for the project.

## Validity

Content validity of the scale was assessed by submitting the objectives that guided the construction of the instrument to two experts. It has been previously mentioned that HORS measures the extent of helping as reflected by interpersonal processes. Therefore, it would seem that psychiatric nurses who have been reported as high achievers in academic and clinical experiences would be better prepared to judge content emphasizing client/nurse interaction.

These behavioral objectives were generated for each of the three phases of helping. Then the experts were requested to articulate each objective with its respective item. The relevancy of the items to the content addressed by the objective was judged by the experts. Finally, the experts determined if the items (client behaviors on the HORS) adequately represented the behaviors contained in the domain of interest.

Two judges were employed. Therefore, an index of content validity (CVI) was used to determine the magnitude of agreement between the two experts.

## Content Validity

Content validity of the scale was assessed by submitting the objectives that guided the construction of the instrument to two judges. The objectives were used as a base for judging the degree that statements (client behaviors) measured the intensity of helping. Therefore, the main concern of the selection process for judges focused on academic and clinical experiences relevant to the aforementioned task. One expert presented a master's degree in medical-surgical nursing. In addition, the expert was prepared at the master's level in psychiatric nursing. The other expert was prepared at the doctoral level, with a clinical specialty in mental health nursing. A four-part instrument was constructed: (1) Strongly Disagree, (2) Disagree, (3) Agree, and (4) Strongly Agree. All items were given a rating of 3 or 4 by both judges. The CVI determined the agreement between the two experts. A CVI of .90 indicated high agreement between the experts.

## Construct Validity

Construct validity determined the extent to which the subjects manifested behaviors specified on the HORS. Construct validity was assessed by employing the following approaches:

Interpersonal processing skills are not limited to nurses prepared in a particular clinical specialty. Medical-surgical nurses as well as psychiatric nurses may be actively involved in human interaction. However, the literature indicates that psychiatric nurses' interpersonal processing skills are more intense than these of other nursing groups. Traditionally, psychiatric nurses have served as consultants at specific points of maturational and situational stress. Therefore, it would seem that a hypothesis could be generated to test the difference in interpersonal processing skills of medical-surgical and psychiatric nurses.

*Hypothesis I*: There will be a significant difference in the mean scores on the HORS for psychiatric and medical-surgical nurses.

A one-way analysis of variance compared the difference between means of the psychiatric and medical-surgical nurses' scores on the HORS. The hypothesis was tested at the .05 level of significance.

A second approach to construct validity focused on measurement of the nurse's (observee's) needs, although the HORS was constructed to measure helping outcomes in nursing. Helping the client to change maladaptive behaviors may be influenced by the need to nurture. If a significant difference is found in the expected direction (i.e., high scores on an instrument that measures nurturance), it can be concluded that some evidence has been obtained for construct validity. Therefore, in order to further assess construct validity, the following hypothesis was tested:

*Hypothesis II*: There will be a positive relationship between psychiatric and medical-surgical nursing scores on the nurturance subscale of the Edwards Personal Preference Schedule (EPPS) (1959) and scores on the HORS.

It would seem that academic and clinical experience would influence nurses' interaction with clients. Nurses with varied academic and clinical experiences participated in the project. It is expected that nurses with higher education (ED) and greater experience (EX) would have higher scores on the HORS. Furthermore, it would seem that nurses who seek higher education and remain in clinical nursing would have a greater need to help (i.e., higher scores on the EPPS variable). The Pearson product-moment correlation coefficient determined the relationship between scores on the EPPS, the HORS, and the ED and EX variables.


# METHOD

The project examined the efficacy of an investigator-constructed direct observational instrument to measure the extent of helping in the following three phases: (1) exploring, (2) understanding, and (3) acting.


## Sample

The sample consisted of registered nurses (volunteers) employed in clinical centers in two Middle Atlantic states. Thirty psychiatric nurses and 30 medical-surgical nurses were selected, using random numbers. The subjects received approval from the director of nursing in addition to that of appropriate managers of the agencies. The rationale for the selection of the two specialties was to include a group that is perceived to be skilled in interpersonal processes and a group that is perceived to be less effective in nurse/client interaction. The selection of the clinical centers was influenced by the judgment of the investigator and the clinical centers' manifested interest in the project. The majority of subjects (46%) were graduates of associate degree programs. Twenty-five percent of the sample were baccalaureate graduates, and 23% were graduates of diploma programs. Six percent of the subjects were prepared at the master's level. Two subjects were male. Subjects' clinical experience ranged from 1 to 44 years.

## Data Collection

Sixty nurses were initially included in the project. However, data gathered from 52 subjects were analyzed. The HORS was constructed to measure helping outcomes in nursing. The literature reveals that the effectiveness of the helper reflects his/her needs. Specifically, the nurse's interaction may be influenced by his/her need to help. Therefore, the nurturance subscale of the EPPS (1959) was employed for data collection. In addition to the time-consuming aspect, some subjects were reluctant to answer some of the questions. Therefore, these subjects were dropped from the project.

Raters were selected by judgment of the investigator and of the administrations of the clinical centers that participated in the project, in addition to the willingness of raters to participate in the project. The 2-hr training session informed the raters of the following: (1) purpose of the project, (2) helping model, (3) HORS, and (4) sampling procedures. In addition, a 2-hr practice (observation) session was provided. All raters showed a high level of readiness for the observation.

Raters and participants (nurses) collaboratively determined the dates and hours that the observations would occur. The two raters began directly observing and recording their concurrent observations on entering the room in which the nurse/client interaction was occurring. The observation lasted 30 min. The raters based their judgments on the nurse's objective for each of the three phases of helping. Then each rater circled one of the 5 points of HORS that represented her perception of the magnitude of helping as manifested by the client's behavior. Following the nurse/client interaction, the nurse being observed completed a Personal Data Form (level of education, clinical unit, and length of experience). In addition, the EPPS measured the nurturance need of each nurse observed.

## RESULTS

### Individual Items

When scores of the individual items were averaged they ranged from 3.40 to 4.09, with standard deviations from .62 to 1.27.

### Reliability

Internal consistency reliability was employed to determine the consistency of the subjects' performance across the items on the HORS. The alpha coefficient was calculated as the estimate of the tool's reliability.

A high alpha resulted for both clinical groups: .963 for the psychiatric group and .970 for the medical-surgical group, indicating strong internal consistency reliability. The item mean for the medical-surgical group (3.65) was greater than the mean for the psychiatric group (3.26).

## Reliability (Interrater)

Two competent raters scored subjects' response's at the same time. The degree of agreement between the two raters was assessed by the Pearson product-moment correlation coefficient. The interrater reliability coefficient was .80 for raters of the psychiatric group and .98 for raters of the medical-surgical group. This finding suggests strong interrater reliability.

## Validity

Content validity of the scale was assessed by submitting to two experts (psychiatric nurses) the objectives that guided the construction of the instrument. The objectives were used as a base for judging the degree that statements (client behaviors) measured the intents of helping. A four-part instrument was constructed: (1) Strongly Agree, (2) Disagree, (3) Agree, and (4) Strongly Disagree. All items were given a rating of 3 or 4 by both judges. The CVI determined the agreement between the two experts. The CVI of .90 indicated high agreement between the experts.

Construct validity determined the extent to which the subjects manifested behavior specified on the HORS. The approaches described below were used to determine construct validity.

*Hypothesis I:* There will be a significant difference in the mean scores on the HORS for psychiatric and medical-surgical nurses.

A one-way analysis of variance (ANOVA) compared the difference between means of the psychiatric and medical-surgical nurses' scores on the HORS. The hypothesis was tested at the .05 level of significance. The group of psychiatric nurses had a mean of 61.38 (SD = 19.03), in comparison to a mean of 75.69 (SD = 16.89) for the medical-surgical nurses (see Table 8.2).

The two groups differed at the .006 level of significance ($F = 8.22$; *df* = 1.50). It was expected that the psychiatric nurses would have a higher mean. However, the mean for medical-surgical nurses was highest. The mental status of the client might have inhibited the psychiatric nurses' performances across the scale. However, since the medical-surgical nurses as a group were more highly educated than the psychiatric nurses, this may account for the result.

*Hypothesis II* (the second approach to assess construct validity): There will be a positive relationship between psychiatric and medical-surgical nurses' scores on the EPPS and on the HORS.

The Pearson product-moment correlation coefficient determined the relationship between scores on the EPPS, the HORS, and personal data (ED and EX). The coefficients for the clinical groups are summarized in Tables 8.3 and 8.4.

**TABLE 8.2** Mean, Standard Deviation, and Analysis of Variance

| | | ANOVA | |
| --- | --- | --- | --- |
| Source | df | Mean Square | F |
| Between | | | |
| Group | 1 | 2661.2581 | 8.219* |
| Error | 50 | 323.7927 | |
| Group | | Mean | SD |
| Psych | | 61.384 | 19.030 |
| M/S | | 75.692 | 16.894 |

\* $p < .006$.

**TABLE 8.3** Coefficient and Significance for Medical-Surgical Nurses

| Variable | ED | EPPS | EX | SCALE |
| --- | --- | --- | --- | --- |
| ED | 1.0000 | 0.2042 | 0.1103 | 0.1562 |
| | | (26) | (26) | (26) |
| | | $p = 0.158$ | $p = 0.296$ | $p = 0.223$ |
| EPPS | 0.2042 | 1.0000 | −0.0187 | −0.3651 |
| | (26) | | (26) | (26) |
| | $p = 0.158$ | | $p = 0.464$ | $p = 0.033$ |
| EX | 0.1103 | −0.0187 | 1.000 | 0.1192 |
| | (26) | (26) | | (26) |
| | $p = 0.296$ | $p = 0.464$ | | $p = 0.281$ |

**TABLE 8.4** Coefficient and Significance for Psychiatric Nurses

| Variable | ED | EPPS | EX | SCALE |
| --- | --- | --- | --- | --- |
| ED | 1.0000 | 0.3092 | −0.1219 | 0.1727 |
| | | (26) | (26) | (26) |
| | | $p = 0.062$ | $p = 0.276$ | $p = 0.199$ |
| EPPS | 0.3092 | 1.0000 | 0.3176 | 0.5704 |
| | (26) | | (26) | (26) |
| | $p = 0.062$ | | $p = 0.057$ | $p = 0.001$ |
| EX | −0.1219 | 0.3176 | 1.000 | 0.5898 |
| | (26) | (26) | | (26) |
| | $p = 0.276$ | $p = 0.057$ | | $p = 0.001$ |

A negative relationship (−.36) was shown among the HORS and EPPS scores for the medical-surgical group. In addition, coefficient values were quite low for ED (.15) and EX (.11). A clear explanation cannot be provided for this finding. The overall length of experience for the medical-surgical nurses was less than that for the psychiatric nurses. However, the overall educational level of the medical-surgical nurses was higher than that of the psychiatric nurses. The low coefficient values indicate that the variables being measured are independent.

The second hypothesis was supported by data from the psychiatric nurse group with the larger positive coefficient, in addition to the high level of significance (.57), ($p = .001$) for the HORS and the EPPS. The HORS and ED variables also showed a larger coefficient (.58), ($p = .001$). Therefore, there is some evidence for construct validity, particularly for the psychiatric group. It has been previously mentioned that the Nurturance scale of the EPPS was used for this investigation. The scores on this scale clustered around the mean for females in both clinical groups, whereas, scores for the Dominance scale were higher for the female subjects. The Nurturance score for one of the two males was quite high.

## CONCLUSIONS

The HORS is based on a practical, systematic, participant model of helping that articulates with the sequential steps in the nursing process. In addition, this model cuts across nursing theoretical boundaries. The instrument offers a strategy for the direct observation of the nurse's and client's collaborative behavior. Furthermore, each of the three steps in the helping process can be measured to determine if helping was worked. The HORS behavioral focus can provide a base for future nursing research or collaborative endeavors with other health professionals.

## REFERENCES

Carkhuff, R. R. (1971). *The development of human resources.* Holt, Rinehart, & Winston.

Carkhuff, R. R. (1983a). *The art of helping.* Amherst, MA: Human Resources Development Press.

Carkhuff, R. R. (1983b). *The art of helping: Trainer's guide.* Amherst, MA: Human Resources Development Press.

Carkhuff, R. R. & Berenson, B. (1977). *Beyond counseling and therapy.* New York: Holt, Rinehart & Winston.

Chaska, N. (1983). *The nursing profession: A time to speak.* New York: McGraw-Hill.

Cronewett, L. (1983). Helping and nursing models. *Nursing Research, 32,* 342-346.

Edwards, A. L. (1959). *Edwards Personal Preference Schedule.* New York: Psychological Corporation.

Egan, G. (1982a). *Exercises in helping skills.* Monterey, CA: Brooks/Cole.
Egan, G. (1982b). *The skilled helper.* Monterey, CA: Brooks/Cole.
Fitzpatrick, J., & Whall, A. (1983). *Conceptual models in nursing.* Bowie, MD: Brady.
Gazda, G., Walters, R., & Childers, W. (1975). *Human relations development.* Boston: Allyn & Bacon.
Hall, L. A. (1963). A center for nursing. *Nursing Outlook, 11,* 805-806.
Jalowiec, A. (1979). *Coping scale.* Chicago: University of Illinois.
Kinlcin, L. M. (1977). *Independent nursing practice with clients.* Philadelphia: J. B. Lippincott.
Long, L., & Phrophet, P. (1981). *Understanding/responding: A communication manual for nurses.* Monterey, CA: Wadsworth.
Rogers, C., Gendin, E., & Traux, C. (1967). *Therapeutic relationship and its impact.* Westport, CT: Greenwood Press.
Roy, C. (1980). The Roy adaptation model. In J. P. Rhiehl & C. Roy (Eds.), *Conceptual models for nursing practice* (2nd ed.). New York: Appleton-Century-Crofts.
Smitherson, C. (1981). *Nursing actions for health promotion.* Philadelphia: F. A. Davis.
Waltz, C. F., Strickland, O. L., & Lenz, E. R. (1984). *Measurement in nursing research.* Philadelphia: F. A. Davis.

# Helping Outcomes: A Rating Scale

Items for this direct observational instrument were derived from three phases of helping that have been identified by Carkhuff (1971). The Carkhuff helping model came out of Carl Rogers's client-centered theory; however, Carkhuff expanded the client-centered approach to include learning theory, with emphasis on problem-solving and reinforcement. Carkhuff felt that health professionals (including nurses) in addition to laypersons can use the systematic helping strategies that are outlined in his model. In addition to Carkhuff's helping model, Egan's (1982) three-phase problem-management helping model also contributed to the formulation of items for this rating scale. Like Carkhuff, Egan (1982, p. 4) believed that a wide variety of health professionals should participate in the helping process using the same facilitative framework. Nurses were clearly listed in addition to other health professionals who need helping skills. The holistic theme of Carkhuff's and Egan's models cuts across nursing theoretical boundaries.

You are expected to use your expertise to judge the extent of helping as measured by the client's behaviors. Base your judgment on the nurse's objective for each helping phase and circle one of the points on the continuum that represents your perception of the magnitude of helping as manifested by the client's behavior: Very Unsuccessful (1); Unsuccessful (2); Minimally Successful (3); Successful (4); Very Successful (5).

## Phase I:   Exploring

The nurse helps the client to explore his/her own problem.

The client:
   1. Explores his/her experiences relevant to the problem.

| 1 | 2 | 3 | 4 | 5 |
|---|---|---|---|---|
| Very Unsuccessful | Unsuccessful | Minimally Successful | Successful | Very Successful |

   2. Explores his/her feelings relevant to the problem.

| 1 | 2 | 3 | 4 | 5 |
|---|---|---|---|---|
| Very Unsuccessful | Unsuccessful | Minimally Successful | Successful | Very Successful |

3. Explores the ways that he/she is living ineffectively.

| 1 | 2 | 3 | 4 | 5 |
|---|---|---|---|---|
| Very Unsuccessful | Unsuccessful | Minimally Successful | Successful | Very Successful |

4. Establishes a working relationship with the nurse.

| 1 | 2 | 3 | 4 | 5 |
|---|---|---|---|---|
| Very Unsuccessful | Unsuccessful | Minimally Successful | Successful | Very Successful |

5. Discloses relevant data.

| 1 | 2 | 3 | 4 | 5 |
|---|---|---|---|---|
| Very Unsuccessful | Unsuccessful | Minimally Successful | Successful | Very Successful |

6. Defines the problem.

| 1 | 2 | 3 | 4 | 5 |
|---|---|---|---|---|
| Very Unsuccessful | Unsuccessful | Minimally Successful | Successful | Very Successful |

## Phase II:  Understanding

The nurse helps the client to understand him/herself better.

The client:
1. Engages in non-defense listening.

| 1 | 2 | 3 | 4 | 5 |
|---|---|---|---|---|
| Very Unsuccessful | Unsuccessful | Minimally Successful | Successful | Very Successful |

2. Recognizes the need to change.

| 1 | 2 | 3 | 4 | 5 |
|---|---|---|---|---|
| Very Unsuccessful | Unsuccessful | Minimally Successful | Successful | Very Successful |

3. Sees wholes instead of fragmented elements of the problem.

| 1 | 2 | 3 | 4 | 5 |
|---|---|---|---|---|
| Very Unsuccessful | Unsuccessful | Minimally Successful | Successful | Very Successful |

4. Sees a behavioral pattern.

| 1 | 2 | 3 | 4 | 5 |
|---|---|---|---|---|
| Very Unsuccessful | Unsuccessful | Minimally Successful | Successful | Very Successful |

5. Identifies self-strengths and weaknesses.

| 1 | 2 | 3 | 4 | 5 |
|---|---|---|---|---|
| Very Unsuccessful | Unsuccessful | Minimally Successful | Successful | Very Successful |

6. Participates in the planning strategy.

| 1 | 2 | 3 | 4 | 5 |
|---|---|---|---|---|
| Very Unsuccessful | Unsuccessful | Minimally Successful | Successful | Very Successful |

7. Establishes goals relevant to the problem.

| 1 | 2 | 3 | 4 | 5 |
|---|---|---|---|---|
| Very Unsuccessful | Unsuccessful | Minimally Successful | Successful | Very Successful |

## Phase III:   Acting

The nurse helps the client to take actions to correct the identified problem.

The client:
1. Operationalizes goals relevant to the problem.

| 1 | 2 | 3 | 4 | 5 |
|---|---|---|---|---|
| Very Unsuccessful | Unsuccessful | Minimally Successful | Successful | Very Successful |

2. Employs unused resources (for example, self-strengths).

| 1 | 2 | 3 | 4 | 5 |
|---|---|---|---|---|
| Very Unsuccessful | Unsuccessful | Minimally Successful | Successful | Very Successful |

3. Uses alternative strategies to achieve goals.

| 1 | 2 | 3 | 4 | 5 |
|---|---|---|---|---|
| Very Unsuccessful | Unsuccessful | Minimally Successful | Successful | Very Successful |

4. Evaluates the effectiveness of goals.

| 1 | 2 | 3 | 4 | 5 |
|---|---|---|---|---|
| Very Unsuccessful | Unsuccessful | Minimally Successful | Successful | Very Successful |

5. Sees discrepancies between goals and actions.

| 1 | 2 | 3 | 4 | 5 |
|---|---|---|---|---|
| Very Unsuccessful | Unsuccessful | Minimally Successful | Successful | Very Successful |

6. Manages situations more effectively.

| 1 | 2 | 3 | 4 | 5 |
|---|---|---|---|---|
| Very Unsuccessful | Unsuccessful | Minimally Successful | Successful | Very Successful |

7. Evaluates the effectiveness of the action program.

| 1 | 2 | 3 | 4 | 5 |
|---|---|---|---|---|
| Very Unsuccessful | Unsuccessful | Minimally Successful | Successful | Very Successful |

# 9

# Measuring Quality of Nursing Care for DRGs Using the HEW-Medicus Nursing Process Methodology

### Elizabeth A. Barrett

*This chapter discusses the HEW-Medicus Nursing Process Methodology, a measure of quality of nursing care in relation to Diagnosis Related Groups (DRGS).*

## BACKGROUND

Why should nursing put a separate price tag on its services? Unless nursing describes and quantifies its specific contribution to patient care, financial solvency is threatened under prospective payment models (Lazona & Stritzel, 1984). Under these reimbursement systems, the variability in intensity of required nursing services, and thus consumption of resources, has not been given sufficient consideration since nursing costs are still calculated on a per diem basis with hotel services (McKibbon & Marshall, 1984).

"Costing out" nursing services gives hospital boards, chief executive officers, and financial officers a stake in common with the nursing department's administrators (Shaffer, 1984). By using nursing costs on a case-mix category basis, budgets could more accurately reflect the monetary requirements needed to provide nursing care to particular types of patients. In addition to the amount of required nursing care, introduction of new treatment modalities, alterations in the physical layout, and location of patient care units requires consideration if nursing costs are to reflect changes (Lazona & Stritzel, 1984). If costs can be defined, charges can be assigned, and nursing can become a revenue-producing department within the hospital's organizational structure (Lazona & Stritzel, 1984).

Data analysis by Cynthia M. Bournazos, M. S.

The literature indicated a consensus among authors that the quantification of nursing services from a revenue perspective is a difficult and complex task (Cohodes, 1982; Feldman & Goldhaber, 1984; Grimaldi & Micheletti, 1982, 1983; Grimaldi, 1984, Halloran, 1980, 1983; Joseph, Shannon & Svendson, 1983; Lazona & Stritzel, 1984; Shaffer, 1984; Vanderzee & Glusko, 1984). However, two essential requirements emerged as themes from the literature: (1) establishment of accuracy of distribution by Diagnostic Related Groups (DRGs)[1]; (2) establishment of quality of nursing care by DRGs.

The advent of prospective reimbursement and particularly DRGs has challenged nursing administrators and researchers to place increased emphasis on quantifying nursing care from a revenue perspective. Awareness of problem situations before they become crises and anticipation and responsiveness to opportunities before they vanish is the key to successful nursing service administration (LeBreton, 1980).

Additionally, Shaffer (1984) maintained that power will come from making nursing the vital link between cost and quality. Beyond the reimbursement implications, focus on patient problems that are specific to case-mix provides potential for increasing quality of care, a vital mission of the institution.

## THE PROBLEM

The problem was defined as development of a methodology to link quality of nursing care raw data for a particular patient to that patient's DRG. Hence, quality scores for particular DRGs were the outcome variable.

This project was a beginning step in establishing the cost-effectiveness of quality nursing care. Achieving quality of patient care at an affordable cost is a critical issue for nursing and health care administrators. The cost of nursing services accounts for a considerable component of total hospital costs (Halloran, 1980), and nursing person-hours in a major medical center may represent approximately 40% of the total hospital person-hours (Davis, 1982).

With prospective reimbursement models, length of stay (LOS) is directly related to the cost of providing care. While many variables impact on LOS, the outcome of this project will facilitate research to test the hypothesis that quality of nursing care explains some of the variance of LOS. Currently, the relationship between quality of nursing care and cost as operationalized by LOS in unknown.

Despite the lack of definitive studies on the effect of nursing care on LOS, there is growing opinion that high-quality nursing care can reduce

[1]It is understood that other bases of determination of case-mix distribution and/or categories could be substituted for DRGs. In this study, a state DRG classification system was utilized. Since the completion of the study, this state has adopted the federal DRG system. The methodology developed in this study is equally applicable to the federal DRG system.

hospital stays (Munson, Beckman, Clinton, Kever, & Simms, 1980). Consistency of contact with patients provided by primary nursing allows nursing practices such as prevention or immediate recognition of complications, patient teaching, discharge planning, early collaboration with clinical nurse specialists, other professionals, and other hospital services. It seems logical that effective nursing care promotes patient outcomes that lead to shorter lengths of hospital stay (Halloran, 1983). However, there remains a critical need to document further that nursing care makes a difference in a patient's recovery process and therefore LOS in the hospital (Hinson, Silva, & Clapp, 1984).

A major obstacle in linking quality of nursing care to DRGs was that most quality monitoring methodologies (as well as patient classification systems) do not uniquely identify specific patient conditions by scores (Jelinek, Haussman, Hegyvary, & Newman, 1974; Haussmann, Hegyvary & Newman, 1976; Lazona & Stritzel, 1984; D. Barhyte, Personal communication, February 1984). Rather, the *nursing unit* (floor, ward) constituted the level of analysis.

This measurement protocol addressed the problem by developing and testing a methodology to score quality monitoring data, as measured by the HEW-Medicus Nursing Process Methodology (H-MNPM) (Jelinek et al., 1974; Haussmann & Hegyvary, 1977; Haussmann et al., 1976) using specific DRGs as the level of analysis. This cost-effective method of using available reliable data for an additional purpose was viewed as a single and interim step in determining the impact of quality of nursing care on LOS. A similar system could be developed to score patient classification data with DRGs as the level of analysis. Such a system would use acuity as the basis for developing DRG nursing resource requirement profiles. Hospitals with reliable and valid patient classification systems and quality monitoring methodologies currently operational have a readily available means for linking the available data to DRGs without further substantial investments of time and money. Hence, development of methodologies whereby acuity and quality data can be linked to cost of nursing care and LOS per DRG are necessary.

The Department of Nursing at a large metropolitan medical center in the Northeast in where this study was conducted has established a track record in relation to commitment to quality of nursing care. In 1981 there were 300 more staff RNs than there were in 1977, and nursing hours increased from 34% to 39% of the total hospital person-hours (Davis, 1982). Since that time, primary nursing has been implemented. RN turnover decreased 10% from 1980 through 1984 (Barrett, 1985). Approximately 70% of the RNs in the Department of Nursing have bachelor's degree's, and about 50% have a B.S.N. as basic preparation for practice (Barrett & Wieczorek, 1984). Concomitantly, quality of nursing care scores have steadily increased (Devereux, 1984).

The investigator was Director of Nursing Standards and Clinical Evaluation at the time the study was conducted.

## VARIABLE MEASURED

The outcome variable was the quality of nursing care score(s) for specific case-mix categories. Quality of nursing care was measured by an assessment of the nursing *process* (H-MNPM); in this project a methodology was developed to utilize case-mix categories, specifically the New York state system of DRGs, as the level of analysis rather than the nursing unit. The *outcome* was the quality-of-care indicator(s) for patients with particular DRGs. The goal of this project was to develop and test a methodology for converting raw data from the H-MNPM into quality scores for patients with *particular DRGs* rather than into quality scores for particular *nursing units*. In future research, quality of nursing care scores for patients can be related to revenue aspects of patient care.

## REVIEW AND ANALYSIS OF LITERATURE REGARDING VARIABLE

While numerous publications have addressed quality of nursing care and its measurement (Barba & Bennett, 1978; Bloch, 1975; Eichhorn, 1979; Haussmann & Hegyvary, 1976, 1977; Haussmann et al., 1976; Hegyvary & Haussmann, 1975; Jelinek et al., 1974; Phaneuf, 1972, 1976; Roeder, 1980; Routhier, 1972; Selvaggi, 1980; Ventura, 1980; Wainwright & Burnip, 1983a; Wandelt & Ager, 1974; Ward & Lindeman, 1979), most instruments lack the methodological rigor that is essential to capture the complex and comprehensive nature of professional nursing care. Donebedian (1970) defined the three classical frameworks for evaluating patient care as structure, process, and outcome. Bloch (1975) argued for consideration of the need to relate process to outcome and maintained that only an evaluation that encompasses both process and outcome has the potential for great impact on the quality of care (p. 258). The two-volume compilation of instruments for measuring health care variables was a major step forward (Ward & Lindeman, 1979), yet instrumentation remains a critical issue (Ventura, Hinshaw, & Atwood, 1981).

Tools that measure nursing care for particular types of patients have frequently not had generalizability. For example, Lindeman and Stetzer (1973) developed a checklist for effectiveness, efficiency, and safety of nursing care for surgical patients during the preoperative period as it impacts on patients during the interoperative period. Questions of reliability and validity were raised (Ward & Lindeman, 1979). Likewise, Woog and Goldman (1975) developed an instrument, Climate of Nursing Home Evaluation, that elicits information on 15 variables pertaining to nursing home environment and nursing home patients. Like many instruments, it offers potential for providing reliable and valid information, yet it is premature to reach conclusions regarding ultimate usefulness (Ward & Lindeman, 1979). This frustrating yet challenging problem continuously confronts quality-of-care researchers.

Few substantive instruments that measure quality of nursing care in a hospital setting and were not limited to a specific patient population were located. Four such tools will be reviewed and critiqued. In each instance, this investigator will expand the discussion presented by Ward and Lindeman (1979) by focusing on difficulties regarding implementation and utility of results in a hospital setting. The tools are Evaluation of Patient Care, Quality Patient Care Scale (Qualpacs), The Phaneuf Nursing Audit, and the HEW-Medicus Nursing Process Methodology (H-MNPM).

## Evaluation of Patient Care

### Discussion and Critique (Ward & Lindeman, 1979)

The instrument, developed and refined over a 2½-year period by Ostrowski and Routhier (Routhier, 1972), collects data encompassing direct and indirect patient care components. A "trained" nurse-interviewer records observations and comments from the patient, patient's family, and nursing staff, along with data from the patient's records over the period of time of the hospital stay. In addition to 100 items of inquiry, observation, and health record audit, 7 open-ended questions elicit patient comments.

Direct patient care elements include admissions procedure, hospital environment, patient's experience, management of psychosocial aspects of care, and discharge planning/assistance for the patient and family. Indirect care components include short- and long-term nursing care plans.

Completion requires 1 to 1½ hr over the period of time from admission to discharge. In the pilot project in a large teaching hospital, arranging a time to meet with the family proved problematic.

Scoring procedures were not provided nor was information on reliability reported. Six persons reviewed the tool in an effort to establish validity of the items.

Comments by Ward and Lindeman (1979) emphasized the need for psychometric attention and raised a question regarding whether or not the instrument primarily measured patient satisfaction rather than quality of nursing care. Additionally, the wording of some items required value judgments. Efforts to define redundancy could eliminate overlap and shorten the instrument.

### Usefulness for Current Project

Since this tool was developed more than 10 years ago, a computer search (of *Index Medicus*) was undertaken to determine further revision and use of the tool. Unfortunately, interim work on the tool does not justify its use for the purposes of this project. Unanswered questions regarding reliability and validity prohibited investment of time and resources into further investigation. There is no assurance that the tool measures quality of nursing care or that measurement is achieved in an accurate, consistent manner. In addition, the logistics of completing the tool at various points throughout the patient's stay, as well as arrangements for collecting data from family, limited the applicability for widespread use of the instrument with large numbers of patients. In addition to the open-ended questions, each item provides for unstructured comments. Such a data collection format presents difficulties in terms of scoring and analysis. Separation of the process from outcome items are additional areas that require attention. Although this tool represented a good beginning, there is no assurance that with further methodological effort the purpose of this project could be achieved by using it in this study.

## Quality Patient Care Scale (Qualpacs)

### Discussion and Critique (Ward & Lindeman, 1979)

This 68-item instrument, designed to be completed in 3 hr by an observer-rater, proposed to measure quality of nursing care being received by a patient in any setting. The authors, Wandelt and Ager (1974), rephrased the items of the Slater's Nursing Performance Rating Scale (Wandelt & Stewart, 1975) to transfer the locus of measurement from the nurse to the patient. Each item was measured on a 5-point rating scale, and any item may be measured more than once during an observation period. The standard of measurement was the care expected of a first-level staff registered nurse. Items were coded to indicate whether direct observation or indirect observation or either of the two methods are required.

Scores were determined for each item by calculating the average of the ratings in all of the cells of the item. The total score was the measure of the quality of nursing care received by the patient and was calculated from the total of the *item* mean scores, not by averaging the six subsection scores. The six categories of care evaluated were psychosocial, individual, psychosocial, group, physical, general, communication, professional implications.

The instrument was pretested in three hospitals in 1969, and the revised instrument was tested in 1970. Evidence of interrater reliability is based on three studies ($r = .74$, $N = 96$ patients; $r = .91$, $N = 6$ patients; $r = .64$, $N = 11$ patients). Kuder-Richardson estimate of reliability of 0.96 was reported for one study in which item, subscale and total score variance and covariance were computed for 55 of the 68 items that had been rated for at least 20 patients. The same sample was used to provide stability coefficients of 0.98 for five patients who were each rated by one observer on two successive days. Content and construct validity were assessed by using observer-raters and four clinical nurse specialists to judge the instrument. However, further psychometric development is required. Additionally, subjectivity and value judgments may bias the data.

## Usefulness for Current Project

The lengthiness of data collection (3 hr) as well as tenuous psychometric evidence of reliability (small samples) and validity did not warrant the selection of this tool for purposes of the current project. However, the ease of scoring as well as the potential for converting the rating choices or Best Care, Between, Average Care, Between, and Poorest Care into a framework for interpretation of the total mean score was methodologically appealing. A current computer search indicated that the instrument has been rather widely used in quality of patient care research (Eichhorn, 1979; Fox & Ventura, 1984; Ventura & Crosby, 1978; Wainwright & Burnip, 1983b).

## The Phaneuf Nursing Audit

### Discussion and Critique (Ward & Lindeman, 1979)

Quality of nursing care was evaluated by information based on seven criteria: application and execution of physician's legal orders, observation of symptoms and reaction, supervision of the patient, supervision of those participating in care, reporting and recording, application and execution of nursing procedures and techniques, promotion of physical and emotional health by direction and teaching, and an overall rating of nursing care.

The 50 items focused primarily on nursing process rather than outcome or structure. About 40 hr are required to "train" raters to evaluate quality of nursing care received by patients in any setting by means of a 30-min audit of the health care record postdischarge. Each criterion is measured by four to six items.

Scores were computed by adding the numerical weights provided for each group of questions; a 3- or 4-point scale was used to record responses to the questions. The total score was the sum of the responses to all 50 items. The total score had five divisions: Unsafe (0-40), Poor (41-80), Incomplete (81-120), Good (121-160), Excellent (161-200). Items were developed deductively from the model of the nursing process developed by Berggren and Zagornik (1968) and inductively from input from nurses and other health professionals. The development of the instrument has been described extensively in Phaneuf's *The Nursing Audit* (1976). However, no information was provided with regard to test-retest, interobserver, or split-half reliability. Nor was statistical information provided regarding the changes from initial testing to testing of the revised instrument. The instrument *appeared* to have validity and has been used in education, practice, and research (Phaneuf, 1972, 1976).

### Usefulness for Current Project

This instrument presented several advantages for use in the current project. First, the postdischarge data collection eliminated the concurrent data collection problem presented by the H-MNPM tool. Since the purpose of this project is to link quality of nursing care to specific case-mix categories, which are usually determined postdischarge, one could question whether concurrent evaluation of quality is representative and comparable to quality of care evaluated after the entire length of hospital stay. However, since postdischarge data collection frequently presents serious issues of validity due to information that is missing in the patient care record, the advantage of retrospective as opposed to concurrent data collection was questionable. Second, provision of an overall score as well as the seven criteria subscores and item scores would be useful for subsequent planned research relating quality of nursing care to other variables of interest. Third, the total score definitions of care, ranging from Safe to Excellent Quality, provided indices of quality that are readily communicated and understood. Finally, the relative ease of data collection and scoring provided more flexibility and less expensive resources than the HEW-Medicus methodology. However, the psychometric sophistication of the HEW-Medicus methodology is not matched by the Phaneuf Audit.

## HEW-Medicus Nursing Process Methodology (H-MNPM)

### Discussion and Critique (Ward & Lindeman, 1979)

This tool measured the quality of nursing care by an assessment of the nursing process defined as the assessing, planning, implementing and evaluating components of care. From a master set of 357 evaluative criteria (Waltz, Strickland, & Lenz, 1984), a computer-generated set of criteria were produced for 32 subobjectives that fall within a framework of six major objectives: The plan of nursing care is formulated; the physical needs of the patient are attended; the nonphysical (psychological, emotional, mental, and social) needs of the patient are attended; achievement of nursing care objectives is evaluated; unit procedures are followed for the protection of all patients; the delivery of nursing care is facilitated by administrative and managerial services. Subobjectives were selected according to patient classification: self-care, partial care, complete care, and intensive care. Alternate forms have varying numbers of items (Waltz et al. 1984).

"The methodology is applied to a nursing unit by reviewing 10 percent of one month's patient census, usually about 20 patients" (Waltz et al., p. 511). Observations should be randomly distributed across days, patients, and day and evening shifts. Interrater reliability of a minimum of 0.85 needs to be established by raters prior to each period of data collection. A computer program was developed to produce "quality indexes" for each of the 32 subobjectives and the 6 objectives for each of the monitored units.

An initial set of 900 items was developed by reviewing existing methodologies. The items were examined for measurability and redundancy, and a revised list of approximately 220 items was used in a pilot study in two hospitals. The criteria were then revised, expanded, and field-tested in 19 hospitals to establish reliability and validity. Item analyses were included in the reliability studies. The claims for construct validity were based on (1) analysis of scores from the 19 hospitals, which indicated that the scores were predictable based on current nursing practices; (2) current trends in nursing education and practice, which led to the hypothesis that components of the nursing process were highly correlated in terms of quality. The hypothesis was supported by analysis of quality scores from the 19 hospitals ($p = .001$). There was little evidence for concurrent or predictive validity. This methodology represented one of the most widely tested means for measuring quality of nursing care, and it featured careful attention to conceptual framework, detail, planning, testing, and evaluation. Ward and Lindeman (1979) noted that although the instrument may be the most expensive in terms of resources, it can make a significant contribution to the nursing profession.

## Usefulness for Current Project

Development of the H-MNPM was a major undertaking; the methodology was subjected to extensive statistical testing. After several revisions and retesting, it was proposed to be a reliable and valid instrument for measuring the quality of the nursing process (Hegyvary, Gortner, & Haussmann, 1976).

Following the review of the literature, the H-MNPM was selected as the instrument for measuring quality of care. The H-MNPM was operational in this investigator's employing institution, which is a 1,212-bed hospital within a major metropolitan medical center. It also appeared to be the most conceptually sound and methodologically sophisticated instrument available to assess quality of nursing care for medical, surgical, obstetric, pediatric, and psychiatric patients. One particular advantage was that patient classification was considered in generation of items. Another advantage was that from the master list of criteria alternate forms were developed according to patient classification and clinical area. The tool has been widely used for quality assurance purposes. As Bloch (1975) noted, the instrument was the result of a major effort to "build upon, refine, and extend the state-of-the-art and it should prove highly useful to those in nursing wishing to evaluate quality of nursing care in institutions" (p. 260). The allocation of considerable resources through HEW grants allowed for the necessary steps in instrument development.

The H-MNPM formed the basis for developing and testing a methodology that used case mix rather than nursing unit as the level of analysis. By using the raw data, quality of care was linked to DRGs rather than to the nursing unit (floor, ward). No studies that described the development of the methodology proposed in this study were located via a computerized literature search. Since the DRG classification system is the basis for prospective payment, which became the law of the land in 1983 (Shaffer,

1984), a method for measuring quality-of-care scores for DRGs seemed essential. Hence, this pilot project used the H-MNPM to build on what exists, for the purpose of developing a system to obtain quality scores for DRGs. Also, use of the raw data that was already available represented a cost-effective means of achieving the DRG quality scores.

Two similar research projects in which patient population was the unit of analysis for the H-MNPM were identified. Haussmann and Hegyvary (1977) began this pioneering research in an effort to relate process and outcomes. Outcome criteria were developed for several patient populations. The correlations were inconsistent, yet selected parts of the nursing process were significantly related to outcomes for each patient population studied (Haussmann & Hegyvary, 1977; Haussmann et al., 1976). While replication and extension of such studies are needed, the expense of data collection and running the required scoring routines is prohibitive with limited financial and human resources. Development of a scoring methodology using the Statistical Package for the Social Sciences (SPSS) would facilitate cost-effective process-outcome studies in the future. Jessie Scott (cited in Haussmann & Hegyvary, 1977) commented on the difficulty of measuring such process-outcome linkages.

Selvaggi (1980) adapted the H-MNPM to obtain quality scores for a high-risk maternity population. To facilitate the study of the relationship of the nursing process to patient outcomes, the same set of questions was used for each subject, and a score was constructed for each of the four dimensions of the nursing process. The computer program used by Haussmann and Hegyvary (1977) for scoring the modified H-MNPM was not available to Selvaggi. She devised a manual-computation scoring process for each dimension of the nursing process for each subject ($N = 147$). Selvaggi found that mean scores on each of the four nursing process variables were higher for units that delivered care via primary nursing versus units that used a functional nursing modality. Other authors have also noted the effectiveness of primary nursing in increasing the quality of nursing care (Felton, 1975; Roeder, 1980; Sellick, Russell & Beckmann, 1983).

## CONCEPTUAL FRAMEWORK

As described by Hegyvary and associates (1976), the nursing process model provided the conceptual framework for the methodology used to measure quality of nursing care with the H-MNPM instrument. Hence, the nursing process model was the conceptual basis underlying the methodology to provide quality scores for patients with particular DRGs. The nursing process model was conceptually defined as the assessment of the patient and family, the planning of care based on needs or problems, the implementation of physical and nonphysical aspects of the care plan, and evaluation of the response to care. The nursing process model was operationally defined by selected criteria that fall within the rubric of 32 subobjectives and 6 major objectives. The model contained aspects of clerical and support services since they impact on the nursing process, especially if nurses engage in those activities (Hegyvary et al., 1976). The operationalization of the framework is presented in Table 9.1.

**TABLE 9.1 Nursing Process Framework**

1.0    The plan of nursing care is formulated.
    1.1    The condition of the patient is assessed on admission.
    1.2    Data relevant to hospital care is ascertained on admission.
    1.3    The current condition of the patient is assessed.
    1.4    The written plan of nursing care is formulated.
    1.5    The plan of nursing care is coordinated with the medical plan of care.

2.0    The physical needs of the patient are attended.
    2.1    The patient is protected from accident and injury.
    2.2    The need for physical comfort and rest is attended.
    2.3    The need for physical hygiene is attended.
    2.4    The need for supply of oxygen is attended.
    2.5    The need for activity is attended.
    2.6    The need for nutrition and fluid balance is attended.
    2.7    The need for elimination is attended.
    2.8    The need for skin care is attended.
    2.9    The patient is protected from infection.

3.0    The nonphysical (psychological, emotional, mental, and social) needs of the patient are attended.
    3.1    The patient is oriented to hospital facilities on admission.
    3.2    The patient is extended social courtesy by the nursing staff.
    3.3    The patient's privacy and civil rights are honored.
    3.4    The need for psychological-emotional well-being is attended.
    3.5    The patient is taught measures of health maintenance and illness prevention.
    3.6    The patient's family is included in the nursing care process.

4.0    Achievement of nursing care objectives is evaluated
    4.1    Records document the care provided for the patient.
    4.2    The patient's response to therapy is evaluated.

5.0    Unit procedures are followed for the protection of all patients.
    5.1    Isolation and decontamination procedures are followed.
    5.2    The unit is prepared for emergency situations.
    5.3    Medical-legal procedures are followed.
    5.4    Unit safety and protective procedures are followed.

6.0    The delivery of nursing care is facilitated by administrative and managerial services.
    6.1    Nursing reporting follows prescribed standards.
    6.2    Nursing management is provided.
    6.3    Clerical services are provided.
    6.4    Environmental and support services are provided.
    6.5    Professional and administrative services are provided.

## MEASUREMENT PROTOCOL

### Construction of the Measure

The H-MNPM was developed through a contract from the Division of Nursing Health Resources Administration, Dept. of Health, Education and Welfare with the Rush-Presbyterian-St. Luke's Medical Center and through them to the Medicus Corporation (Jelinek et al., 1974). The first phase of the project reviewed state-of-the-art nursing research regarding quality of nursing care and subsequently developed a methodology for monitoring quality of care (Jelinek et al., 1974). The second phase consisted of a national trial of the methodology in 19 hospitals of differing size and characteristics (Haussman et al., 1976). The relationship between nursing process, as measured by the quality-monitoring methodology, and nursing outcome criteria for six patient conditions was the focus of the third phase of the study (Haussmann & Hegyvary, 1977).

Currently, the Medicus Corporation is revising the instrument, and following testing of the updated version, it will be available through Medicus, most likely in 1987 (J. Nollman, personal communications, January 22, 1986). Although many of the criteria continue to reflect current nursing practice, additions and deletions are needed to incorporate changes that have occurred over the past 15 years.

### Objectives

The major objective of this study was to use existing reliable raw data collected for monitoring quality of nursing care on a nursing unit in order to obtain scores indicative of quality of nursing care for specific case-mix categories of patients. Later, the relationship between DRG quality-of-care scores and LOS can be determined. Also, additional scoring procedures that will allow for greater flexibility and meaningful interpretation than is currently available with the ANS COBOL program could be developed. This project provided for an additional use of the H-MNPM data for research purposes only. It did *not* change the currently implemented methodology for monitoring quality of nursing care on particular nursing units.

Since the completion of the project, this investigator's institution has purchased from Medicus software for the IBM Personal Computer that processes and analyzes patient classification and quality monitoring data. Several new reports are available, such as quality versus staffing and trending reports.

### Administration

The tool was administered in the manner currently operational in this investigator's institutions. That is, data collection procedures remained the same. Before each data collection period, a 7.5-hr orientation for data collection is given, and interrater reliability is established. Although 0.85

agreement among data collectors is the minimal acceptable level of interrater reliability, the current range is from .90 to .98 (Creegan, personal communication, March 1984). During the data collection period, master's-prepared nursing staff educators (clinical resource nurses) randomly select patients for monitoring. For the current project, use of these data provided for a cost-effective and reliable means of data collection. Haussman and Hegyvary (1977) noted that the most significant variable related to this instrument is observer training and repeated testing for interrater reliability.

## Collection of Additional Data

The project was approved by the institutional review board Research Activities Committee. The cooperation of the medical records department made it possible for this investigator to pursue this project as designed.

Patient names and identification of specific versions of the tool used for data collection during 1984 were obtained from a control sheet. The purpose of the control sheet was to avoid monitoring the same patient twice on successive days. The control sheet was essential to link data to a particular patient because neither names nor identification numbers appeared on the data collection instrument in order to protect confidentiality.

Second, patient names, monitoring data, and nursing units were used to access, via microfiche, patient identification numbers from Medical Records. The identification numbers were used to retrieve the patient's DRG from computerized reports that provide this information.

Third, when the number of cases per DRG was determined, two DRGs having the highest number of cases were selected for investigation in this study. Quality data were retrieved from the original data collection answer sheets for those patients with the DRGs that were being considered in this study.

Fourth, the following information was recorded: patient identification number, DRG, and raw data scores for each item monitored during data collection. Patient names were not used in order to assure confidentiality.

## Scoring

For purposes of this project, data could be analyzed and scored using the SPSS (Nie, Hull, Jenkins, Steinbrenner, & Bent, 1975) rather than the ANS COBOL program, which was used to provide quality indices for nursing units. The small sample size did not warrant development of the SPSS procedure; rather, data were manually manipulated. The scoring methodology, however, is the same for all three ways that data could be analyzed (COBOL, SPSS, manual).

During the initial instrument development of the H-MNPM, applying statistically developed weights to the criteria in generating subobjective scores produced no significant differences in quality rankings compared with rankings derived from scores that were unweighted (Jelinek et al., 1974). Later it was proposed that empirical weights be developed by statistical correlation methods involving item-total correlations. Although problems involving computational issues might be overcome, it was decided to abandon the idea of weighting items because problems of interpretation and comparison of scores over time and across nursing units would be enormous (Haussman et al., 1976).

In the scoring procedure, "each criterion score is the ratio of positive responses based on the number of valid observations for the criterion" (Haussman et al., 1976, p. 11). In other words, all criteria within a subobjective were treated equally. They were not weighted in terms of importance to the particular objective being addressed by the subobjective. A score for each subobjective and objective was produced. However, since a varying number of subobjective items were included in the alternate forms of the instrument, objective scores were based on an average of subobjective scores, each of which was weighted by the number of items used to measure that subobjective. The same methodology was used to produce scores in the current project, where the unit of analysis was the particular case-mix category. However, in this study, scores were produced for only the first four objectives and subobjectives. Moreover, in none of the literature reviewed was a mechanism for providing a total score described, nor was this investigator able to find discussion regarding the pros and cons of producing a total score.

The SPSS system would provide a cost-effective and flexible methodology for empirically investigating additional scoring procedures. In addition to producing a total score, which has the advantage of a single number to indicate quality of care, other scores can be provided. Specifically, it has been noted that whereas assessment of the quality of care must consider support services simultaneously, "it is important that the core of nursing care not be confounded with the evaluation of non-clinical support activities. The nursing process structure of this methodology permits such review" (Haussman et al., 1976, p. 7). Thus, the first *four* objective scores could be combined to provide an index of quality of *nursing* care. This score could be compared with the total index score, which would consider the *six* subobjectives. Variability by case-mix category could also be explicated for the two total scores: (1) assessing, planning, implementing, and evaluating quality of nursing care; (2) assessing, planning, implementing, and evaluating quality of nursing care, unit procedures, and administrative and managerial services. It is understood that such additional scoring procedures in no way eliminate the need for the detail provided by objective and subobjective scores.

Although this is a criterion-referenced test, wide variability in scores, in addition to lack of a cutoff score to substantiate achievement of quality, suggests a norm-referenced interpretation (Waltz et al., 1984). Interpreting data and providing meaningful feedback to nurse managers and administrators present problems. For example, is an increase in any particular score from 70 to 73 clinically or statistically significant? What score indicates "unsafe" practice? How can changes in scores over time be interpreted without large-scale trend analysis or time-series analysis studies? The basic question is, what does any particular score mean in terms of a quality indicator? Although these questions are the focus for an additional follow-up study, the literature has not sufficiently addressed the issue of interpretation of scores. For purposes of this project, percentage scores were used.

Additional scoring procedures were not completed in this phase of the current project. Rather, a score for the first four objectives and subobjectives was obtained. These were scores for patients with a particular DRG rather than scores for a nursing unit.

## PRIOR ASSESSMENT OF RELIABILITY AND VALIDITY

### Reliability

During the developmental phase of this tool, significant revision of the criteria resulted from methodological procedures. These included marginal distributions to assess discriminating power of the criteria, interitem correlations to estimate degree to which criteria were correlated within subobjectives, item-to-item correlations to identify redundant criteria, and cluster analysis to determine subobjective cohesiveness. These extensive measures seem to have produced an internally consistent and reliable instrument (Jelinek et al., 1974; Haussman et al., 1976; Waltz et al., 1984).

### Validity

The authors claimed that the most important fact about the structure of the instrument was its level of detail. They proposed that no other existing methodology for monitoring quality of nursing care is based on an operational definition of the nursing process to this degree of specificity (Haussmann et al., 1976).

Demonstration of content validity began with a comprehensive review and selection of state-of-the-art nursing process criteria (Jelinek et al., 1974; Waltz et al., 1984). Following the Phase I testing at two hospitals, a follow-up study was conducted in Phase II at 19 hospitals (Haussman et al., 1976; Jelinek et al., 1974). Data (high correlations, $p = .001$) on parts of the nursing process that experts deemed should be related have been presented as evidence of contruct validity, and limited data have supported predictive validity (Betz, Dickerson, & Wyatt, 1980; Waltz et al., 1984). Both of these areas are ripe for further investigation. Hospitals that have accumulated large data bases over time have sufficient sample sizes to conduct construct validity studies using factor analysis. Projects such as this investigator is conducting are forerunners to studies that may substantiate construct and predictive validity.

# RESULTS

## Findings

Using data collected for the purpose of producing quality-of-care scores for nursing units (floors, wards), a methodology was developed whereby quality scores were produced for selected DRGs. From the patients monitored during the period when DRG data was available, sample size for the highest-volume DRG was 43. Since this sample size was inadequate for appropriate reliability and validity testing, the findings are presented but not interpreted. It is recommended that data collection continue until adequate sample size allows for repeating the testing procedures used in this study. In addition, factor analysis could be used to test for construct validity, and the variance of factor scores would be appropriate means of reliability testing. If the sample is not large enough to warrant factor analysis ($N = 300$), cluster analysis would also be appropriate.

For this project the highest-volume DRGs were selected for reliability and validity testing. Normal Mature Newborn ($N = 43$) and Schizoaffective Psychosis, Manic-Depressive Psychosis (a single DRG category, $N = 20$) constituted the sample.

## Reliability

Interrater reliability for the current project was .94. In addition to this 94% rate of agreement among data collectors, item-to-total correlations were computed to test for homogeneity of the criteria in each dimension of the nursing process (objectives 1, 2, 3, 4). The range for Normal Mature Newborn was .32 to .89 (Table 9.2); the range for Schizoaffective Psychosis, Manic-Depressive Psychosis was .00 to .94 (Table 9.3). Only subobjectives 1.1, 1.3, 2.3, 3.3, and 3.7 for Schizoaffective Psychosis, Manic-Depressive Psychosis had item-to-total correlations below .30. Alpha coefficients for the Normal Mature Newborn were .49, .14, .72, and .20 for objectives 1 through 4, respectively. Alpha coefficients for Schizoaffective Psychosis, Manic-Depressive Psychosis were .32, .13, .47, and .31 for objectives 1 through 4, respectively. (See Table 9.4).

Due to small sample size, interpretation should be made cautiously, and no conclusions can be drawn. Reporting is for informational purposes only.

**TABLE 9.2** Item-Total Correlations: Normal Mature Newborn (*N* = 43)

| Subobjective/objective | 1.0 | 2.0 | 3.0 | 4.0 |
|:---:|:---:|:---:|:---:|:---:|
| 1.1 | .32 | | | |
| 1.2 | .34 | | | |
| 1.3 | .77[a] | | | |
| 1.4 | .64 | | | |
| 1.5 | .53 | | | |
| 2.1 | | * | | |
| 2.2 | | * | | |
| 2.3 | | .87[b] | | |
| 2.5 | | * | | |
| 2.6 | | * | | |
| 2.7 | | .89[c] | | |
| 2.8 | | .44[d] | | |
| 3.3 | | | * | |
| 3.4 | | | .61[b] | |
| 3.6 | | | .89[e] | |
| 4.1 | | | | .88 |
| 4.2 | | | | .65[c] |

[a]*N* = 31; [b]*N* = 23; [c]*N* = 29; [d]*N* = 18; [e]*N* = 12.
\* No variance in subobjective scores.

**TABLE 9.3** Item-Total Correlation: Schizoaffective Psychosis, Manic-Depressive Psychosis (*N* = 20)

| Subobjective/objective | 1.0 | 2.0 | 3.0 | 4.0 |
|:---:|:---:|:---:|:---:|:---:|
| 1.1 | .15 | | | |
| 1.2 | .58 | | | |
| 1.3 | .13 | | | |
| 1.4 | .75 | | | |
| 1.5 | .70 | | | |
| 2.1 | | .65[a] | | |
| 2.2 | | .31[b] | | |
| 2.3 | | .00[c] | | |
| 2.5 | | .76[d] | | |
| 2.6 | | .56[e] | | |
| 2.7 | | .33[f] | | |
| 3.1 | | | .58 | |
| 3.2 | | | .51[g] | |
| 3.3 | | | .29 | |
| 3.4 | | | .42[g] | |
| 3.5 | | | .49[h] | |
| 3.6 | | | .53 | |
| 3.7 | | | .25[i] | |
| 4.1 | | | | .65 |
| 4.2 | | | | .94[c] |

[a]*N* = 18; [b]*N* = 17; [c]*N* = 15; [d]*N* = 10; [e]*N* = 12; [f]*N* = 14; [g]*N* = 19; [h]*N* = 9; [i]*N* = 16.

**TABLE 9.4** Alpha Coefficients
for Two DRG Categories

| Category | Alpha |
|---|---|
| DRG 90 | |
| Objective 1.0 | .32 |
| Objective 2.0 | .13 |
| Objective 3.0 | .47 |
| Objective 4.0 | .31 |
| DRG 318 | |
| Objective 1.0 | .49 |
| Objective 2.0 | .14 |
| Objective 3.0 | .72 |
| Objective 4.0 | .20 |

DRG 90: Schizoaffective Psychosis,
Manic-Depressive Psychosis; DRG 318:
Normal Mature Newborns.

## Validity

Although issues of validity of particular criteria (items) need to be reconsidered with the changes in nursing practice, including primary nursing as a method of delivering care, no attempt was made to assess item content validity as a measure of the extent to which the item was a measure of the content domain. Since the instrument was not altered, the basic validity remains intact. To address predictive validity in this project would have been premature. However, providing a methodology that will identify quality of nursing care for particular populations will lay groundwork for future validity studies.

In a beginning effort to establish validity of the scoring methodology whereby quality-monitoring data were linked to the patient's DRG rather than to the nursing unit, scores were compared for the normal newborn nurseries (nursing unit) with scores for normal newborn patients (DRG) (Table 9.5, Figure 9.1). Since not all subobjective items are included in the various versions of the H-MNPM instrument, objective scores are based on an average of subobjective scores, each of which was weighted by the number of items used to measure that subobjective. The scores are not expected to be identical since DRG sample ($N = 43$) is a subset of data within the larger sample ($N = 64$) representing the nursing units. Differences in sample size are primarily due to inability to retrieve DRG data for all patients. In addition, some patients in the normal newborn nurseries had DRG classifications other than normal newborn (DRG 318). However, scores were similar and supported the validity of the DRG scoring methodology. Since most patients in the normal newborn nurseries were within the same DRG, this comparison was used to validate comparability of the two scoring systems. Note that scores are computed for objectives 1 to 4 without consideration of clerical and support services.

Since the psychiatric units have considerable variability regarding DRG classification, a similar comparison was not appropriate for Schizo-affective Psychosis, Manic-Depressive Psychosis (Table 9.6).

In summary, the results indicated that the proposed methodology is workable. However, the procedures used in this study need to be repeated with a sample size that is adequate for establishing reliability and validity. Factor analysis and/or cluster analysis are alternate means for establishing construct validity; the variances of factor scores or theta coefficients would provide appropriate estimates of reliability.

## SUMMARY, CONCLUSIONS, AND RECOMMENDATIONS

The purpose of this project was to develop a method to measure quality of nursing care for diagnosis-related groups (DRGs). Specifically, a methodology was designed for using raw data obtained via the HEW-Medicus Nursing Process Methodology (H-MNPM) to produce quality scores for patients with particular DRGs. In this study, case mix rather than nursing unit, as in the customary H-MNPM procedure, became the level of analysis.

As described by Haussman and associates (1976), the nursing process model provides the conceptual framework for the methodology used to measure quality of nursing care with the H-MNPM instrument. Hence, the nursing process model was the conceptual basis underlying the methodology to provide quality scores for patients with particular DRGs. The model was operationally defined by 357 criteria that are within the rubric of 32 subobjectives and 6 major objectives. The model contained aspects of clerical and support services since they impact on the nursing process, especially if nurses engage in those activities (Haussman, Hegyvary, & Newman, 1976).

For purposes of this project the quality monitoring data were linked to the patient rather than to the nursing unit. Information obtained from medical records was used to identify the patient's DRG according to the New York state system. Next the highest-volume DRG categories were determined. Quality monitoring of raw data was used to obtain DRG scores for selected DRGs for the subobjectives and objectives. Each score was the ratio of positive responses based on the number of observations for that criterion.

Data concerning DRG classification was available for only a 1-year period. Approximately 1,550 patients were monitored during this period and represented numerous DRGs. Small sample size per DRG was inadequate for appropriate reliability and validity testing. However, reliability and validity of items were previously established during instrument development (Jelinek et al., 1974).

**TABLE 9.5 Comparison of Quality Scores for Normal Newborn Units with Normal Mature Newborn DRG**

| Objectives and subobjectives | Average score Unit 1/Unit 2 | DRG 318 |
|---|---|---|
| 1.0 The plan of nursing care is formulated. | 77 | 85 |
|   1.1 The condition of the patient is assessed on admission. | 94 | 96 |
|   1.2 Data relevant to hospital care is ascertained on admission. | 94 | 93 |
|   1.3 The current condition of the patient is assessed. | 65 | 61 |
|   1.4 The written plan of nursing care is formulated. | 69 | 86 |
|   1.5 The plan of nursing care is coordinated with the medical plan of care. | 70 | 94 |
| 2.0 The physical needs of the patient are attended. | 97 | 99 |
|   2.1 The patient is protected from accident and injury. | 99 | 100 |
|   2.2 The need for physical comfort and rest is attended. | 98 | 100 |
|   2.3 The need for physical hygiene is attended. | 94 | 96 |
|   2.5 The need for activity is attended. | 100 | 100 |
|   2.6 The need for nutrition and fluid balance is attended. | 100 | 100 |
|   2.7 The need for elimination is attended. | 97 | 99 |
|   2.8 The need for skin care is attended. | 50[a] | 100 |
| 3.0 The nonphysical (psychological, emotional, mental, and social) needs of the patient are attended. | 68 | 57 |
|   3.3 The patient's privacy and civil rights are honored. | 88 | 100 |
|   3.4 The need for psychological-emotional well-being is attended. | 82 | 84 |
|   3.6 The patient's family is included in the nursing care process. | 56 | 33 |
| 4.0 Achievement of nursing care objectives is evaluated. | 80 | 89 |
|   4.1 Records document the care provided for the patient. | 87 | 90 |
|   4.2 The patient's response to therapy is evaluated. | 69 | 85 |

[a]No Score on unit 1.

Interrater reliability for the current project was .94. In addition to this 94% rate of agreement among data collectors, item-total correlations were computed to test for homogeneity of the criteria in each dimension of the nursing process and ranged from .00 to .94. In addition, alpha coefficients were also computed and ranged from .13 to .72. Given adequate sample size, factor analysis could be used to test for construct validity, and the variance of factor scores would be appropriate means of reliability testing. Ongoing data collection will allow for such studies. In this small sample, normal newborn DRG scores (a subset of data obtained for the units) were compared to the nursing unit scores for the normal newborn nurseries. Scores were similar and thus support the validity of the DRG scoring methodology. Additionally, DRG quality scores were computed for Schizoaffective and Manic-Depressive Psychoses.

Factor analysis and/or cluster analysis are alternate means for establishing construct validity for large samples. The variances of factor scores or theta coefficients would provide appropriate estimates of reliability. The low correlations seem to be related to the lack of variability in ranges of scores. If this proves to be the situation when the sample size has been increased, then other measures of reliability that do not assume as much variation in scores, such as interclass correlation or gamma or kappa, may be more appropriate.

Case-mix quality of nursing care scores are one way to demonstrate that nursing care makes a difference in the patient's recovery process and contributes to hospital revenue generation. For hospitals that have implemented the H-MNPM, a beginning methodology has been developed for cost-effectively using raw data to compute quality scores for DRGs.

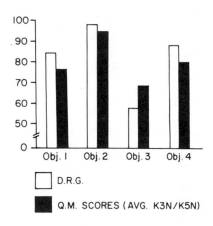

**FIGURE 9.1** Comparison of quality scores for normal newborns: Nursing unit versus DRG. Obj. 1, The plan of nursing care is formulated; Obj. 2, The physical needs of the patient are attended; Obj. 3, The nonphysical needs of the patient are attended; Obj. 4, Achievement of nursing care objectives is evaluated.

**TABLE 9.6** DRG Quality Scores for Schizoaffective Psychosis, Manic-Depressive Psychosis

| Objectives and subobjectives | DRG 90 |
| --- | --- |
| 1.0 The plan of nursing care is formulated. | 87 |
| 1.1 The condition of the patient is assessed on admission. | 85 |
| 1.2 Data relevant to hospital care is ascertained on admission. | 85 |
| 1.3 The current condition of the patient is assessed. | 95 |
| 1.4 The written plan of nursing care is formulated. | 85 |
| 1.5 The plan of nursing care is coordinated with the medical plan of care. | 91 |
| 2.0 The physical needs of the patient are attended. | 80 |
| 2.1 The patient is protected from accident and injury. | 88 |
| 2.2 The need for physical comfort and rest is attended. | 96 |
| 2.3 The need for physical hygiene is attended. | 81 |
| 2.5 The need for activity is attended. | 95 |
| 2.6 The need for nutrition and fluid balance is attended. | 52 |
| 2.7 The need for elimination is attended. | 29 |
| 3.0 The nonphysical (psychological, emotional, mental, and social) needs of the patient are attended. | 72 |
| 3.1 The patient is oriented to hospital facilities on admission. | 47 |
| 3.2 The patient is extended social courtesy by the nursing staff. | 63 |
| 3.3 The patient's privacy and civil rights are honored. | 79 |
| 3.4 The need for psychological-emotional well-being is attended. | 82 |
| 3.5 The patient is taught measures of health maintenance and illness prevention. | 52 |
| 3.6 The patient's family is included in the nursing care process. | 83 |
| 3.7 Psychological-emotional well-being is attended. | 86 |
| 4.0 Achievement of nursing care objectives is evaluated. | 94 |
| 4.1 Records document the care provided for the patient. | 96 |
| 4.2 The patient's response to therapy is evaluated. | 89 |

# REFERENCES

Barba, M., & Bennett, B. (1978). The evaluation of patient care through use of ANA's standards of nursing practice. *Supervisor Nurse*, 1978, *9*, 42, 45-46, 49-50.

Barrett, E. A. M. (1985). *RN turnover: State of the art*. Unpublished manuscript, The Mount Sinai Hospital Department of Nursing, New York.

Barrett, E. A. M., & Wiecozorek, R. R. (1984). *Professional nurse profile: Phase I report*. Unpublished manuscript, The Mount Sinai Hospital Department of Nursing, New York.

Berggren, H. J., & Zagornik, A. D. (1968). Teaching nursing process to beginning students. *Nursing Outlook, 16,* 32-35.

Betz, M., Dickerson, T., & Wyatt, D. (1980). Cost and quality: Primary and team nursing compared. *Nursing and Health Care, 1,* 150-157.

Bloch, D. (1975). Evaluation of nursing care in terms of process and outcomes. *Nursing Research, 24,* 256-263.

Cohodes, D. R. (1982). Problems in measuring the cost of illness. *Evaluation and the Health Professions, 5,* 381-392.

Davis, S. (1982). The Mount Sinai Hospital: Success in the competition for survival. *The Mount Sinai Journal of Medicine, 49,* 265-268.

Devereux, P. (1984). *Quality of nursing care.* Unpublished manuscript, The Mount Sinai Hospital Department of Nursing, New York.

Donebedian, A. (1970). Patient care evaluation. *Hospitals, 44,* 131-136.

Eichhorn, N. L. (1979). Evaluation of a primary nursing system using the quality patient care scale. *Journal of Nursing Administration, 9,* 11-15.

Feldman, J., & Goldhaber, F. I. (1984). Living with DRGs. *The Journal of Nursing Administration, 14,* 19-22.

Felton, G. (1975). Increasing the quality of nursing care by introducing the concept of primary nursing: A model project. *Nursing Research, 24,* 27-32.

Fox, R. N., & Ventura, M. R. (1984). Internal psychometric characteristic of the quality patient care scale. *Nursing Research, 33,* 112-117.

Grimaldi, P. L. (1984). Cost concepts and contribution margins. *Nursing Management, 15,* 14-17.

Grimaldi, P. L., & Micheletti, J. A. (1982). RIMS and the cost of nursing care. *Nursing Management, 13,* 12-22.

Grimaldi, P. L., & Micheletti, J. A. (1983). *Diagnosis related groups: A practitioner's guide.* Chicago: Pluribus Press.

Halloran, E. J. (1980). *Analysis of variation in nursing workload by patient medical and nursing condition.* Unpublished doctoral dissertation, University of Illinois at the Medical Center, Chicago.

Halloran, E. J. (1983). The cost dimension of the national joint practice commission demonstration project. *Nursing and Health Care, 4,* 307-313.

Haussmann, R. K. D., & Hegyvary, S. T. (1976). Field testing the nursing quality monitoring methodology: Phase II. *Nursing Research, 25,* 324-331.

Haussmann, R. K. D., & Hegyvary, S. T. (1977). *Monitoring quality of nursing care: Part III* (DHEW Publication No. HRA 77-70). Washington, DC: U.S. Government Printing Office.

Haussmann, R. K. D., Hegyvary, S. T., & Newman, J. F. (1976). *Monitoring quality of nursing care: Part IV* (DHEW Publication No. HRA 76-7). Washington, DC: U.S.Government Printing Office.

Hegyvary, S. T., Gortner, S. R., & Haussmann, R. K. D. (1976). Development of criterion measures for quality of care: The Rush-Medicus experience. In *Issues in Evaluation Research* (pp. 106-114) (No. G-124 2m) Kansas City, MO: American Nurses Association.

Hegyvary, S. T., & Haussmann, R. K. D. (1975). Monitoring nursing care quality. *Journal of Nursing Administration, 5,* 17-26.

Hinson, I., Silva, N., & Clapp, P. (1984). An automated Kardex and care plan. *Nursing Management, 15,* 35-43.

Jelinek, R. C., Haussmann, R. K. D., Hegyvary, S. T., & Newman, J. F. (1974). *A methodology for monitoring quality of nursing care* (DHEW Publication No. HRA 76-25). Washington, DC: U.S. Government Printing Office.

Joseph, E., Shannon, K., & Svendson, G. (1983). *A DRG and prospective pricing action plan for nursing.* Chicago: Care Communications.

Lazona, T. G., & Stritzel, M. M. (1984). Nursing care requirements as measured by DRG. *The Journal of Nursing Administration, 14,* 15-18.

LeBreton, P. P. (1980). Measuring a nursing services department's effectiveness. *Nursing and Health Care, 1,* 158-164.

Lindeman, C. A., & Stetzer, S. L. (1973). Effect of preoperative visits by operating room nurses. *Nursing Research, 22,* 4-16.

McKibbin, R., & Marshall, J. (1984, March). *DRG refinement for nursing care. Preliminary description of Health Care Financing Administration grant.* Kansas City, MO: American Nurses Association, Center for Research.

Munson, F., Beckman, J., Clinton, J., Kever, C., & Simms, L. (1980). *Nursing assignment patterns users manual.* Washington, DC: AUPHA Press.

Nie, N. H., Hull, C. H., Jenkins, J. G., Steinbrenner, K., & Brent, D. H. (1975). *SPSS: Statistical Package for the Social Sciences.* New York: McGraw-Hill.

Phaneuf, M. C. (1972). *The nursing audit: Profile for excellence.* New York: Appleton-Century-Crofts.

Phaneuf, M. C. (1976). *The nursing audit* (2nd ed.). New York: Appleton-Century-Crofts.

Roeder, M. A. (1980). Patient care plans and the evaluation of nursing process. *Supervisor Nurse, 11,* 57-58.

Routhier, R. W. (1972). Tool for the evaluation of patient care. *Supervisor Nurse, 3,* 17-27.

Sellick, K. J., Russell, S., & Beckmann, J. L. (1983). Primary nursing: An evaluation of its effect on patient perception of care and staff evaluation. *International Journal of Nursing Studies, 20,* 265-273.

Selvaggi, L. M. (1980). *Effects of nursing modality on quality care: Evaluation of nursing process and patient outcomes.* Unpublished doctoral dissertation, University of Miami, Coral Cables, FL.

Shaffer, F. (1984). Nursing power in the DRG world. *Nursing Management, 15,* 28-31.

Vanderzee, H., & Glusko, G. (1984). DRGs, variable pricing, and budgeting for nursing services. *The Journal of Nursing Administration, 14,* 11-41.

Ventura, M. (1980). Correlation between the quality patient care scale and the Phaneuf audit. *International Journal of Nursing Studies, 17,* 155-162.

Ventura, M., & Crosby, F. (1978). Preparing the nurse observer to use the quality patient care scales: A modular approach. *Journal of Continuing Education in Nursing, 9,* 37-40.

Ventura, M., Hinshaw, A. S., & Atwood, J. (1981). Instrumentation: The next step. *Nursing Research, 30,* 257.

Wainwright, P., & Burnip, S. (1983a). Burford: A model for nursing: *Nursing Times, 79,* 36-38.

Wainwright, P., & Burnip, S. (1983b). Qualpacs: The second visit. *Nursing Times, 79,* 26-27.

Waltz, C. F., Strickland, O. L. & Lenz, E. R. (1984). *Measurement in nursing research.* Philadelphia: F. A. Davis Co.

Wandelt, M. A., & Ager, J. (1974). *Quality Patient Care Scale.* New York: Appleton-Century-Crofts.

Wandelt, M. A., & Stewart (Slater), D. (1975). *Slater Nursing Competencies Rating Scale.* New York: Appleton-Century-Crofts.

Ward, M. J., & Lindeman, C. A. (Eds.). (1979). Instruments for measuring practice and other health care variables (Vols. 1 & 2). Hyattsville, MD: U.S. Department of Health, Education & Welfare. (DHEW Publication Nos. 78-53, 78-54).

Woog, P., & Goldman, E. (1975). The utilization of educational research in an allied field. *Evaluation, 2,* 78-80.

# 10

# Measuring Attitudes Towards Cost-Effectiveness in Nursing

## Doris R. Blaney and Charles J. Hobson

*This chapter discusses the Blaney/Hobson Nursing Attitude Scale and the Behaviorally Anchored Rating Scale, measures of attitudes of nurses toward cost-effectiveness.*

The purpose of this project was to develop a reliable and valid tool for measuring the attitudes of nurses toward cost-effectiveness in nursing practices and procedures.

Today hospitals are confronted with an overwhelming combination of interrelated external pressures that demand more cost-effective operations in order to provide service. A number of the more significant pressures are included in Figure 10.1.

A model was developed that illustrates the nurse's role as the key person who influences the patient's progress toward discharge. Within the model, nurses unquestionably perform an indispensable role in managing patients in a more cost-effective manner. Figure 10.1 shows the focal position occupied by nurses, which offers a number of challenges and opportunities to assume a leadership role as "patient care manager" in developing and implementing cost-effective nursing practices and procedures.

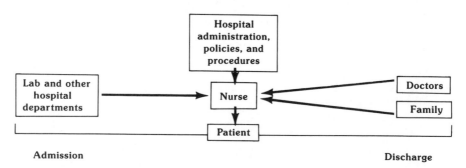

**FIGURE 10.1** Model of the nurse's central role in patient care, processing, and management.

Unfortunately, many nurses are currently ill-equipped to handle the demands and requirements of emerging cost-effectiveness programs and strategies. In the past, cost considerations were rarely an issue in providing quality patient care, and most nurses received little or no systematic exposure or formal education in cost concepts or cost-effective nursing. Perhaps more problematic is the pervasive perception among nurses that a concern with cost-effective practices will inevitably result in lower-quality patient care. In summary, many nurses currently have a relatively uninformed and less than positive attitude toward cost-effectiveness.

The attitude model chosen for this study was that of Fishbein and Ajzen (1972, 1975), which indicates that attitudes are largely based on beliefs about the attitude object. This model emphasizes the critical connection between attitudes and behavior and stresses that attitudes can be developed and changed by focusing on beliefs about the attitude object.

In terms of the present study, the Fishbein and Ajzen model suggests that the exhibition of cost-effective nursing behaviors must ideally be preceded by the development of a favorable attitude toward cost-effectiveness and the generation of appropriate behavioral intentions. Furthermore, the model indicates that the basic attitude can be developed and fostered by focusing attention on positive and personally relevant beliefs concerning cost-effectiveness in nursing.

Attitudes are formed and changed as a result of basic learning processes, leading first to the development of beliefs concerning the attitude object and then to the attitude itself. Five specific research-documented mechanisms for attitude formation and change are participation in decision making, position discrepency, fear reduction, fear arousal, and providing new information (Steers, 1984).

In this project, a continuing education seminar was developed that utilized each of these five mechanisms in an attempt to foster a positive attitude toward cost-effectiveness among nurses. The evaluation of this program provided the framework within which the focal attitude questionnaire was psychometrically tested.

## PURPOSE OF THE MEASURE

The primary purpose or objective of this questionnaire was to provide a reliable and valid tool for measuring the attitude of nurses toward cost-effectiveness in nursing practices and procedures. A 10-item questionnaire was developed.

## METHODS

The study was structured as a quasi-experimental design known as the "non-equivalent control group design," (Campbell & Stanley, 1963), as shown in Figure 10.2.

|                              | Time 1                  | Time 2              | Time 3                  |
|------------------------------|-------------------------|---------------------|-------------------------|
| Experimental group (Training)| Attitude measurement    | Training session    | Attitude measurement    |
| Control group (No training)  | Attitude measurement    |                     | Attitude measurement    |

**FIGURE 10.2** Nonequivalent control group design.

In a 750-bed midwestern hospital, eight similar nursing units were utilized; four units received the attitude training and four units did not receive the training. A total of 156 RNs participated. Within the framework of this design, reliability was assessed with coefficient alpha and test-retest reliability. Construct validity was determined by examining (a) changes in attitude scores as a function of training and (b) the relationships between attitudes and job behaviors.

## RESULTS

### Sample Characteristics

A total of 156 nurses participated in this study. Basic demographic data were collected from all participants, including sex, age, nursing education, years of work experience, and average hours worked per week.

In terms of sex, 96% of the sample was female, with only 4% male. Five age categories were utilized with the following response percentages: 20 to 24 (29.1%), 25 to 29 (22.5%), 30 to 34 (13.2%), 35 to 39 (13.2%), 40 and over (21.9%). Nursing education consisted of three categories with the following associated percentages: associate degree (79.5%), diploma (12.6%), bachelor's degree (7.9%). Work experience in nursing was represented by the following five separate categories along with the associated response percentages: less than 1 year (21.2%), 1 to 4 years (50.3%), 5 to 9 years (11.9%), 10 to 14 years (10.6%), 15 or more years (6.0%). Finally, average hours worked per week was coded using three categories with the following percentages: 20 to 29 (12.7%), 30 to 40 (42.7%), over 40 (44.7%).

### Administration and Scoring

The attitude scale is administered in the form of a questionnaire with Likert rating scales. The computation of overall attitude scale scores involves first reverse-scoring the 5 negatively worded items and then summing the responses on all 10 items on the questionnaire. The response format is a 1 to 5 scale from Strongly Disagree to Strongly Agree, thus producing a range of total score values from 10 to 50. Higher scores indicate a more positive attitude, with a score of 30 representing the midpoint or neutral point on the scale. For the entire sample at time 1, prior to the training program, the mean attitude score was 33.19, with a standard deviation of 6.13. This suggests a slightly positive mean attitude toward cost-effectiveness in nursing.

## Reliability

In assessing the reliability of the 10-item attitude questionnaire, two separate analyses were conducted: one involving coefficient alpha; and the second, test-retest reliability.

### Coefficient Alpha

Prior to beginning the present study, the initial version of the questionnaire was administered to a group of 85 university students in order to assess coefficient alpha and make any necessary item revisions. A value for coefficient alpha of .82 was obtained, and subsequent analyses indicated that two items were detracting from the scale's internal consistency. These two items were slightly revised, producing the final revision of the questionnaire, which can be found at the end of this chapter.

In the main study, coefficient alpha for the revised questionnaire was computed at two times, before and after the training program, with an interval of approximately 2 months between administrations. Prior to the training program, an analysis of the responses of 156 nurses in both the experimental and control groups yielded a coefficient alpha of .75. The second administration involved 135 nurses and produced a coefficient alpha of .80.

These results are slightly lower than the .82 computed in the student pilot group. However, the data were collected in a more realistic setting, using actual working nurses, and thus the obtained values are probably more accurate estimates of the scale's true reliability. Nevertheless, the standard minimum acceptable level for coefficient alpha of .80 recommended by Nunnally (1978) was attained in the second administration and nearly so in the first administration.

Further developmental work on the measure was suggested by the item analyses. Specifically, item 10 on the revised questionnaire detracted from the overall scale reliability and should be revised prior to future use. Additionally, one might consider lengthening the scale to 15 or 20 items as a way to improve its reliability, since scales with fewer items are likely to have lower internal consistency reliability (Nunnally, 1978; Waltz, Strickland, & Lenz, 1984).

### Test-Retest Reliability

Test-retest reliability was assessed in the control group by correlating attitude scale scores collected at Time 1 (prior to the training program for the experimental group) with scores collected at Time 3 (after the training program). The interval between the two administrations was approximately 2 months, and the number of nurses involved in the control group was 67. The computed test-retest reliability coefficient was a disappointingly low .43. However, during the 2-month interval between administrations in early 1985, the topics of nursing and hospital cost-effectiveness were very much in the national and local news and hotly debated and discussed issues. Thus, it is possible that attitudes were fluctuating during the period, producing the low test-retest reliability coefficient. The 2-month period between administrations is much longer than the recommended 2-week period between test-retest administrations. Therefore, the lengthened period between administrations allowed more time for history effects on retest scores, which can reduce test-retest reliability coefficients.

To investigate this possibility, two strategies were undertaken. First, interviews were conducted with the control group members to explore potential changes in attitudes, and second, an additional test-retest reliability analysis was conducted in a separate sample of 54 nurses, involving an interval of 2 weeks.

Interview results confirmed the hypothesis of changing attitudes and feelings toward cost-effectiveness in nursing attitudes during the 2-month period between administrations. With dramatic new information and perspectives appearing in the press on an almost daily basis, attitudes were fluctuating as a consequence. Further support for this argument is provided by the test-retest reliability coefficient of .81 computed in the separate sample with only a 2-week interval between administrations.

## Validity

Initial attempts to establish the construct validity of the 10-item questionnaire included an assessment of (1) hypothesized improvements in attitude scores as a function of the training program and (2) hypothesized attitude-behavior relationships.

### *Attitude Improvements*

It was hypothesized that if the questionnaire does in fact measure attitude toward cost-effectiveness, then the training program designed to improve the attitude should result in (1) more favorable attitudes in the experimental (trained) group after the training session and (2) more favorable attitudes in the experimental than in the control (untrained) group after the session.

In the experimental group, consisting of 68 nurses, the mean attitude score prior to the training program was 32.79; the mean score after the program increased to 36.13. A correlated $t$-test between these two means produced a $t$-value of 5.10 ($df = 67$; $p < .001$). This significant $t$-value indicates that the training did result in more favorable attitudes toward cost-effectiveness.

Additional evidence supporting the construct validity of the scale was obtained by comparing the mean attitude scores in the experimental and control groups after the training program. As hypothesized, the experimental group mean of 36.13 was significantly higher than the control group mean of 33.43, $t = 2.49$ ($df = 132$; $p < .01$).

## Attitude-Behavior Relationship

As discussed earlier, attitudes are theoretically related to behaviors directed toward the attitude object. Thus, one would hypothesize that attitude's toward cost-effectiveness in nursing should correlate positively with actual cost-effective nursing behaviors as reported by the subjects' head nurses.

Job performance scales were developed for three critical cost-related dimensions of nursing practice: (1) supply utilization practices, (2) patient goal setting, and (3) patient scheduling. Using job-related input from a committee of staff nurses, head nurses, and nursing administrators, behaviorally anchored rating scales (BARS) were developed for each of the three performance dimensions (Schwab, Heneman, & Decotiis, 1975). The BARS consisted of 9-point scale with specific behavioral anchors or examples to represent the 2, 5, and 8 levels. The three BARS used in this study can be found at the end of this chapter.

Head nurses in both the experimental (trained) and control (untrained) groups were asked to evaluate their staff (who participated as subjects in the study) on the three BARS prior to the training and again after the program. Scores on the three dimensions were summed to provide a composite index of cost-effective performance for each individual nurse. Scores could range from a low of 3 to a high of 27, with larger scores indicating more cost effective job performance.

The test-retest reliability of the composite BARS scale was assessed in the control (untrained) group using an interval of approximately 2 months. A reliability coefficient of .68 was obtained, based on the responses of 75 nurses. The magnitude of this coefficient, while marginally acceptable, suggests that more developmental work on the BARS is needed. Also, more extensive training on scale utilization by the head nurses seems warranted.

The validity of the composite BARS scale was not empirically assessed. Given the nature of the developmental procedures and the focus on specific job behaviors, BARS are generally assumed to be content-valid measures of performance. In future research with this scale, empirical verification of its validity is needed.

The hypothesis advanced in this study was that attitude scores should be positively related to performance scores. If such a positive relationship were found, this would be interpreted as further support for the construct validity of the attitude scale. In the sample as a whole ($N = 156$) the correlation between total score on the attitude scale and composite performance behavior rating (an additive combination of the three separate behaviorally anchored rating scale scores) was $r = .15$, $p < .05$. Though modest in magnitude, this positive correlation provides some evidence of the scale's construct validity.

Additional validity evidence was obtained by comparing mean composite behavioral scores, as rated by the head nurses, in (1) the experimental group before and after the training and (2) the experimental and control groups after the training program. In the experimental group, the behavioral mean ratings before and after the session were 11.23 and 15.30, respectively. A correlated $t$-test between these two means produced at $t$-value of 8.98 ($df = 68$; $p < .001$). In comparing the experimental and control groups, the mean behavioral ratings were 15.30 and 11.28, respectively, and were found to be significantly different, $t = 5.06$ ($df = 146$; $p < .001$).

Taken as a whole, the results presented in this section provide preliminary evidence for the construct validity of the 10-item attitude scale. In all instances, findings were consistent with hypothesized relationships and support the validity of the scale as a measure of attitude's toward cost-effectiveness in nursing.

## IMPLICATIONS FOR NURSING

The attitude scale developed for this study has resulted in the availability of a psychometrically promising scale to measure nursing attitude's toward cost-effectiveness, clearly a factor critical to the success of any comprehensive effort to control nursing costs. A rigorous design framework was presented to evaluate the impact of a nursing continuing education program, resulting in strong and clear-cut statistical evidence of program success in the current study.

Although the preliminary evidence in this study supports the reliability and validity of the scale developed to measure attitude's toward cost-effectiveness in nursing, further development and testing of the instrument is warranted. The addition of more items to the 10-item scale could enhance its reliability and validity.

## REFERENCES

Campbell, D. T., & Stanley, J. C. (1963). *Experimental and quasi-experimental designs for research*. Chicago: Rand McNally.

Fishbein, M., & Ajzen, I. (1972). Attitudes and opinions. *Annual Review of Psychology, 23*, 487-544.

Fishbein, M., & Ajzen, I. (1975). *Belief, attitude, intention, and behavior: An introduction to theory and research*. Reading, MA: Addison-Wesley.

Nunnally, J. (1978). *Psychometric theory* (2nd ed.). New York: McGraw-Hill.

Schwab, D. P., Heneman, H. G., & Decotiis, T. A. (1975). Behaviorally anchored rating scales: A review of the literature. *Personnel Psychology, 28*, 549-562.

Steers, R. M. (1984). *Introduction to organizational behavior* (2nd ed.). Glenview, IL: Scott, Foresman.

Waltz, C. F., Stirckland, O. L., & Lenz, E. R. (1984). *Measurement in nursing research.*. Philadelphia: F. A. Davis.

# Instrument A
# Blaney/Hobson Nursing Attitude Scale*

## REVISED NURSING QUESTIONNAIRE

*Directions:* Please respond to the following statements dealing with the issue of cost-effectiveness in nursing practices and procedures by indicating the extent to which you disagree or agree with each one. Please *circle* your response.

| | Strongly Disagree | Disagree Somewhat | Neither Agree Nor Disagree | Agree Somewhat | Strongly Agree |
|---|---|---|---|---|---|
| 1. The introduction and use of cost-effective practices and procedures will improve overall nursing effectiveness. | SD | D | N | A | SA |
| 2. The introduction and use of cost-effective nursing practices and procedures will benefit me personally. | SD | D | N | A | SA |
| 3. Operating a unit in order to make a profit is wrong. | SD | D | N | A | SA |
| 4. I look forward to the introduction and use of cost-effective practices and procedures in nursing. | SD | D | N | A | SA |
| 5. The introduction and use of cost-effective nursing | | | | | |

practices and
procedures will
result in a
decrease in the
quality of
patient care.                    SD        D        N        A        SA

6. The introduction
and use of cost-
effective
practices and
procedures will
benefit the
nursing profession
as a whole.                      SD        D        N        A        SA

7. The thought
of introducing
cost-
effectiveness
into nursing
makes me uneasy.                 SD        D        N        A        SA

8. Hospital nursing
units should not
be concerned
with making or
losing money.                    SD        D        N        A        SA

9. The introduction
and use of cost-
effective nursing
practices and
procedures will
benefits patients.               SD        D        N        A        SA

10. Cost-
effectiveness
should not
influence
the way in
which nurses
provide patient care.            SD        D        N        A        SA

# Instrument B
# Behaviorally Anchored Rating Scale

## PERFORMANCE DIMENSION: GOAL SETTING AND PATIENT CARE PLAN

Nurse's Name: _____

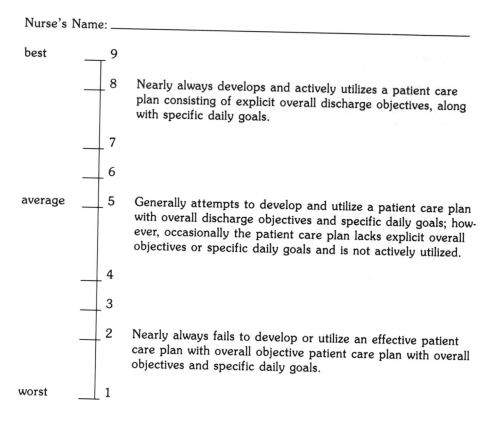

best — 9

8     Nearly always develops and actively utilizes a patient care plan consisting of explicit overall discharge objectives, along with specific daily goals.

7

6

average — 5     Generally attempts to develop and utilize a patient care plan with overall discharge objectives and specific daily goals; however, occasionally the patient care plan lacks explicit overall objectives or specific daily goals and is not actively utilized.

4

3

2     Nearly always fails to develop or utilize an effective patient care plan with overall objective patient care plan with overall objectives and specific daily goals.

worst — 1

## PERFORMANCE DIMENSION: EFFICIENT SUPPLY UTILIZATION

Nurse's Name: _____

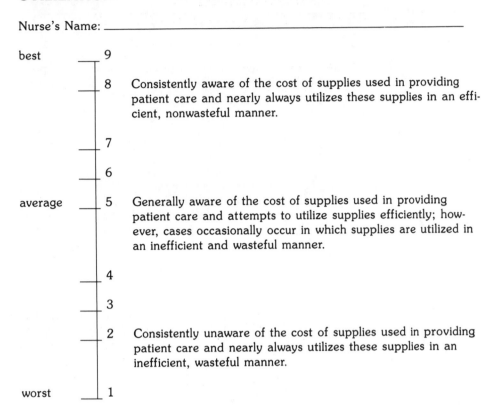

best     9

8    Consistently aware of the cost of supplies used in providing patient care and nearly always utilizes these supplies in an efficient, nonwasteful manner.

7

6

average    5    Generally aware of the cost of supplies used in providing patient care and attempts to utilize supplies efficiently; however, cases occasionally occur in which supplies are utilized in an inefficient and wasteful manner.

4

3

2    Consistently unaware of the cost of supplies used in providing patient care and nearly always utilizes these supplies in an inefficient, wasteful manner.

worst    1

## PERFORMANCE DIMENSION: OPTIMAL SCHEDULING

Nurses's Name: _____

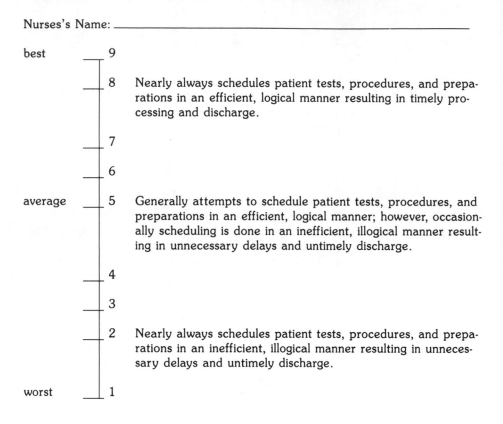

best ___ 9

___ 8    Nearly always schedules patient tests, procedures, and prepa-
         rations in an efficient, logical manner resulting in timely pro-
         cessing and discharge.

___ 7

___ 6

average ___ 5    Generally attempts to schedule patient tests, procedures, and
                 preparations in an efficient, logical manner; however, occasion-
                 ally scheduling is done in an inefficient, illogical manner result-
                 ing in unnecessary delays and untimely discharge.

___ 4

___ 3

___ 2    Nearly always schedules patient tests, procedures, and prepa-
         rations in an inefficient, illogical manner resulting in unneces-
         sary delays and untimely discharge.

worst ___ 1

# 11

# Measuring Clinical Decision Making in Nursing

## Helen M. Jenkins

*This chapter discusses the Clinical Decision Making in Nursing Scale, a measure of nurses' clinical decision making capabilities.*

Appropriate and effective decision making has long been a desired element in the curricula of baccalaureate nursing programs; however, to date there have been few ways to assess this process. The purpose of this chapter is to present a tool, the Clinical Decision Making in Nursing Scale (CDMNS), that can be used to assess and evaluate clinical decision making in nursing.

Decision making, as a skill to be learned, can be enhanced by education and practice. In any given nursing program it is hoped that students are taught decision-making skills and are encouraged to make their own clinical decisions, establishing habit patterns that will carry over into professional use. Decision making is often mentioned as a theme or part of the theoretical framework for nursing curricula. Examination of the curriculum may reveal themes having to do with decision making, but whether or not students perceive their own decision-making patterns is often assumed or misinterpreted. Therefore, the investigator's aim was to examine decision making as an element of curricular process by developing a self-report measure to assess how students saw themselves making clinical decisions. Hypotheses tested focused on differences that might occur among students from sophomore to senior levels, with an expectation of upward progression of CDMNS scores.

## SHORT DESCRIPTION OF LITERATURE RELATED TO THE TOOL

Nursing today is confronted with complex legal, professional, and educational problems for which effective decision making is needed at all levels of practice. Gill (1979) defined decision making as one of the most critical elements for nurse leaders, and del Bueno (1983), maintained that clinical decision making is "a highly desirable skill that most educators talk about, that many managers complain is nonexistent, but that neither is absolutely sure how to teach or evaluate" (p. 7). Studies conducted in nursing have focused on simulations (Grier, 1976; McDonnel, Kramer, & Leak,1972; Verhonick, Nichols, Glor, & McCarthy, 1968) or on work situations, especially those conducted in the 1960s by Kelly (1964, 1966), Hammond (1966), and Hammond, Kelly, Schneider, and Vancini (1966). These early studies seldom have been replicated, although hypothetical case studies like those of Corbett and Beveridge (1980), Hansen and Thomas (1968), and Grier (1976) continue to be used.

A large body of literature concerned with rational decision making exists within the mathematical and managerial arenas. Mathematical probability models explain decision making and have contributed greatly to operations research, allowing decision makers to handle quantities of complex information in a systematic way (Montgomery & Adelbratt, 1982; Svenson, 1979). Managerial models have concentrated more on the social interaction of individuals within organizations (Cyert, Feigenbaum, & March, 1971; Ference, 1970; Taylor & Dunnett, 1974). Most of the tools available to assess decision making are focused on rational or normative models and are universally supported with data from male samples. Because there seemed to be little fit between existing models and the aims of the study, the author developed and tested a tool that could be applied to clinical decision making in nursing.

## CONCEPTUAL BASIS FOR THE TOOL

In Western culture people are believed to be rational, and much has been written about rational decision making. For example, over the past three decades decision-making literature has encompassed numerous sources, including systems-oriented, normative-based decision models. Normative structures seemed to be preferred – that is, how decision making "should" be done. Although details for models presented in the literature varied, viewing decision making as a series of steps was fairly consistent. The model chosen to develop the tool was used because it suggested a way of examining the qualitative features of decision making and because it could easily accommodate quantitative measures.

The conceptual basis for the tool was derived from Janis and Mann's *Decision Making: A Psychological Analysis of Conflict, Choice, and Commitment* (1977). To develop a decision-making theory about conflict situations, they looked at normative structures and arrived at seven criteria assumed to be ideal for making decisions. Janis and Mann have stated that when an individual meets all criteria adequately, a state of "vigilant information processing" has occurred, and the decision maker's objectives have an excellent chance of being implemented. Their criteria came from an extensive review of literature on effective decision making and include the following:

The decision maker, to the best of his ability and within his information processing capabilities

1. thoroughly canvasses a wide range of alternative courses of action;
2. surveys the full range of objectives to be fulfilled and the values implicated by the choice;
3. carefully weighs whatever he knows about the costs and risks of negative consequences, as well as the positive consequences, that could flow from each alternative;
4. intensively searches for new information relevant to further evaluation of the alternatives;
5. correctly assimilates and takes account of any new information or expert judgment to which he is exposed, even when the information or judgment does not support the course of action he initially prefers;
6. reexamines the positive and negative consequences of all known alternatives, including those regarded as unacceptable, before making a final choice;
7. makes detailed provisions for implementing or executing the chosen course of action, with special attention to contingency plans that might be required if various known risks were to materialize. (Janis & Mann, 1977, p. 11)

These seven criteria were examined critically to determine how they could provide the basis for a tool to measure clinical decision making.

## PROCEDURES FOR CONSTRUCTION AND REVISION OF THE TOOL

Janis and Mann's (1977) seven criteria were condensed into four categories to simplify their procedural ordering. Criteria 1 and 2 remained stable. Criteria 3, 6, and 7 refer to risks and benefits and thus were combined into one category. Criteria 4 and 5, concerning information search and acquisition were considered together. The process produced four categories of decision making: (a) search for alternatives or options, (b) canvassing of objectives and values, (c) evaluation and reevaluation of consequences, and (d) search for information and unbiased assimilation of new information.

Items that applied to each of the four categories were sought from decision-making and nursing decision-making literature; these eventually became subscales for the CDMNS. Grouping items together was important, as it allowed rationales to be developed for each category. For example, in the Search for Alternatives or Options subscale, one factor influencing decision making is past experiences, especially in the way we search for options. Most authors, including those in nursing, (e.g., Holle & Blatchley, 1982; Marriner, 1977) agree that we use habitual patterns to approach this task and tend to use the same seta of actions to make similar decisions. As items were developed, rationales from the literature were written for the other three categories in like manner.

Representative items were written in simple terms, avoiding qualifiers or words likely to be misunderstood. Both negative and positive items were included, and insofar as possible, items were constructed to be applicable to clinical decision making.

A preliminary test was conducted with 32 senior nursing students in order to clarify directions and format and to isolate misunderstood material. Following this administration a debriefing session was conducted with the students. That process yielded suggestions for correction of overlaps and options for refinement and improvement. Twenty-three items were discarded, and the resultant 44 items them comprised the tool.

A pilot test of the tool was carried out with 10 additional baccalaureate nursing students from each level (sophomore, junior, and senior) who were actively involved in clinical experiences. No student taking the preliminary or pilot test was involved in the final testing. Scores were coded and computed. Four items with low item-to-total coefficients were discarded.

## ADMINISTRATION AND SCORING

Items on the CDMNS are rated from 5 (Always) to 1 (Never) by the nurse or nursing student to reflect perceptions of his/her own behavior while caring for clients. Item ratings are summed to obtain a total score. The final tool has 40 items. Therefore, a potential score range of 40 to 200 exists, with higher scores indicating higher perceived decision making.

## METHODOLOGY FOR TESTING RELIABILITY AND VALIDITY

### Content Validity

Content validity was established in several ways:

1. Items were based on literature from normative decision making and nursing decision making (initially 67 items).
2. A preliminary test of the tool improved clarity and congruity within each item and subscale.
3. A panel of five nurse experts in baccalaureate education rated each item with a specification matrix and gave each item several scores, based on representativeness, sense, appropriateness, and degree of independence from other items. The matrix yielded a total score for each item. All items that received a total score of 77% or greater were rated good and were retained. Items scoring 70 to 76% were rated as fair and evaluated critically for inclusion or exclusion. Items scoring less than 70% were excluded.

## Pilot-testing of the Instrument

Formal testing of the tool took place near the end of the semester with generic students who were engaged in clinical experiences. The available population consisted of about 250 students. Of these, 111 students chose to participate (27 sophomores, 43 juniors, 41 seniors).

Using the Statistical Package for the Social Sciences (SPSS) subprograms, reliability was assessed throughout the testing phases by means of Cronbach's alpha. These procedures measure internal consistency and can be considered the mean of all split – half coefficients (O'Muircheartaigh & Payne, 1978). When pilot scores were calculated, resulting Cronbach's alpha was 0.79 for 44 items. Four items having the lowest coefficients were dropped, and Cronbach's alpha for the remaining 40 items was 0.83 ($N = 111$).

No significant differences in results were found among levels of students except for Subscale A, Search for Alternatives or Options. The Multiple Range Scheffe test determined the means between which significant differences existed. It was found that seniors differed from juniors, with the greatest differences between means, and that sophomores did not differ significantly from either group, having a mean higher than that of the juniors but lower than that of seniors. Using analysis of covariance procedures, no effects related to age or full-time work experience were noted.

The results of no differences in total scores were not as expected because if decision making was being effectively taught, then there ought to be some perceptions by students that would vary from sophomore to senior. It is likely that students, in general, do not perceive themselves as decision makers in the fairly restricted environment in which they are placed. Perhaps the opportunities to make decisions are being unknowingly restricted. Stress seems to play a large part in students' ability to make and be responsible for decisions. It is also possible that students do not have accurate perceptions of their decision-making processes or that social desirability may have influenced students' responses on the tool to the extent that differences were not noted.

There may have been some problematic concerns in using a normative model. Some basis exists for the presumption that totally rational decision making is not possible in the real world – that we can never gather enough information, calculate outcomes with certainty, or predict all of the variables that impact on the decision (Steinbruner, 1974). Nurses are limited in using a purely rational approach because of situational and temporal influences.

Tool construction focused on decision subprocesses, since the literature stressed them as separate constructs. This separation is artificial, and in real life one does not proceed through decision phases in this fashion. The mental processes involved in making decisions are almost simultaneous, complex, and multifaceted.

Recommendations and suggestions for future studies follow, based not only on the results discussed but related to the broad curriculum questions with which the measure was concerned. It is recommended that

1. More studies about the nature and characteristics of decision making be done. We know little about how information gathering, data use, cues, contexts, and time all interact during decision making.
2. Exploratory observational studies be done to supply the qualitative point of view to clinical decision making that could decrease the potential for the influence of social desirability on scores, as is the case with self-report.
3. Usual learned decision-making styles be investigated to see if normative procedures for measurement are preferred.
4. Studies be done to correlate decision making with self-esteem.
5. Samples from other nursing populations be tested with the CSMNS to compare results with the findings thus far (Jenkins, 1985b).

There are also several important implications (Jenkins,1985a). Nurse educators need to help students become aware of broad curricular aims and objectives. If decision making is a desired thread in the framework of the curriculum, it should be emphasized. Decision-making patterns for student nurses should be used early and consistently throughout their program so that effective decision making is truly an outcome of the process. Nursing programs must provide students with opportunities and context in which decision making can occur. As del Bueno (1983) stated, there cannot be "too much practice in the development of effective decision making" (p. 7). We must give students permission to risk making their own decisions. The atmosphere for decision making should be one that is open, one in which risk taking is rewarded, and one in which the teacher can also be a risk taker (Berman, 1968). Students today face a complex and demanding profession. They are unlikely to be successful without systematic preparation and experience for making effective decisions.

## REFERENCES

Berman, L. M. (1968). *New priorities in the curriculum.* Columbus, OH: Merrill.

Corbett, N. A., & Beveridge, P. (1980). *Clinical simulations in nursing practice.* Philadelphia: W. B. Saunders.

Cyert, R. M., Feigenbaum, E. H., & March, J. G. (1971). Models in a behavioral theory of the firm. In J. Dutton & W. Starbuck (Eds.), *Computer simulation of human behavior (pp.246-259).* New York: Wiley.

del Bueno, D. J. (1983). Doing the right thing: Nurses' ability to make clinical decisions. *Nurse Educator,8,* 7-11.

Ference, T. P. (1970). Organizational communications systems and the decision process. *Management Science, 17,* B-83-96.

Gill, S. A. (1979). Leadership guidelines for decision making. *Imprint, 26*(3), 29-31,44.

Grier, M. (1976). Decision making about patient care. *Nursing Research, 25,* 105-110.

Hammond, K. R. (1966). Clinical inference in nursing: II. A psychologist's viewpoint. *Nursing Research, 15,* 27-38.

Hammond, K. R., Kelly, K., Schneider, R. J., & Vancini, M. (1966). Clinical inference in nursing. *Nursing Research, 15,* 134-138.

Hansen, A., & Thomas, D. (1968). A conceptualization of decision making. *Nursing Research, 17,* 436-443.

Holle, M., & Blatchley, M. (1982). *Introduction to leadership and management in nursing.* Monterey, CA: Wadsworth.

Janis, I. C., & Mann, L. (1977). *Decision making: A psychological analysis of conflict, choice, and commitment.* New York: Free Press.

Jenkins, H. M. (1985a). Improving clinical decision making in nursing. *Journal of Nursing Education, 24,* 242-243.

Jenkins, H. M. (1985b). A research tool for measuring perceptions of clinical decision making. *Journal of Professional Nursing, 1,* 221-229.

Kelly, K. J. (1964). An approach to the study of clinical inference in nursing. *Nursing Research, 13,* 314-322.

Kelly, K. J. (1966). Clinical inference in nursing. *Nursing Research, 15,* 23-26.

Marriner, A. (1977). The decision making process. *Supervisor Nurse, 8,* 58-67.

McDonnel, C., Kramer, M. & Leak, A. (1972). What would you do? *American Journal of Nursing, 72,* 296-301.

Montgomery, H., & Adelbratt, T. (1982). Gambling decisions and information about expected value. *Organizational Behavior and Human Performance, 29,* 39-57.

O'Muircheartaigh, C. A., & Payne, C. (1978). *Exploring data structures.* New York: Wiley.

Steinbruner, J. D. (1974). *The cybernetic theory of decision.* Princeton, NJ: Princeton University Press.

Svenson, O. (1979). Process descriptions of decision making. *Organizational Behavior and Human Performance, 23,* 86-112.

Taylor, R. N., & Dunnett, M. D. (1974). Relative contribution of decision-maker attributes to decision processes. *Organizational Behavior and Human Performance, 12,* 286-298.

Verhonick, P. J., Nichols, G. A., & McCarthy, R. (1968). I came, I saw, I responded: Nursing observation and action survey. *Nursing Research, 17,* 38-44.

# The Clinical Decision Making in Nursing Scale*

Directions:   For each of the following statements, think of your behavior while caring for clients. Answer on the bases of what *you are doing now in the clinical setting.* There are no "right" or "wrong" answers. What is important is your assessment of how you ordinarily operate as a decision maker in the clinical setting. None of the statements cover emergency situations.

Do not dwell on responses. Circle the answer that comes closest to the way you ordinarily behave.

Answer all items. About 20 minutes should be required to complete this exercise, but it it must be taken from the classroom, a 24-hour time limit will be imposed for its return.

## SCALE FOR THE CDMNS

Circle whether you would likely behave in the described way:

A – Always: What you consistently do every time.
F – Frequently: What you usually do most of the time.
O – Occasionally: What you sometimes do on occasion.
S – Seldom: What you rarely do.
N – Never: What you never do at any time.

*Sample statement:* I mentally list options before making a decision. *Key*:
A   Ⓕ   O   S   N
The circle around response F means that you usually mentally list options before making a decision.
*Note*: Be sure you respond in terms of what you are doing in the clinical setting *at the present time.*

1. If the clinical decision is vital and there is time, I conduct a thorough search for alternatives.
2. When a person is ill, his or her cultural values and beliefs are secondary to the implementation of health services.
3. The situational factors at the time determine the number of options that I explore before making a decision.
4. Looking for new information in making a decision is more trouble than it's worth.
5. I use books or professional literature to look up things I don't understand.

*Copyright 1983

6. A random approach for looking at options works best for me.
7. Brainstorming is a method I use when thinking of ideas for options.
8. I go out of my way to get as much information as possible to make decision.
9. I assist clients in exercising their rights to make decisions about their own care.
10. When my values conflict with those of the client, I am objective enough to handle the decision making required for the situation.
11. I listen to or consider expert advice or judgment, even though it may not be the choice I would make.
12. I solve a problem or make a decision without consulting anyone, using information available to me at the time.
13. I don't always take time to examine all the possible consequences of a decision I must make.
14. I consider the future welfare of the family when I make a clinical decision which involves the individual.
15. I have little time or energy available to search for information.
16. I mentally list options before making a decision.
17. When examining consequences of options I might choose, I generally think through "If I did this, then..."
18. I consider even the remotest consequences before making a choice.
19. Consensus among my peer group is important to me in making a decision.
20. I include clients as sources of information.
21. I consider what my peers will say when I think about possible choices I could make.
22. If an instructor recommends an option to a clinical decision making situation, I adopt it rather than searching for other options.
23. If a benefit is really great, I will favor it without looking at all the risks.
24. I search for new information randomly.
25. My past experiences have little to do with how actively I look at risks and benefits for decisions about clients.
26. When examining consequences of options I might choose, I am aware of the positive outcomes for my client.
27. I select options that I have used successfully in similar circumstances in the past.
28. If the risks are serious enough to cause problems, I reject the option.
29. I write out a list of positive and negative consequences when I am evaluating an important clinical decision.
30. I do not ask my peers to suggest options for my clinical decisions.
31. My professional values are inconsistent with my personal values.
32. My finding of alternatives seems to be largely a matter of luck.
33. In the clinical setting I keep in mind the course objectives for the day's experience.
34. The risks and benefits are the farthest thing from my mind when I have to make a decision.
35. When I have a clinical decision to make, I consider the institutional priorities and standards.
36. I involve others in my decision making only if the situation calls for it.
37. In my search for options, I include even those that might be thought of as "far out" or not feasible.
38. Finding out about the client's objectives is a regular part of my clinical decision making.

39. I examine the risks and benefits only for consequences that have serious implications.
40. The client's values have to be consistent with my own in order for me to make a good decision.

Thank you for being a participant in this study. Do you have any ideas about decision making in nursing that were not covered by the scale that you would like to share? You can speak to specific items or give any general comments you would like to. Feel free to use this last page or the back of the answer sheet.

# 12

# Developing a Measure of Clinical Decision Making Through the Use of a Clinical Simulation Film

*Donna Ketchum Story*

*This chapter discusses a clinical decision-making measure to be used with a simulation film.*

## PURPOSE

Making and implementing nursing decisions is the core of nursing. In recent decades, researchers have endeavored to provide knowledge to enhance decision making. The analytically oriented researchers have focused on delineation and collection of information and of alternative solutions, and evaluation and choice from among the aternatives. The behaviorally oriented researchers, on the other hand, have focused on recognition and definition of the problem and implementation of the decision (Ward & Tversky, 1967).

The curricula of baccalaureate nursing programs vary in depth and breadth of content in the decision-making domain. Although the attribute of precise clinical decision-making skill is frequently listed as a terminal program objective, there is little evidence that this attribute is measured (National League of Nursing, 1983).

In clinical nursing, administration, and education, decision making is required of nurses at all levels, and the increasing complexity of problems requires an awareness of the domain of decision making. There is an expectation that nurses be able to make decisions with a high degree of versatility and flexibility (Kaioth, 1977).

Without a measure of the complexity of the decision, the domain of decision making cannot be adequately addressed and nursing educators cannot alter the curricula to meet the learning needs of students.

# REVIEW OF THE LITERATURE

The process of subjecting clues to mental screening against different models of knowledge such as anatomical, physiological, and pathological to arrive at a diagnostic inference was recommended by Erikson (1964). He described this process of "clinical thinking" as effectiveness in decision making (pp. 49-50). The process of clinical inference in nursing was studied by Hammond (1966). He recommended that nurses be competent in seeking information and have a thorough background in theoretical knowledge to conduct the search for cues and evaluate the evidence.

More recent researchers examined additional factors of decision making. Grier (1976) studied the process of making nursing decisions to determine if the intuitive decision was in agreement with the decision made using quantitative techniques. Aspinall (1979) studied the use of a decision tree to assist nurses in utilizing theoretical knowledge in conducting the search for clues and evaluating evidence in the diagnostic process. Decision-making behaviors were also studied. Using the Vroom and Yetton model of decision methods, Taylor (1978) presented a mechanism through which nurse managers could examine and improve their decision-making behavior. Corcoran (1983) concluded that information processed in decision making is contingent on the demands of the task. Nursing behavior of an expert practitioner involves the capacity to structure complex problems so that appropriate decisions can be made. Brodrick and Ammentorp (1979) examined the methodology of measuring information content and manipulating nursing subject matter.

## Teaching Decision Making

Kubo, Chase, and Leton (1971) employed a motion picture test to examine decision making. The teaching film was used as a basis for developing an essay examination. The examination tested students' ability to identify problems from cues given by the patient. Students were asked to identify cues and problems and to develop a nursing care plan.

McIntyre, McDonald, Bailey, and Clause (1972) developed a written simulated clinical nursing test to assess decision-making skills of nurses. The researchers acknowledged that their test revealed knowledge, not performance.

Schneider (1979) developed a film-based test for the purpose of evaluating clinical competence. The 16mm sound film presented a patient situation that required students to respond to actual behavior rather than to a description of behavior. The test included questions on the adequacy of the performance of the nurses in the film, the appropriateness of the nurses' responses to the patient, and alternate methods of achieving patient-care goals. The 60-item test was based on six levels of the cognitive domain. Bloom's (1956) Taxonomy of Educational Objectives was used in developing the blueprint for construction of the test. Although Kropp and Stoker (1966) and Mandrillo (1969) reported the futility of construction of multiple choice questions over the categories of synthesis and evaluation, Schneider (1979) decided to attempt to construct some items at those levels.

The test items were examined for item difficulty. One expected finding was that item difficulty was unrelated to the cognitive process. Mean difficulty and discrimination indices were computed for the 30 items at the higher cognitive levels – analysis and evaluation – and for the 30 items at the lower cognitive levels: knowledge, comprehension, and application. There was very little difference between the higher and lower categories.

Almost one-half of the items had a difficulty level of between 50 and 79%. Item difficulty was unrelated to the cognitive process level. For example, one analysis item had a difficulty level of 64.8% whereas a lower-level item, a comprehension item, had a difficulty level of 42.3 % (Schneider, 1979, p. 33).

Biserial correlations were computed for each item and indicated the relationship between the item and the test part or between the item and the total score. Biserial correlations indicate the discriminating ability of the correct answer.

The Kuder-Richardson Formula 20 (KR20) was used to measure the reliability of the test. The reliability coefficient for the total test was .764. When the items are homogeneous, the numerical value of KR20 will be greater (Magnusson, 1966).

Content validity was obtained through the use of subject matter experts, maternity nursing car textbooks, and periodicals. Construct and concurrent validity were obtained by theorizing a relationship between performance on a criterion behavior checklist and the test. The top 25% of the checklist scores were correlated with the top 25% of the test scores, and the bottom 25% of the checklist scores were correlated with the same bottom percentage of the test scores. The correlation was similar to the total correlation of the test scores to the checklist of criterion behavior.

## Measurement

Errors in the measurement process may be constant or random. Selltiz, Wrightsman, and Cool (1976) describe a constant error as "one introduced into the measurement by some factor that systematically affects the characteristic being measured or the process of measurement" (p. 168). The constant error is contrasted with a random error, which is described as "due to those transient aspects of the person, of the situation or measurement, or of the measurement procedures that are likely to vary from one measurement to the next, even though the characteristics being measured have not changed" (Selltiz et al., 1976, p. 169). Constant errors affect validity. Random errors, which are transient in nature, affect both reliability and validity.

Reliability refers to the consistency with which a device or method assigns scores to subjects. Validity refers to the determination of whether or not a device or method is useful for the purpose for which it is intended (Waltz & Bausell, 1981, p. 60).

Constant errors are the most difficult to detect. The constant error of measurement is made when a subject responds in a manner that is socially acceptable.

Random errors can occur as a result of transient personal factors affecting the subject, such as not feeling well or being distracted by some other activity. Transient personal factors may be accounted for by repeating the instrument or by using another instrument and comparing the results. There is an inverse relationship between the amount of random error introduced into measurement and the reliability of the measurement. The higher the reliability of the measurement, the less random error is introduced into the measuring procedure (Waltz, Strickland, & Lenz, 1984, p. 65).

Techniques for determining reliability consist of a comparison of two sets of data obtained under the same conditions. Reliability is usually determined by using one or more of four procedures: test-retest, alternate form, split-half or odd-even, and average intercorrelations. The test-retest design requires that the same test or instrument be used with the same population with a short interval between the first and second administrations. The two sets of data are correlated to determine the coefficient. An alternate-form design requires the development of two equivalent forms of the test. Both forms are administered to the same population, and the scores are correlated. The split-half, or odd-even, design is used when it is not practical to design two forms of the test or to use the test-retest method. Generally, one half of the scores are the even-numbered items and the other half are the odd-numbered items. The results are expressed as split-half coefficients. The average intercorrelations design of reliability is the Kuder-Richardson procedure. Each item is correlated against every other item on the test, and the average intercorrelations obtained. The Kuder-Richardson procedure is limited to research that uses instruments or tests with right and wrong answers (Kovacs, 1985, p. 94)

## CONCEPTUAL BASIS FOR THE MEASURING TOOL

The conceptual framework for this study was drawn from two separate areas: decision making and measurement.

The conceptual framework for this study uses the theory that decision making forms a phase of the nursing process (Yura & Walsh, 1978, p. 117). The nursing process, a designated series of actions intended to fulfill the purposes of nursing, is composed of many theories from a variety of disciplines. These theories include the general systems theory, information theory, communication theory, decision and problem-solving theories, and theories of perception and human need (Banathy, 1968, pp. 3-4; Lee, 1971, p. 7; Maslow, 1970, p. xxv; Yura & Walsh, 1978, p. 439).

Through the nursing process the nurse has the means to collect, designate meaning to, and make inferences about information. Lancaster and Beare (1982) described the search process for locating information about possible alternatives, including factors that affected the search. Viewing the selections of a nursing action as a decision-making process focuses attention on the application of concepts of decision theory to nursing.

The classical test theory identified by Lord and Novick (1968), Stanley (1971), and Nunnally (1978) serves as as basis for the model used for assessing random measurement error. The classical test theory is a logical foundation for the method used by this study for the derivation of psychometric data and for estimating the reliability of empirical measurements. The measurement technique of magnitude estimation is being tested for use in the social sciences for the measurement of complexity of decisions.

For this study, a scale to measure the magnitude of the degree of complexity of decisions was developed from an achievement test. The paper-and-pencil test is combined with a simulated clinical setting. The standardized simulated achievement test was constructed by H. Schneider (1979).

## ASSUMPTIONS

For the purpose of this study the following are assumed:

1. The situation depicted parallels one likely to have been encountered by most baccalaureate nursing students in the course of their education.
2. Nurses have been seen performing the kinds of activities customarily expected in that situation.
3. The dialogues between the nurse and patient and the physician were extensive enough to permit judgments to be made.
4. Content from a variety of disciplines (sociological, psychological, and physiological) related to the situation.
5. The quality of the film's sound and photography was such that the extraneous noise and subject matter did not interfere with an examinee's performance on the test.
6. Lack of knowledge of obstetric nursing did not affect the performance on the test.

# METHODOLOGY

An instrument to measure the magnitude of the degree of complexity of specific decisions in a simulated clinical setting was developed. The final instrument was based on a decision-making exercise. A decision-making exercise "allow one to assess subject's performance at the higher levels of the learning taxonomies and are especially valuable for this reason" (Waltz & Bausell, 1981, p. 87).

A nursing action that involves a nursing decision was provided to the subjects through the use of a 16mm movie film. The movie depicted a real situation, that of a woman in labor and the birth of her baby. The situation was presented to the subjects, who were then asked to make a decision based on their own rationale for the choice.

The most often used method of observation and data collection in the behavioral sciences is the test or scale (Kerlinger, 1973). A scale is a set of symbols or numerals constructed in such a manner that the symbols or numerals can be assigned by rule to individuals (or their behaviors) to whom the scale is applied, the assignment of the numerals being indicated by the individual's possession of the attribute being measured. The relative simplicity of the magnitude-judgment method permits the production of a scale to measure social stimuli, such as attitude, or complexity of task (Stevens, 1960). The method asks a judge to estimate the complexity of a task relative to a set of tasks previously evaluated as average by that judge.

Scaling by the magnitude-estimation method requires (a) identification of the variable, a set of social stimuli, (b) training of the judges to give proportional judgments and a population of appropriate subjects.

## Description of Method

The first step was developing an instrument that used the magnitude-estimation measurement technique to obtain a complexity-of-decision score for each test item. The instrument was then administered to subjects to obtain reliability coefficients.

## Development of the Instrument

A nursing performance simulation instrument, using magnitude scaling, that permits a score of the magnitude of the degree of complexity of decision making was developed in the following manner:

1. The variable of decision making was operationalized. A broad definition of decision complexity was constructed. Although the definition was deliberately broad, it contained only one conceptual definition (Hinshaw & Field, 1974). For this study, decision making was explained as follows: There are a number of factors that influence the difficulty of the decision. You have probably noted that some decisions are easier to

make, and others are more difficult. You will see and read about some decisions. Among the decisions, which would you consider to be average in difficulty?

2. The judges were trained to give proportional judgments on the stimuli. Several methods of training have been used (Hinshaw, 1975; Hinshaw & Field, 1974). The training needs to emphasize that the judge think in proportional terms. The training session is crucial to the study because the production of a magnitude scale is dependent on the use of the proportional judgment technique.

3. A search for a simulated clinical situation was initiated. the goal of the search was to find a clinical situation that would require some decision making on the part of the subject. It was essential that the situation be the same for each subject. A paper-and-pencil test based on a depicted obstetrical clinical situation presented through a 16mm film was selected. Harriett Schneider (1979) developed a paper-and-pencil test using a filmed obstetrical clinical situation. Further, Schneider established reliability and validity on the test. The blueprint of the test indentified the cognitive domain of each question (Bloom, 1956). Schneider's Nursing Test Based on a Filmed Clinical Situation in Labor and Delivery was used to elicit decisions regarding specific nursing actions. Only the 29 items that test the cognitive levels of application, evaluation, and synthesis were used (Schneider, 1979).

4. Two judges were given a selection of six nursing care items that were related to the clinical situations in labor and delivery from Scheider's test. The judges were asked to rate the item for greater or lesser complexity in decision making. Each judge was given the items independent of the other judge.

5. Each judge was asked to determine which one of the six items was of average complexity of decision making. The item selected as average was assigned the number 100.

6. Each judge then was asked to rate each of the other five items one at a time in relation to the nursing care item they determined to be average. The judge was asked to rate the decision as twice as difficult, half as difficult, one-third as difficult, five times as difficult. Judges were to use proportional terms.

7. Then each judge independently rated each test item, assigning a number describing the degree of complexity of decision making, using 100 as average.

8. The mean of the assigned numbers determined the degree of complexity of decision making for each item.

## Reliability of the Instrument

An interrater reliability was completed between the assigned scores of the judges. A Pearson correlation coefficient of .72 was obtained. Reliability in the form of stability was estimated though the test-retest technique. The test-retest reliability coefficient was found to be .84.

## Validity of the Instrument

Content validity of the instrument was determined through a content validity index (CVI). The CVI is the proportion of items rated as Quite/Very Relevant by two judges. Two judges independently rated each of the 29 statements, with the relevance of the statement to the domain under study. Each judge independently rated the relevance of each statement, using a 4-point rating scale: 1, Not Relevant; 2, Somewhat Relevant; 3, Quite Relevant; and 4, Very Relevant (Waltz & Bausell, 1981). The CVI was .82.

The content validity of the test items had previously been established by Schneider (1979).

## ADMINISTRATION AND SCORING

Following the development of the instrument it was administered in the following fashion:

1. Subjects were volunteers who were students in an RN completion program. Subjects were shown the film "Birthday through the Eyes of the Mother" and asked to answer the 29 selected items from the Nursing Test Based on Filmed Clinical Situation in Labor and Delivery.
2. The subject's score on each correctly answered test item was the scored value of the degree of complexity of the decision making.
3. Each subject had a scored value of the degree of complexity of decision making used for specific nursing care situations.

A Kuder-Richardson reliability of .4899 was obtained on the 29-item test. An alpha coefficient of .61 was obtained.

## FINDINGS

The range of the correct responses was from 20 to 9. The mean of the right-wrong answers was 13.95, with a standard deviation of 3.18.

The mean of complexity of the scale was 77.84, with a standard deviation of 15.66. The range of scores was 47.5 to 100.

Logarithmic transformations of the data allowed the use of statistics requiring linear additive assumptions. The pattern of the complexity of the decision was of primary interest. Therefore, the geometric mean was obtained from the logarithmic transformations. The mean of the complexity of the scale was 7.04, with a standard deviation of .2. The range of scores was 6.586 to 7.372.

The coefficient of determination between the correct answers and the logarithmic transformations was $r^2 = .934$. The coefficient of correlation was estimated to be .966, with a standard error of the estimate of .051.

## IMPLICATIONS FOR NURSING

Society expects nurses to be able to make decisions with a high degree of versatility and flexibility. Yet many nurses cannot handle the decision situations they face in their clinical practice (Taylor, 1978).

Without a measure of how well the phases of decision making are being learned, nursing educators are unable to meet the needs of their students. Graduates who failed to learn the attributes of decision making as students utilize the decision making they learned at an earlier time. They may have learned the decision making they use by modeling parents, teacher, and peers. Unfortunately, competent decision-makers often do not reveal what goes on quite automatically in their heads, so the models may be inadequate. The result is that most nurses learn by trial and error, and although this is a functional way to learn, it means poor decisions may be made while learning proceeds. In addition, inappropriate decisions may be still made later because the learning did not proceed far enough or fast enough.

In many situations, both personal and professional, the penalty for making a poor decision is insignificant. However, it is the decision with significant consequences that is of concern. The decision matters if the patient is a victim of a poor decision-maker. Ignorance can cause problems; poor decision-makers do little to solve them.

Research suggests the usefulness of focusing on the process by which decisions are made. Nurse educators must be made aware of the need to strengthen the connection between the analytical tools and behavior insights of decision making taught in the nursing education program.

The study demonstrates the use of magnitude-estimation techniques in the study of complexity of decisions. The magnitude-estimation techniques are used to produce ratio scales of the variables. Logarithmic transformations were applied. The data were not subjected to linear statistics. It was possible to examine the averaged data as well as to work with individual scores. A tool was produced that measures the complexity of a clinical decision. The magnitude-estimation technique may be a way to measure subjective phenomena in nursing. The technique can increase the precision of measurement by producing a ratio-level scale.

With a tool to measure the magnitude of the complexity of a decision, the nurse educator can examine and teach the decision-making process. Graduates who learned decision-making skills as students will use those skills in practice.

## REFERENCES

Aspinall, M. J. (1979). Use of a decision tree to improve accuracy of diagnosis. *Nursing Research, 28*, 182-185.

Banathy, B. (1968). *Instructional systems*, Palo Alto, CA: Fearon.

Bloom, B. (Ed.). (1956). *Taxonomy of educational goals, Handbook I: Cognitive domain.* New York: David McKay.

Broderick, M. E., & Ammentorp, W. M. (1979). Information structures: An analysis of nursing performance. *Nursing Research, 28*, 106-110.

Corcoran, S. A. (1983). *Decision making by nurses concerning drug administration plans to control pain.* Unpublished doctoral dissertation, University of Minnesota, Minneapolis.

Erikson, E. (1964). *Insight and responsibility.* New York: W. W. Norton.

Grier, M. R. (1976). Decision making about patient care. *Nursing Research, 25*, 105-109.

Hammond, D. (1966). Clinical inference in nursing: A psychologist's viewpoint. *Nursing Research, 15*, 27-28.

Hinshaw, A. S. (1975). *Professional decisions: A technological perspective.* Unpublished doctoral dissertation, University of Arizona, Tucson, AZ.

Hinshaw, A. S., & Field, M. (1974). An investigation of variables that underlie collegial evaluation. *Nursing Research, 23*, 292-300.

Kaioth, S. (1977). *A study to determine the effects of the design and operation of nursing systems model on the quality of patient care plans.* Unpublished doctoral dissertation, Florida State University, Tallahassee, FL.

Kerlinger, F. N. (1973). *Foundations of behavioral research* (2nd ed.). New York : Holt, Rinehart & Winston.

Kovacs, A. (1985). *The research process: Essentials of skill development.* Philadelphia: F. A. Davis.

Kropp, R. & Stoker, H. (1966). *The construction and validation of tests of the cognitive processes as described in the taxonomy of educational objectives.* Tallahassee, FL: Florida State University, Institute of Human Learning and Department of Educational Research and Testing.

Kubo, W., Chase, L., & Leton, J. (1971). A creative examination. *Nursing Outlook, 19*, 524.

Lancaster, W., & Beare, P. (1982). Decision making in nursing practice. In J. Lancaster & W. Lancaster (Eds.), *Concepts for advanced nursing practice: The nurse as a change agent* (pp. 147- 170). St. Louis: C. V. Mosby.

Lee, W. (1971). *Decision theory and human behavior.* New York: John Wiley.

Lord, F. M., & Novick, M. R. (1968). *Statistical theories of mental test scores.* Reading, MA: Addison-Wesley.

Magnusson, D. (1966). *Test theory.* Reading, MA: Addison- Wesley.

Mandrillo, M. (1969). *A comparative study of cognitive skills of the graduating baccalaureate degree and associate degree nursing students.* Unpublished doctoral dissertation, Teachers College, Columbia University, New York.

Maslow, A. (1970). *Motivation and personality.* New York: Harper & Row.

McIntyre, H., McDonald, F., Bailey, J., & Clause, K. (1972). A simulated clinical nursing test. *Nursing Research, 21*, 429.

National League for Nursing. (1983). *Criteria for the evaluation of baccalaureate and higher degree programs in nursing.* New York: Council of Baccalaureate and Higher Degree Programs.

Nunnally, J. C. (1978). *Psychometric theory* (2nd ed.). New York: McGraw-Hill.

Schneider, H. (1979). *Evaluation of nursing competence.* Boston: Little, Brown.

Selltiz, C., Wrightsman, L., & Cook, S. (1976). *Research methods in social relations* (3rd. ed.). New York: Holt, Rinehart & Winston.

Stanley, J. C. (1971). Reliability. In R. L. Thorndike (Ed.), *Educational measurement* (pp. 356-442). Washington, DC: American Council on Education.

Stevens, S. S. (1960). The psychophysics of sensory function. *American Scientist, 48*, 226- 253.

Taylor, A. G. (1978). Decision making in nursing: An analytical approach. *Journal of Nursing Administration, 8*(11), 22-30.

Waltz, C., & Bausell, R. (1981). *Nursing research: Design, statistics and computer analysis.* Philadelphia: F. A. Davis.

Waltz, C., Strickland, O., & Lenz, E. (1984). *Measurement in nursing research*. Phila-
delphia: F. A. Davis.
Ward, E., & Tversky, A. (1967). *Decision making: Selected readings*. Harmonsworth,
Middlesex, England: Penguin.
Yura, H., & Walsh, M. (1978). *The nursing process: Assessing, planning, implementing,
evaluating* (3rd ed.). New York: Appleton-Century Crofts.

# Sample of a Clinical Decision-Making Measure Developed for Use with a Specific Film Description of Sample Film

The film *Birth through the Eyes of the Mother* follows the labor process and birth of an infant as it would be seen by the mother in this case a woman named Maureen. The camera angle is as if it were in the position of the mother's eyes. In other words, it is about 4½ to 5 feet above the ground. All of the script is in the form of people talking to the mother and her response. There is no narration of the film, and there are no pictures of the mother. The film begins with the mother walking down the hall to the labor admission area. The nurse is giving her directions, and asking her questions about the beginning of her contractions. When the patient is on the admission table and positioned for an examination, her knees appear on either side of the screen, and the nurse's face approaches the camera. The film advances the time by looking at the clock at intervals. There are only three or four characters in the film, the mother, the nurse or nurses and the unseen patient. The patient does not have a support person for the labor and birth process. The actions of the characters are natural and appear to be unrehearsed. The actions of the nurse are those that would be seen by many mothers. The doctor also appears in a natural role. His information and directions to the mother are the same as that given many times in an actual labor and delivery situation.

## Questions used with the film *"Birthday through the Eyes of the Mother.*

1.  The nurse asked Maureen a question that was based on the assumption that Maureen
    1.  had attended an antepartal clinic.
    2.  was anxious about the outcome of the pregnancy.
    3.  had been timing her contractions.
    4.  was knowledgeable about what to expect in subsequent stages of labor.

2.  The nurse asked Maureen all of the following questions shortly after her admission. While all of the questions would be useful in establishing a nursing care plan, which one could justifiably have been postponed?
    1.  "Have you been exposed recently to a communicable disease?"
    2.  "Are you leaking any fluid?"
    3.  "How much weight did you gain during your pregnancy?"
    4.  "Do you expect to breast – or bottle – feed your baby?"

3.  Which of these occurrences soon after Maureen was admitted would probably have diminished her confidence in the personnel?
    1.  The nurse did not immediately notify the doctor of Maureen's arrival on the unit.

    2.   Neither a doctor nor a nurse stayed with Maureen continuously.

    3.   No one provided Maureen with information about the infant's condition.

    4.   Maureen was asked the same questions by both the nurse and the doctor.

4.  The doctor seemed to make several assumptions in relation to Maureen's labor and delivery. Which of them was most apparent?
1. That Maureen was going to have a larger-than-average baby.
2. That Maureen was going to have anesthesia.
3. That Maureen's intrapartum course was going to be prolonged.
4. That Maureen was going to require medication only at the end of the first stage of labor.

5.  While Maureen was being shaved, it would have been desirable for the nurse to say,
1. "Although you will experience some discomfort when the hair grows back, shaving is a necessary procedure."
2. "Women usually complain of a tickling sensation as the hair regrows, but it shouldn't pose any great problems for you."
3. "It's common to be embarrassed because the shaving involves a private area, but it will help to promote the safety of the birth process."
4. "We're pretty lucky not having to shave every day, aren't we?"

6.  Maureen made several comments in relation to the enema she was about to have. Which comment, if Maureen had made it, would indicate that the nurse did not prepare her adequately for the enema?
1. "I thought I was going to drop the baby."
2. "I had an enema as a child, but I've had none since then."
3. "I won't be able to hold the fluid if I have a contraction."
4. "I don't understand why an enema is so important."

7.  The nurse's approach to Maureen while she was in labor appeared to be based on Maureen's
1. socioeconomic status.
2. prior experience with nurses and doctors.
3. acceptance of the nurse as a helping person.
4. preparation for childbirth.

8.  All of the following are desirable nursing measures for mothers in early labor. Which one did the nurse caring for Maureen carry out?
1. Telling the mother to relax between contractions.
2. Encouraging the mother to relax between contractions.
3. Waiting for the mother's contraction to be over before continuing with a procedure.
4. Reassuring the mother about the baby's condition.

9.  A judgment that is warranted about the doctor's sitting on Maureen's bed is that it was
1. unsafe because patients may view such behavior as being unprofessional.
2. unwise because patients may view such behavior as being unprofessional.
3. acceptable as a means of establishing a closer relationship with a patient.
4. permissible on a maternity unit, though it would not be on other hospital units.

10. After the doctor noticed that Maureen's legs were shaking, he told her that the "shaking and shivering would get worse afterwards." Which judgment of the doctor's comment is accurate? (Assume that this is Maureen's first baby.)
    1. Since chills occur less frequently after delivery today than was once true, it was an inappropriate response.
    2. Since multiparas are more susceptible to chills that are primiparas, it was an inappropriate response.
    3. Since emotionally stable patients develop chills more frequently than do emotionally labile ones, it was a premature response.
    4. Since excessive body fluid precipitates chills following delivery, it was a premature response.

11. Which of these observations about Maureen's care is most justifiable in relation to the giving of medications to her?
    1. Personnel failed to give her information about the intended effects of the medications.
    2. Measures were not taken by the nurse to allay discomfort between medications.
    3. There was a hesitancy on the part of staff to administer any medication.
    4. She was made to feel that she would be violating the principles of prepared childbirth if she were to be medicated.

12. While the doctor was examining Maureen's rectum, which of these actions by the nurse was especially undesirable in terms of Maureen's emotional needs?
    1. Leaving Maureen's lower abdomen and legs exposed.
    2. Standing in back of the doctor rather that next to Maureen.
    3. Failing to explain to Maureen what was being done.
    4. Neglecting to confer with the doctor promptly about the extent of Maureen's discomfort.

13. While Maureen was being examined by the doctor, the nurse failed to provide for
    1. proper positioning of Maureen for the procedure.
    2. disposal of the equipment used by the doctor.
    3. adequate draping of Maureen's legs.
    4. visibility of the area.

14. Maureen's comments during labor should lead one to conclude that she was
    1. unusually anxious.
    2. anticipating a prolonged labor.
    3. eager for the presence of another person.
    4. favorably impressed with the medical and nursing staffs.

15. While Maureen was in labor, the nurses giving her care failed to provide for
    1. a quiet environment conducive to rest and relaxation.
    2. instructions in how to work with contractions
    3. physical comfort measures.
    4. equipment to promote safety.

16. The nurse coached Maureen in breathing techniques. Which judgment of the nurse's approach and method is accurate?

1. The approach was appropriate, and the method was acceptable.
2. The approach was appropriate, but the method was unacceptable.
3. The approach was inappropriate, but the method was acceptable.
4. The approach was inappropriate, and the method was unacceptable.

17. Which of these statements accurately assesses the reaction of personnel to Maureen when she was experiencing discomfort associated with contractions?
    1. The doctor was more responsive to her than were the nurses.
    2. The nurses were more supportive of her than was the doctor.
    3. There was essentially no difference between the behavior of the doctor and the nurses toward her.
    4. The actions of the admitting nurse were more like those of the doctor than were those of the nurse who cared for her later.

18. The clock in Maureen's room was visible at various times. On the basis of the passage of time gleaned from the film, which of these judgments of the length of Maureen's labor as a primigravida is warranted?
    1. Maureen's labor appeared to fit the normal pattern.
    2. The first stage of Maureen's labor was within normal limits, but the second stage assumed to be prolonged.
    3. The first stage of Maureen's labor was unusually long, but the second stage was within the normal range.
    4. There was insufficient data to allow a conclusion about the duration of Maureen's labor.

19. On the basis of the information provided in the film, the probable rationale for the use of forceps with Maureen was to
    1. adhere to medical policy.
    2. shorten the second stage of labor.
    3. facilitate delivery of a large baby.
    4. prevent perineal tears.

20. A procedure usually carried out immediately after delivery of the placenta that was not seen in the film was
    1. administering an oxytocic.
    2. performing the "Crede" maneuver.
    3. discontinuing the intravenous infusion.
    4. evaluating the amount of blood loss.

21. The one aspect of the baby's management in the delivery room that could most justifiably be criticized was that he was
    1. not given to this mother soon enough.
    2. held by the doctor with only one hand.
    3. placed on his mother's abdomen prior to delivery of the placenta.
    4. examined rather superficially for congenital anomalies.

22. At the end of the film, when Maureen commented, "The baby was inside me for nine months and now here he is," the doctor answered, "You did a good job." Which of these assessments of his comment is justifiable?
    1. It was made before the patient's remark was clarified.
    2. It immediately reinforced positive behavior in the patient.
    3. It was a complimentary acknowledgment of the patient's reaction.
    4. It reinforced the reality of the baby's arrival for the patient.

23. Which of these interpretations is most justifiable about the nurse-doctor relationship in the film?
    1. There appeared to be an interaction commonly called "professional" between them.
    2. There seemed to be a feeling of mutual respect between them.
    3. There was little or no communication between them.
    4. There did not seem to be any independent action on the part of doctors or nurses in relation to the patient's management.

24. Which of these generalizations should a nurse have about the effect of doctor-nurse relationships on patients like Maureen in a situation such as the one depicted in the film?
    1. If any disagreement between doctors and nurses is perceived by the patient, it might be interpreted by the patient as a potential threat to her.
    2. Patients in labor are so self-centered that they are unaware of doctors' and nurses' behavior.
    3. An attitude of joviality and lightheartedness on the part of doctors and nurses contributes to an anxiety-free experience for the patient.
    4. The behavior of doctors and nurses as individuals is more important than the relationships between and among them.

25. From both verbal and nonverbal interactions between Maureen and the nurses, it is reasonable to infer that
    1. there was a lack of affective feelings evident in their relationships with Maureen.
    2. the nurses' behavior toward Maureen is typical of the way most nurses treat maternity patients regardless of their marital status.
    3. the calmness exhibited by the nurses is synonymous with acceptance of Maureen as a person.
    4. there was an absence of judgment on the part of Maureen and the nurses.

26. The film does not tell whether Maureen has had a baby previously or whether she has ever seen a delivery. If personnel had had such information, it would have been most useful as the
    1. basis for teaching, since knowing where the patient "is" allows the nurse to be more helpful.
    2. means by which the nurse could review and reiterate pertinent information.
    3. frame of reference for establishing a nursing care plan.
    4. mechanism by which a meaningful nurse-patient relationship could be established.

27. An assumption seemed to be made by personnel about Maureen and her baby. This assumption was that Maureen
    1. was disappointed in the baby's sex.
    2. needed help in coming to a decision about the baby's future.
    3. was uncertain about her ability to take care of the baby.
    4. planned to keep the baby.

28. The most obvious omission in the film was any reference to Maureen's
    1. feelings about giving birth.
    2. relationship with the baby's father.

   3. decision about the feeding of her baby.
   4. general health status.

29. If a group of primigravidas were to view the film, what general effect might be expected?
   1. Anxiety, because many points about labor and delivery were not covered.
   2. Satisfaction of curiosity, because some aspects of having a baby were made evident.
   3. Disappointment, because only the mother's role was shown.
   4. Disillusionment, because the joy of childbearing was not made explicit and the pain was.

# PART III
# Measuring Educational Outcomes

# 13

# Measuring Assertive Behavior in Registered Nurses as an Outcome of a Continuing Education Program

*Paulette Freeman Adams and Linda Holbrook Freeman*

*This chapter discusses the Assertiveness Behavior Inventory Tool, a measure of assertive behavior in nurses.*

## PURPOSE

The purpose of this study was to measure assertive behavior of registered nurses over a period of time as an outcome of a continuing education program.

## CONCEPTUAL BASIS

Over the past 5 years, the researchers have conducted numerous continuing education programs on assertive behavior for nurses. These programs were developed out of a recognition that many nurses did not value their rights as persons or as professionals in practice.

From the literature review it became apparent to the researchers that the measurement of outcome behaviors of an assertive–behavior program was essential to determining the effectiveness of a continuing education offering. The literature documented a precedent for evaluating a one-time continuing education program on assertiveness with nurse participants (Faulk, 1984). Faulk's study reported a difference in the pre- and posttest scores on assertiveness in a 1 month follow-up survey. No control group was used for comparison in the study.

Since the early 1970s numerous professional articles have been published related to assertiveness and assertive training programs. Among the better–known works are Alberti and Emmons (1970), Galassi and Galassi (1976), Kazdin (1976), and Lange and Jakubowski (1976). Most of the early literature focused on the type of program or training methods that should be used in developing assertive behavior rather than on the measurement of assertive behavior. Brown and Brown (1980) investigated the historical trends in assertiveness training literature, using content analysis, and found articles prior to 1970 to be mostly case studies and descriptions of programs. Experimental studies began to appear in the early 1970s.

Both nursing and other professional literature has abounded in books and articles related to assertiveness behavior training for nurses (Burgess, 1979; Chenevert, 1978; Clark, 1978; Cohen, 1983; Donnelly, 1978, 1979; Gluck & Charter, 1980; Grissum & Spengler, 1976; Hutchins & Colburn,1979; Ryan-Merritt, 1982; Whitman,1982). Several authors have addressed the need to prepare the nursing student in assertive behavior to become an effective professional nurse (Donner & Goering, 1982; Pardue, 1980).

Grissum and Spengler (1976) have emphasised the socialization process women are subjected to as children, pointing out the submissive role girl children are expected to follow. These authors see a continuation of much of this expected behavior in schools of nursing. Most nurses may leave their educational programs without learning assertive behaviors. Burgess (1979) states that "until nurses practice collective assertiveness as a profession and strive for professional self-actualization they will not be recognized for the impact they are making daily in the lives of others (p. 6)."

In summary, the nursing literature primarily emphasizes the need for assertiveness training for nurses but documents sparse efforts at determining the effectiveness of programs addressing the topic of assertiveness, that is, the measurement of assertive behavior as an outcome. Therefore, the researchers have determined that this study is important in order to add to the literature measurement of assertive behavior of registered nurses over a period of time as an outcome of a continuing education program.

The theoretical framework for the continuing education program on assertive behavior was derived from Alberti and Emmons (1970) behavioral therapy model which views becoming assertive as a learning process for self-directed development, and from the cognitive-behavioral model of Lang and Jakubowski (1976), which addresses cognitive restructuring. The continuing education program is constructed to include cognitive awareness of various behaviors, group exercises, self-disclosure, and self-assessment.

## METHODOLOGY

Methodology for the study addressed the following research question: Is there a difference in the level of assertive behavior reported by registered nurses on the researcher-developed instrument, Assertive Behavior Inventory Tool (ABIT), before participation in an assertiveness workshop and 4 months after participation in the workshop? The researchers formulated a composite theoretical definition of assertive behavior based on the work of Alberti and Emmons (1970). This definition included (a) acting in one's own best interest, (b) standing up for oneself, (c) expressing honest feelings, and (d) exercising one's own rights without denying the rights of others.

The researchers then operationalized a definition of assertive behavior: the score obtained on the ABIT.

As part of the methodology for the study the researchers decided to continue the workshop on assertiveness as it had been presented, to test the ABIT for reliability and validity, and to measure the level of assertive behavior over a period of time, using the ABIT. The continuing education program was conducted for the target population in a one-time, 5-hr. session.

## TOOL DEVELOPMENT

Although the workshops were called Assertive Behavior for Nurses, the tool used for these programs actually inventoried three types of behaviors – assertive, nonassertive, and aggressive.

Tools found in the literature did not seem appropriate for the purpose to be accomplished in the study – measurement of assertive behavior in registered nurses over a specified time period. A widely used tool is one developed by Alberti and Emmons (1970). This tool is a 35–item inventory that assesses assertive, nonassertive and aggressive behavior. Alberti and Ammons have stated that no measures of reliability and validity have been obtained for this tool, nor do they intend to obtain any such measures. Galassi, DeLo, Galassi, and Bastien (1974) developed the College Self-Expression Scale: A Measure of Assertiveness. This tool is a 50–item inventory designed to measure assertiveness in college students. However, 30 of the items require reverse scoring, which indicates that these items measure either nonassertive or aggressive behavior. A number of items in this tool address areas specific to college students, such as interactions with roommates and parents. The Rathus (1973) Assertiveness Schedule is a 30–item tool developed to measure assertiveness. It too has items requiring reverse scoring, which indicates that several items measure non-assertive and aggressive behaviors. Most of the items did not address situations a career woman such as a registered nurse would encounter. The Rathus tool has been standardized on college populations. Gay, Hollandsworth, and Galassi (1975) developed the Adult Self-Expression Scale, a 48–item tool designed to measure assertiveness in the general adult population. All of these tools were for general population use but have been tested primarily with college-age groups and therapy groups. The researchers needed to develop a tool that would reflect (a) the usual work setting of registered nurses, (b) life events common to the general population, and (c) measurement of only assertive behaviors.

The tool that was originally developed by the researchers was called Assertiveness Inventory (AI) and inventoried assertive, nonassertive, and aggressive behaviors. For the present study it was decided by the researchers to eliminate items on the tool that reflected nonassertive and aggressive behaviors and to have a tool that contained only items describing assertive behaviors. This new tool was named Assertive Behavior Inventory Tool (ABIT). The items in the ABIT met the following criteria: (a) the items reflect assertive behaviors in both work and home settings, (b) the items reflect common life events that occur at home and at work, and (c) the inventory can be completed quickly and easily.

## REVISION AND TESTING OF THE ABIT FOR RELIABILITY AND VALIDITY

The original Assertiveness Inventory, which included 44 items on assertive, nonassertive, and aggressive behaviors, along with definitions of the three behaviors, was sent to 25 judges, all of whom had knowledge of the concept of assertiveness. The judges were asked to label each item on the tool as assertive, nonassertive, or aggressive behavior. Twenty-three responses (92%) were received. The responses were tallied for each item. Only items that 16 judges (70%) agreed described assertive behavior were retained in the first revision. Twenty-five of the original 44 items were retained as describing assertive behaviors. The tool with these remaining 25 items was sent to two judges (raters). These judges were asked to identify the extent to which each item on the tool reflected assertive behavior. The scale used to rate the items included four options: not relevant, somewhat relevant, quite relevant, and very relevant.

The content validity index as described in Waltz, Strickland, and Lenz (1984) was used to determine the interrater agreement. There were no items that both judges rated 1 or 2, not or somewhat relevant. There were no items that Judge 1 rated 3 or 4 and Judge 2 rated 1 or 2. There were two items that Judge 1 rated 1 or 2 and Judge 2 rated 3 or 4. There were 23 items (92%) that both judges rated 3 or 4, quite or very relevant. Therefore, the content validity index was 92, which represented the proportion of items rated 3 or 4 by both judges.

The ABIT reflected the following specifications:

1. General description: Given a written list of items describing assertive behavior, the participant will indicate the extent to which that behavior is exhibited by the participant.

2. Stimulus attributes

   Each item describes an assertive behavior.
   Items are grouped according to where they occur – at work or away from work.
   Each item is a complete sentence.

3. Response attributes

> The subject may select from responses that describe how frequently the participant exhibits the behavior if known.
> The responses are displayed in a Likert scale.
> Only one response is appropriate for each item.
> There is no correct or wrong response.

## Administration and Scoring

Participants completing the ABIT indicated how often the assertive behavior occurs, using a 5–point rating scale: Almost Always, Often, Seldom, Almost Never, and Don't Know. The responses are given a score of 4 through 0 with 4 (Almost Always) representing the most assertive response and a score of 1 (Almost Never) representing the least assertive response. The response Don't Know is given a value of 0. Item scores are summed to obtain the tool scale score. The maximum score that can be obtained on the ABIT is 96. The higher the score, the more assertive are the behaviors reported by the participant.

The researchers administered the tool to a convenience sample of 45 registered nurses working in an acute care agency located in an urban area. These nurses were chosen because they were representative of the population that would be exposed to the assertive–behavior program. Following a 2-week period, the test was readministered to this sample in order to correlate the scores from the two administrations of the tool. The 2-week period was believed to be a sufficient length of time to reduce the effect of testing and a short enough period to reduce the effects of history and maturation, thus reducing the threats to internal validity. Only the subjects completing both tests were included in the data analysis. The test–retest reliability of the instrument was 0.78.

The ABIT thus addressed the problems of existing tools previously cited. The ABIT included only items related to assertive behavior, was tested for reliability and validity, and was specific to the nurse population.

## PILOT STUDY

A quasi-experimental design was used to conduct a pilot study using the ABIT in a continuing education program for registered nurses. The study population was a convenience sample of registered nurses employed in acute care agencies owned by a for-profit corporation and located in a another metropolitan area. The sample included a treatment group of 27 participants, 21 of whom completed the 4-month retest. The control group included a convenience sample of 35 registered nurses employed in similar agencies, that is acute care agencies owned by a for-profit corporation and located in another metropolitan area.

The University of Louisville Human Studies Committee determined that the study was exempt from the requirement for review. Each participant received a letter outlining the purpose of this study and a guarantee of voluntary participation and confidentiality in reporting the results. The researchers were not able to link the identity of the participants with their responses on the ABIT. The ABIT had only an identifying number. A list matching the participant names with the tool number was secured by a staff member in the School of Nursing and was destroyed at the completion of the study.

## MAJOR FINDINGS AND RESULTS

The findings revealed a wide range of scores on the inventories for both groups. The control group mean score was 73.5 (SD = 11.9) on the pretest, with minimum and maximum scores of 45 and 93; and 72.6 (SD = 10.9) on the posttest, which had a minimum score of 55 and maximum score of 95. The treatment group mean was 70.1 (SD = 11.1) on the pretest, with a minimum score of 54 and a maximum score of 90. The posttest mean was 71.5 (SD = 9.6) for the treatment group, with minimum and maximum scores of 51 and 90.

A $t$-test for independent samples was computed to test for statistically significant differences in the pretest mean scores of the treatment and control groups. The $t$-test results revealed a $p$-value of .33, with 41 degrees of freedom. Therefore, there was no significant difference between the pretest mean scores of the treatment and control groups.

A paired $t$-test for dependent samples was run to test for statistically significant differences between the pre- and posttest mean scores of the treatment group and the control group. The $t$-test resulted in a $p$-value of .64, with 20 degrees of freedom, for the treatment group; and a $p$-value of .70, with 21 degrees of freedom, for the control group. There was no statistically significant difference in the level of assertive behavior in either the treatment or control group over time.

The findings of the study indicated that a one-time workshop did not make a difference in the level of assertive behavior reported by registered nurses over a designated period of time and that cognitive restructuring for assertive behavior may require reinforcement on a continuing basis.

## IMPLICATIONS FOR THE NURSING PROFESSION AND MEASUREMENT OF NURSING OUTCOMES

The findings in this study raise questions about how effective one-time continuing education programs are in changing professional behaviors that socialize nurses into professional roles.

Future research should be expanded to a larger sample size, both to test the internal consistency reliability of the ABIT and to address the research question. In addition, a future study could include three groups in the sample – the one-time, 5-hr-session treatment group, the control group, and a multiple–session (three 5-hr sessions) treatment group.

Since construct validity is useful in measures of affect, an additional study needs to be conducted using an experimental manipulation approach (Waltz et al., 1984).

## REFERENCES

Alberti, R., & Emmons, M. (1970). *Your perfect right.* San Luis Obispo, CA: Impact.

Brown, S., & Brown, L. (1980). Trends in assertion training research and practice: A content analysis of the published literature. *Journal of Clinical Psychology,36,* 265-269.

Burgess, G. R. (1979). Nurses as women. *Nursing Leadership,2*(4), 26-28.

Chenevert, M. (1978). *Special techniques in assertiveness training for women in the health profession.* St. Louis: C. V. Mosby.

Clark, C. C. (1978). *Assertive skills for nurses.* Wakefield, MA. Contemporary Publishing.

Cohen, S. (1983). Programmed instruction. Assertiveness in nursing: Part I. *American Journal of Nursing, 6,* 911-928.

Donnelly, G. F. (1978). The assertive nurse. *Nursing '78, 8*(1), 65-69.

Donnelly, G. F (1979). Assertiveness workbook: When assertiveness exacts a price. *RN, 42*(10), 28-31.

Donner, G., & Goering, P. (1982). Helping nurses learn assertiveness. *Journal of Nursing Education, 3,* 14-19.

Faulk, L. (1984). Continuing education program evaluation for course improvement, participant effect and utilization in clinical practice. *Journal of Nursing Education, 4,* 139-146.

Galassi, J. P., DeLo, J. S., Galassi, M. D., & Bastien, S. (1974). The College Self-Expression Scale: A measure of assertiveness. *Behavioral Therapy, 5,* 165-171.

Galassi, M. D. & Galassi, J. P. (1976). Assertion: A critical review. *Psychotherapy: Theory, Research, Practice, 15*(1), 16- 29.

Gay, M., Hollandsworth, J. G., & Galassi, J. P. (1975). An assertiveness inventory for adults. *Journal of Counseling Psychology, 22,* 340-344.

Gluck, M., & Charter P. (1980). Personal qualities of nurses implying need for continuing education to increase interpersonal and leadership effectiveness. *Journal of Continuing Education for Nurses, 11*(4), 29-36.

Grissum, M., & Spengler, C. (1976). *Women power and health care.* Boston: Little, Brown.

Hutchins, H., & Colburn, L. (1979). An assertiveness training program for nurses. *Nursing Outlook, 6,* 394-397.

Kazdin, A. E. (1976). Effects of covert modeling, multiple models, and model reinforcement on assertive behavior. *Behavioral Therapy, 7,* 211-222.

Lange, A., & Jakubowski, P. (1976). *Responsible assertive behavior.* Champaign, IL: Research Press.

Pardue, S. F. (1980). Assertiveness for nursing. *Supervisor Nurse, 11*(2), 47-50.

Rathus, S. (1973). A 30 item schedule for assessing assertive behavior. *Behavioral Therapy, 4,* 398-406.

Ryan-Merritt, M. (1982). A teaching strategy for evaluating assertive behavior change. *Journal of Nursing Education, 9,* 13-16.

Waltz, C. F., Strickland, O. L., & Lenz, E. R. (1984). *Measurement in nursing research.* Philadelphia: F. A. Davis.

Whitman, M. (1982). Toward a new psychology for nurses. *Nursing Outlook, 1,* 48-52.

# Assertiveness Behavior Inventory Tool

## WORK

|  | ALMOST ALWAYS | OFTEN | SELDOM | ALMOST NEVER | DON'T KNOW |
|---|---|---|---|---|---|

1. I tell others of my special skills.
2. I suggest new policies, procedures and solutions.
3. I tell co-workers when I disagree with their opinions in a calm, reasonable way.
4. I tell co-workers when they have done a good job.
5. I can let co-workers know when they did something wrong in a calm, reasonable way.
6. I can express anger at work without being "out of control."
7. I express my ideas when serving on a committee.
8. I do not hesitate to ask a doctor a question about a patient.
9. I ask my co-workers for help in a very direct way.
10. I can refuse assignments at work that I do not want to do.

## AWAY FROM WORK:

11. I express my real feelings to the family.
12. I can tell a friend I think he/she is being unfair.
13. When I walk into a room, I can introduce myself first.
14. I can speak up in a line at the store and indicate I am next to be waited on.
15. I can say no to family members without feeling guilty.

ALMOST ALWAYS

OFTEN

SELDOM

ALMOST NEVER

DON'T KNOW

16. I request help with household chores because I feel all family members should share the workload.

17. I am able to say no to requests made by friends.

18. When a salesperson tries to sell me something I don't want, I tell him no the first time.

19. I have confidence in my judgments about everyday life.

20. I am able to compliment family members.

21. I am able to let family members know I disagree with their opinions without becoming angry.

22. I can express my preferences for an evening of entertainment to my friends.

23. I allow other people to express their opinions even if I disagree.

24. I can maintain eye contact when talking to people.

# 14

# Examining Simulated Clinical Performance

*Blossom Gullickson*

*This chapter discusses the Simulated Clinical Performance Examination Measurement Tool, a measure of the clinical competence of nursing students.*

Valid and reliable evaluation tools that measure the clinical competence of nursing students remain a prevalent and persistent need. The focus of this study was to develop a clinical performance examination using the criterion-referenced measurement framework and simulation to measure the clinical competence of beginning nursing students in a baccalaureate program at the conclusion of the first clinical nursing course.

## SIMULATED CLINICAL PERFORMANCE EXAMINATION

The evaluation of a nursing student's clinical competence continues to be a concern of nurse educators as documented in the literature and by individual nursing instructors' observations and experience. A variety of methods have been proposed as ways to evaluate the nursing student's competency in the clinical setting. However, major problems prevail in the evaluation methods used in many nursing programs, causing frustration to both faculty and students. The major areas of concern are

1. Subjectivity in the clinical observations by instructors.
2. Student learning experiences that are not comparable.
3. Undefined standards of performance.
4. Simultaneous learning by and evaluation of students.
5. The dual role of instructor in the clinical setting as teacher and evaluator.
6. Lack of application of principles of testing.
7. Accountability for competence in nursing graduates.

Recently the idea of "examination" of student learning in meeting clinical objectives, and particularly the concept of performance examination, has been proposed. Nurse educators as well as educators in the other health professions have begun to develop clinical performance examinations to assess clinical competence. Also, recently the criterion-referenced framework for measurement of student learning and the use of simulation in evaluation have alerted and prompted educators to develop measurement tools incorporating these concepts. Consequently, a valid and reliable simulated, criterion-referenced performance examination to be used in the evaluation of a nursing student's clinical competence has become of interest and value to nurse educators – particularly since demands have increased for more accountability to assure the public and profession that nursing graduates possess the knowledge and competence to provide skillful and sensitive nursing care.

## LITERATURE REVIEW

The struggle for a more valid and reliable measurement of the clinical competence of nursing students continues to persist (Lenburg, 1979; Wood, 1982; Woolley, 1977). Accountability for student learning has prompted nurse educators as well as educators in the other health professions to delve further into the question of how to accurately measure a student's clinical competence (Lenburg, 1979; Morgan & Irby, 1978; Morgan, Luke, & Herbert, 1979; Newble, Elmslie, & Baxter, 1978; Popham, 1978b). Although not entirely a new idea, the timing of the resurgence and further development of criterion-referenced measurement is very opportune and facilitates the future development of clinical measurement tools to evaluate the competence of nursing and other health profession students. Criterion-referenced measurement is defined as the determination of an individual's performance in relation to a preestablished standard (criterion) with respect to a clearly defined behavioral domain. Behaviors that are representative of this domain comprise the performance test (Berk, 1980; Lenburg, 1979; Popham, 1978a; Waltz, Strickland, & Lenz, 1984). The student competes with the standard and not with the performance of others. The rationale for selection of the criterion-referenced measurement framework is discussed in the literature (Bower, 1974; Krumme, 1975; Lenburg, 1979). According to Waltz and associates (1984), this framework can be used effectively in testing the application of knowledge and skills, particularly in the evaluation of clinical nursing skills.

The complexity of the actual clinical setting and the simultaneous interplay among the cognitive, affective, and psychomotor domains complicates the measurement (Field, Gallman, Nicholson, & Dreher, 1984). By employing the strategy of simulation, variables can be better controlled, thereby promoting more objectivity and consistency in the measurement of each student's performance. An appropriate relationship between a high degree of realism in the simulation which promotes validity and the control of variables which promotes reliability needs to be determined (Thorndike, 1971). Guidelines for the development of a simulation with acceptable authenticity and control of variables are described by several authors (Barrows, 1971; Lincoln, Layton, & Holdman, 1978; Morgan & Irby, 1978). The potential for using simulation in clinical measurement exists and may be an effective approach to this perplexing issue. Time, energy, cost, and adequacy of resources are important considerations when, determining whether to proceed with the development of a simulated clinical performance examination (Barrows, 1971; Kolb & Shugart, 1984; McBride, Littlefield, & Garman, 1981; McDowell, Nardini, Negley, & White, 1984). The benefits of simulation along with the criterion-referenced measurement include the reduction of subjectivity common in presently used methods of clinical evaluation, identification of the standard of performance with defined critical behaviours, establishment of a more controlled testing situation, and a specified time for testing. According to Lenburg (1979), initial efforts toward the development of a tool to be used at the conclusion of the first semester in the nursing major are more feasible and manageable prior to other efforts in the more advanced nursing courses.

During the development of a clinical performance examination, the same rigorous planning and construction of the test is required as for any other type of examination, whether written or performance-oriented. Selection of a measurement framework and conceptual model, definition of the content domain, sampling from the domain of observable and measurable behaviors, specification of the method for writing behaviors, delineation of the method for administration of the examination, and setting the performance standards for interpretation of scores are the essential initial steps in the process. Documentation of validity and reliability and carrying out a pilot test are the final steps in the first phase of development of such a measurement tool (Lenburg, 1979; Popham, 1978b; Wyman & Ferman, 1977; Waltz et al., 1984).

Setting performance standards for interpretation of scores continues to be a process fraught with questions. Methods for setting standards have been classified as judgmental, empirical, or combination models and are reviewed by various measurement specialists. A primary concern relates to the setting of the performance standard either too high or too low for the clinical examination. The goal is the accurate classification of the performance of students as to whether or not they meet the standard of competence. Ebel's (1979) judgemental method of rating each behavior as to relevance and difficulty is one acceptable method to use when setting the standard for interpretation of scores in a performance examination (Berk,

1980; Breyer, 1983; Hambleton & Powell, 1983; Popham, 1978b; Shaycoft, 1979; Waltz et al., 1984).

Documentation of the validity and reliability of a measurement tool is fundamental in the development of a useful and worthy instrument. Content validity is a primary concern and needs to be determined prior to other forms of validity. The indices of content validity and item-objective congruence can be calculated after content experts judge if each behavior is relevant and is an indicator of the objective. Besides these initial efforts in the estimation of validity, other statistical procedures to determine concurrent validity by correlating simulated clinical performance examination scores with instructor evaluation in the actual clinical setting, as well as eventually construct and/or decision validity using the contrasted-group approach, would establish further the validity of a performance measurement tool. A primary issue in establishing reliability pertains to the tool's consistency classifying nursing students as achieving or not achieving the set standard of performance. Interrater reliability, the method of two raters observing the students at the same time, can be estimated by using the parametric statistic of the Pearson $r$ correlation coefficient, the nonparametric statistic of Kendall's tau or Spearman's rho, and/or nonparametric statistic of $P_0$ and kappa with consideration of the underlying assumptions for each procedure and the level of measurement. A salient question in reference to interrater reliability is, do the evaluators rate the performance of each student from a similar perspective? Videotape to increase rater reliability through training sesions has been proposed and found effective by Loustau et al. (1980).

Internal consistency, which is the consistency of performance by the nursing students on any one behavior in the tool as related to performance on any other behavior, is another method in attempting to estimate reliability that can be calculated using Cronbach's alpha coefficient. According to Krumme (1975) and Popham (1978b) the question can be raised as to the appropriateness of determining internal consistency reliability on a criterion-referenced clinical tool more precisely. Acceptable methods to be used in estimating the validity and reliability of a simulated, criterion-referenced clinical performance examination are described in the literature (King, 1979; Krumme, 1975; Lenburg, 1979; Martuza, 1977; Popham 1978b; Shaycoft, 1979; Waltz et al., 1984).

## PURPOSE

The specific purpose of this measurement study was to develop a simulated, criterion-referenced clinical performance examination to measure the clinical competence of a beginning nursing student in a baccalaureate program at the conclusion of the first clinical nursing course in the care of postoperative adult patients.

# CONCEPTUAL FRAMEWORK

The conceptual framework that guided the development of this measurement tool had two main components:

1. Concept of examination
2. Lenburg's (1979) constellation of 10 basic concepts.

The primary considerations in the concept of examination are as follows:

1. A time for learning precedes the testing time.
2. The examination is developed in as precise, consistent, and objective a manner as possible.
3. A specified time for the examination is announced.
4. The content and conditions of the examination are identified.
5. The examination is given in as objective and consistent a manner as possible.
6. A framework for interpretation of test scores has been predetermined.

These principles can be applied to a performance examination testing clinical competence of a nursing student as well as any other type of examination given in nursing.

Lenburg's (1979) constellation of basic concepts delineates the interrelatedness, complexity, and integration of the essential concepts fundamental to the development and implementation of a performance examination. The 10 basic concepts, diagrammed as 10 lines all crossing at a center point and depicting a continuum, spells out the polarities as follows: testing-teaching; areas of care-procedures; critical elements-steps in procedure; objectivity-subjectivity; sampling-total content; comparability-incomparability; acceptability-ideal; systemized conditions-spontaneous arrangements; flexibility-rigidity; and consistency-inconsistency (Lenburg, 1979, p. 77).

According to Lenburg, a thorough analysis of each concept contributes to the proper development and implementation of a performance examination.

# ASSUMPTIONS

The following assumptions formed the basis for the development of this simulated, criterion-referenced, clinical performance examination.

1. Criterion-referenced measurement is the most effective framework for a clinical performance examination.

2. Simulation is a viable strategy to be used in a clinical performance examination.
3. The accepted general principles used in testing can be applied to a clinical performance examination.
4. Examination of a nursing student's clinical competence is necessary and important in order to evaluate attainment of the educational objectives of the nursing program.
5. A time for student learning and a designated time for student evaluation is essential in order to provide a conducive environment for student learning and evaluation of competence.
6. The nursing instructor's role as evaluator occurs at the time of the clinical performance examination, which is separate from the teaching role.

## DEFINITIONS

Key concepts and the domain from which critical behaviors are sampled were defined to provide guidance in the development of the measurement tool.

### Key Concepts

1. *Clinical competence* involves possessing sufficient knowledge and skill in nursing and being able to demonstrate the ability to apply this knowledge and skill to a clinical nursing situation.
2. *Criterion-referenced measurement* is the determination of a student's performance in relation to a preestablished standard (criterion) that includes behaviors representative of a clearly defined behavioral domain (Waltz et al., 1984, p. 159).
3. *Simulation*, as defined by Kolb and Shugart (1984),(p. 84). is "the creation of a situation which imitates some aspect of reality."
4. *Simulated clinical performance examination* is a test that requires the student to demonstrate the application of theory in a simulated clinical situation by actually carrying out a representative sample of behaviors in a defined domain in the presence of an evaluator using a measurement tool with a preestablished standard of competence.

### The Content Domain

The domain from which the critical behaviors are sampled is a clinical nursing situation that requires demonstration of application of knowledge and skills in the care of a convalescing postoperative adult patient with a total hip replacement. The domain includes the nursing process, oral and written communication, helping relationship, psychomotor skills, and postoperative care, which are defined as follows.

*Nursing process* is a problem-solving approach used to meet the nursing needs of patients. The four major steps are assessment, planning, implementation, and evaluation. The collection of data and establishment of nursing diagnoses consists of the assessment phase. Establishing goals, setting priorities, and determining nursing interventions comprise the planning phase. Carrying out the plan of care is the implementation phase. Determining the achievement of goals, response of the patient to the care, and consideration of modifications in the plan of care comprise the evaluation phase.

*Communication* is an interchange of information and feelings during an interaction between a nurse and a patient. Communication occurs in verbal and nonverbal forms. Verbal communication consists of the spoken language and takes place at various times during the interaction. Nonverbal communication consists of facial expression, posture, gestures, physical distance, and touch and takes place more consistently. The process includes a message sent, a message received, and feedback response of the receiver. In addition, written communication, which consists of documentation of the patient, is another form used by the nurse.

A *helping relationship* is a dynamic interpersonal process that enhances and facilitates the patient's ability to function. Demonstration of empathy, acceptance of the patient, and willingness of the nurse to provide care are essential attributes. Attending and responding to the feelings and concerns expressed through words or actions by the patient are integral aspects of a helping relationship.

*Psychomotor skills* are the techniques concerned with nursing actions and are based on accepted principles. Application of the principles related to each technical skill and the sensitive manner in which the skill is carried out are essential for demonstration of competence.

*The postoperative period* includes the immediate period during which the patient is recovering form the anesthetic. The convalescing period is the time that the patient is making further progress toward his/her recovery. During the convalescing period the major goals are to maintain the body's functioning and to prevent any complications.

Five objectives to be tested were derived from these definitions in the domain are:

1. Student demonstrates use of the nursing process in the delivery of nursing care.
2. Student demonstrates effective use of oral and written communication skills.
3. Student demonstrates use of a helping relationship with the patient.
4. Student performs the psychomotor skills according to accepted principles and procedure using the proper supplies.
5. Student demonstrates application of knowledge essential in meeting

the nursing needs of an adult postoperative patient.

Critical behaviors related to each objective were written using Lenburg's (1979) 12 criteria as guidelines (pp. 142 – 143). A total of 140 behaviors comprises the performance examination.

## METHODOLOGY

### Creation of a Simulation

A simulation with consideration of problem, setting, and scenario was created (Morgan & Irby, 1978, p. 126). The problem selected for the nursing care situation was the care of an adult postoperative patient with total hip replacement patient because all of the students had the theoretical knowledge discussed in the classroom, had the opportunity to practice the related psychomotor skills in the classroom skills laboratory, and had cared for this type of patient in the actual clinical area. The setting for the simulation included three separate rooms. The preparation site had materials such as the patient's chart and medication profile, the nursing care plan, the nurse's worksheet, a medical dictionary, and drug and laboratory references. The student had 45 min. to study the situation and prepare the worksheet, which had the following headings: (a) subjective and objective data, (b) nursing diagnoses, (c) goals of care, (d) priorities of goals of care, (e) nursing interventions, and (f) evaluation. The performance site included a patient's hospital unit, medication area, and an area with supplies required to care for the patient. The student had 45 min to demonstrate competence in the care of a postoperative patient. The termination site was the room where the student documented the care given on a treatment form and charted in the nurses' notes, using the problem-oriented method. Also, on the worksheet that the student had developed initially, the student recorded during the termination phase the evaluation of the care given. In addition, the student gave a verbal report on an audiocassette tape as a way of "reporting off duty." The student had 45 min to complete the charting, worksheet, and verbal report, which were evaluated on the basis of the related criteria in the measurement tool at the conclusion of the day's testing.

Initially, as part of the scenario of the patient situation, the patient's demographics, preoperative health status, operative results, and the immediate postoperative recovery were outlined. Then the precise timing of the meeting of the student and simulated patient and the activities the student would be expected to perform were developed. Also, a script to guide the simulated patient was written to further clarify the scenario. A retired nurse was selected to role-play an elderly patient who had had total hip replacement surgery, and she was oriented to the role through verbal information, tour of the examination setting, and written information for study prior to the role playing. A properly trained simulated patient promotes better control of variables, allows repeated performances to be scheduled, and contributes to the consistency in the performance examination.

## Subjects

The subjects were 20 baccalaureate nursing students enrolled in a private liberal arts college nursing program who were at the conclusion of the first clinical nursing course. The students were requested to participate in the pilot study with an explanation that all test scores would be confidential and that the test scores would not affect their final grades. Of 21 students, 20 agreed to be a part of the convenience sample. Demographics were as follows:

1. Female:   17
2. Male:   3
3. Age:   20 to 27 years

Education prior to entering the first clinical nursing course was as follows:

1. Nineteen students had completed 1 to 4 years in college.
2. One student had already graduated from college.

The method used in the orientation of students entailed introduction to the concept of a simulated clinical performance examination, objectives to be tested, the specific patient problem, setting for the examination, standard of performance, time limitations, and the date/time of the examination. Written information was given during the first week for the students in the clinical setting and again 2 weeks prior to the examination dates, along with a time for questions. The purpose of the orientation was to facilitate the student's performance during the examination. Likewise, the evaluators were oriented to their role with written information, discussion sessions, a tour of the examination setting, and doing nine psychomotor-skills examinations simultaneously and comparing the ratings, followed by discussion. A specific orientation on the use of the measurement tool was conducted for the evaluators. The meaning of the ratings Yes and No were clarified. Each behavior that was checked as Yes indicated that the behavior was performed, and if checked No, the behavior was not performed in a manner expected of a nursing student in the beginning-level clinical nursing course.

## Content Validity

Content validity was promoted by the manner in which the behaviors and the tool were constructed, using Lenburg's (1979) framework and criteria as well as Waltz and colleagues' (1984) steps in the development of criterion-referenced measures. Initially, six experts – who included two nurse educators, two clinical orthopedic practitioners, one university professor responsible for education nursing instructors, and a graduate student with expertise in orthopedic nursing and taking education classes – rated each behavior on the relevance of each item to the objective, using a 4-point scale, and rated whether each behavior was a measurement of that objective. The experts also recorded any behaviors that they felt were not included in the tool. Changes were made in the tool based on their ratings. Next, on the revised tool two nurse educators with subject matter expertise were requested again to rate each behavior as described above. Then the index of content validity and index of item-objective congruence, an index cut-off score was set at 0.75 to differentiate between valid and nonvalid behaviors. Any behaviors below 0.75 in the tool were scrutinized and revised as indicated.

## Administration and Scoring

The tool is completed by an observer, usually the nursing instructor, who rates each behavior identified on the tool according to whether the student performed (rated Yes) or did not perform (rated No) the expected behavior. The tool is completed during the student's actual performance.

To set the cut-off score Ebel's judgmental method was used: Two educators with content expertise and one clinical orthopedic specialist were asked to rate each behavior along two dimensions, relevance and difficulty (Waltz et al., 1984, pp. 179-180). Based on these calculations, the cut-off score was set at 85%.

## Reliability Procedures

When the simulated clinical performance examination was administered, the two evaluators observed each student simultaneously and rated the behaviors as Yes or No and used the comment columns only for clarification of a rating. Based on the data collected, interrater reliability and internal consistency reliability of the tool were calculated.

## RESULTS

The index of content validity, which is the proportion of items given a 3 (Quite Relevant) and 4 (Very Relevant) rating by both content experts was calculated. Items for objectives related to communication skills, helping relationships, psychomotor skills, and postoperative care received content validity indices of 1.0. Items for the objective related to nursing process received a content validity index of 0.97.

The index of item-objective congruence, which is the agreement between content experts of whether each behavior is a measurement of the related objective, is summarized in Table 14.1. The results ranged from 0.72 to 1.0, with four behaviors below the index cutoff score of 0.75. The experts were in agreement that the 112 behaviors (of 140) were measures of the objective, but 24 behaviors were on the borderline and 4 behaviors were not measures of the objective.

The interrater agreement procedure resulted in Pearson's correlation coefficients between raters' scores of .88, .92, .87, .84, and .65 for objectives 1 through 5, respectively. The interrater reliability for the entire test was .96. These interrater reliabilities indicate a high level of agreement between the raters for the entire test and for Objectives 1 through 4 but a lower level of agreement for Objectives 5.

**TABLE 14.1** Content Validity – Item-to-Objective Congruence

| Objective | Index of item–objective congruence (value range, −1.00 to +1.00) |
|---|---|
| Nursing process | 1.0   = 24 items |
|  | 0.75 =   5 items |
|  | 0.72 =   1 item |
| Communication skills | 1.0   = 22 items |
|  | 0.75 =   5 items |
|  | 0.72 =   2 items |
| Helping relationships | 1.0   =   4 items |
|  | 0.75 =   9 items |
| Psychomotor skills | 1.0   = 33 items |
|  | 0.72 =   1 item |
| Postoperative care | 1.0   = 29 items |
|  | 0.75 =   5 items |
| Predetermined index cutoff score | 0.75 |

**TABLE 14.2** Internal Consistency Reliability

| Test and subset | Alpha coefficients | |
|---|---|---|
|  | Rater 1 | Rater 2 |
| Entire test | .91 | .88 |
| Objective 1 | .80 | .73 |
| Objective 2 | .83 | .77 |
| Objective 3 | .79 | .75 |
| Objective 4 | .82 | .75 |
| Objective 5 | .54 | .23 |

The index of internal consistency reliability using the alpha coefficient is summarized in Table 14.2. The alpha coefficients indicate that Rater 1 has consistently higher values than Rater 2. Also, the alpha coefficients are low for Objective 5 for both raters, but the obtained alpha coefficients on the entire test and Objectives 1 through 4 indicate a high degree of internal consistency reliability.

Based on this pilot study, the performances by the students were not classified by the raters as achieving the preestablished standard of performance of 85% of the total number of behaviors. The issue of setting the performance standard too high became a primary concern, since the students did not meet the preestablished cutoff score. Analyzing the test scores in order to determine an acceptable standard of performance became paramount.

## DISCUSSION

Although the simulated, criterion-referenced performance examination is not the only alternative in evaluating the clinical competence of nursing students, the conclusions from this measurement project indicate that the development and implementation of this type of measurement tool is not only feasible but a project worthy of serious consideration in order to have more valid and reliable measurement. Four conclusions are outlined.

1. Criterion-referenced measurement is an effective framework for the development of a valid and reliable clinical performance examination.
2. A simulation can be created to represent a portion of the real world that can be used as the common stimulus for measurement of a nursing student's competence.
3. The concept of examination can be applied to develop and implement a clinical performance examination just as for a written theoretical examination.
4. In terms of cost, the supplies and equipment required were minimal with an available and equipped classroom skills laboratory. Cost for faculty time for the development of the tool can be met through faculty development funds and grants. Minimum payment for the person playing the simulated role can be made initially from the special funds or grants and eventually could become a part of the nursing department's budget.

The meaning of the results needs to be explored further. Although the indexes of validity and reliability are generally high for this occasion and group of students, the estimation of validity and reliability needs to be substantiated further. Particular attention should be drawn to Objective 5 for its lower interrater reliability and the low alpha coefficient for internal consistency. In other words, the raters did not agree well, and the students got lower scores. Consequently, analysis of the behavior of the students, raters, and the person in the simulated patient role is indicated. Are the students learning the content being tested by Objective 5? Are the raters having more difficulty observing and evaluating the behavior? What is the behavior of the patient, the cues given by the patient, in relation to Objective 5? In addition, Rater 1 has consistently higher internal consistency reliability indexes than Rater 2. Is this a question of orientation of the raters? Can other means of orientation change any inherent differences in the way the raters evaluate any given situation? Also, a question needs to be raised regarding the appropriateness of the 85% cutoff score based on the student scores. Rethinking can revolve along the following lines:

- Was the information given adequate for the students to be able to perform to the best of their ability?
- Did the students have problems getting into the role in the simulated situation?
- Does the beginning level of the students mean their learning is still fragmented to the point that they have difficulty combining abilities to demonstrate competence at the level of 85% of these behaviors? Is the problem related to application of knowledge to a specific patient situation? Are the expectations realistic for a beginning student?

Limitations of this measurement tool include the following:

1. A convenience sample of 20 nursing students in one baccalaureate program is adequate for the pilot test, but a larger random sample is required to generalize the applicability of the tool in other nursing school programs.
2. Reliability and validity estimates are based on this one occasion and group of students and need to be repeated on each administration of the tool.
3. The patient situation is a simulated one and is not in the actual clinical setting.
4. The measurement tool is designed to evaluate the clinical competence of a beginning nursing student only.
5. The clinical performance examination is limited to demonstration of application of knowledge and skills in the care of a convalescing postoperative adult patient.

For the continued development of this measurement tool the determination of concurrent, construct, and decision validity is recommended. As for recommendations for the administration of the test, four seem pertinent at this time. First, other evaluators who have not been as involved in the evaluation of and the planning of learning experiences for beginning-level nursing students, or in providing input into this tool, need to be oriented and use this tool in order to have additional estimates of reliability. Second, the question of the length of the test is an issue. Is a 45 min performance too long a time from the students' and evaluators' perspectives? Since there were numerous opportunities during the simulation for the evaluators to observe the behaviors, could the tool be refined? On the other hand, the students do need adequate time to demonstrate competence. Another concern is the fatigue factor of the evaluators and students, which affects reliability. Third, the placement or physical distance of the evaluators from the students can be a factor in the student's ability to perform at the optimum level. Ideally, a one-way mirror would be helpful to promote a more natural place for the interaction to occur between the student and patient. Fourth, in order for students to receive feedback from the performance examination and have an opportunity for additional practice and improving their skills, giving the examination several weeks prior to the end of the semester is an option worthy of consideration.

The implications of this measurement project concern nursing students, nurse educators, the nursing profession, and the recipients of nursing care. In a criterion-referenced measurement tool, the students are not compared with the performance of others, which allows the student to compete with the identified standard, places the responsibility of learning on the student, and promotes more cooperation among students to help each other learn. Nurse educators are challenged and accountable for the development of valid and reliable tools to measure educational outcomes. Nursing is a practice-oriented profession that necessitates the testing of competency in all three domains of learning. A simulated, criterion-referenced clinical performance examination can be developed and has the potential to test the cognitive, affective, and psychomotor domains of learning. With the use of more valid and reliable tools to measure the competence of nursing students during their educational programs, the public may have increased confidence in the ability of nursing graduates to provide knowledgeable, skillful, and sensitive nursing care.

## REFERENCES

Barrows, H. (1971). *Simulated patients (programmed patients)*. Springfield, IL: Charles C. Thomas.

Berk, R. A. (Ed.). (1980). *Criterion-referenced measurement: The state of the art*. Baltimore: John Hopkins University Press.

Bower, F. L. (1974). Normative- or criterion-referenced evaluation. *Nursing Outlook, 22*(8), 449-502.

Breyer, F. J. (1983). Setting passing scores. *Nursing and Health Care, 4*(9), 518-522.

Ebel, R. L. (1979). *Essentials of educational measurement*. Englewood Cliffs, NJ: Prentice-Hall.

Field, W., Gallman, L., Nicholson, R. & Dreher, M. (1984). Clinical competencies of baccalaureate students. *Journal of Nursing Education, 23*,(7), 284-293.

Hambleton, R. K., & Powell, S. (1983). A framework for viewing the process of standard setting. *Evaluation and the Health Professions. 6*(1), 3-24.

King, E. (1979). Determining and interpreting test validity, reliability and practicality. *Nurse Educator, 4*(3), 6-11.

Kolb, S., & Shugart, E. (1984). Evaluation: Is simulation the answer? *Journal of Nursing Education, 23*(2), 84-86.

Krumme, U. (1975). The case for criterion-referenced measurement. *Nursing Outlook, 23*(12), 764-770.

Lenburg, C. (1979). *The Clinical Performance Examination.* New York: Appleton-Century-Crofts.

Lincoln, R., Layton, J., & Holdman, H. (1978). Using simulated patients to teach assessment. *Nursing Outlook, 26*(5), 316-320.

Loustau, A., Lentz, M., Lee, K., McKenna, M., Hirako, S., Walker, W., & Goldsmith, J. (1980). Evaluation student's clinical performance: Using videotape to establish rater reliability. *Journal of Nursing Education, 19*(7), 10-17.

Martuza, V. (1977). *Applying norm-referenced and criterion-referenced measurement in education.* Boston: Allyn & Bacon.

McBride, H., Littlefield, J., & Garman, R. (1981). A simulation method of measuring psychomotor nursing skills. *Evaluation and the Health Professions, 4*(3), 295-305.

McDowell, J., Nardini, D., Negley, S., & White, J. (1984). Evaluating clinical performance using simulated patients. *Journal of Nursing Education, 23*(1), 37-39.

Morgan, B., Luke, C., & Herbert, J. (1979). Evaluating clinical proficiency. *Nursing Outlook, 27*(8), 540-544.

Morgan, M., & Irby, D. (1978). *Evaluating clinical competence in the health professions.* St. Louis: C. V. Mosby.

Newble, D., Elmslie, R., & Baxter, A. (1978). A problem-based criterion-referenced examination of clinical competence. *Journal of Medical Education, 53*, 720-726.

Popham, W. J. (1978a). *Criterion-referenced measurement.* Englewood Cliffs, NJ: Prentice-Hall.

Popham, W. J. (1978b). Measurement requisites for competency assurance in the health professions. *Evaluation and the Health Professions, 1*(1), 9-15.

Shaycoft, M. (1979). *Handbook of criterion-referenced testing: Development, evaluation, and use.* New York: Garland STPM Press.

Thorndike, E. L. (Ed.). (1971). *Educational Measurement* (2nd ed.). Washington, DC: American Council of Education.

Waltz, C., Strickland, O., & Lenz, E. (1984). *Measurement in nursing research.* Philadelphia: F. A. Davis.

Wood, V. (1982). Evaluation of student nurse clinical performance – a continuing problem. *International Nursing Review, 29*(1), 11-18.

Wolley, A. S. (1977). The long and tortured history of clinical evaluation. *Nursing Outlook, 25*(5), 308-315.

Wyman, J., & Ferman, K. (1977). Developing a criterion-referenced tool. *Nursing Outlook, 25*(9), 584-586.

# Simulated Clinical Performance Examination Measurement Tool

Student _____     Date _____

Score _____ Pass/Fail _____     Evaluator _____

*Purpose*: The purpose of the tool is to measure the clinical competence of a beginning nursing student in a baccalaureate program at the conclusion of the first clinical nursing course in the care of a convalescing postoperative adult patient in a simulated clinical situation. The student demonstrates competence by applying the knowledge and skills learned in a fundamental theoretical course as related to the five objectives identified in the tool.

*Directions*: Place a check in the column labeled *Yes* if the behavior was performed. Place a check in the column labeled *No* if the behavior was not performed. Use the comment column only for clarification of an unusual circumstance. Complete the checklist during the student's actual performance. Student's written and audiocassette test materials are to be evaluated at the completion of the testing time.

*Definition*: As used in this tool, the term *Yes* affirms that the behavior as identified was performed in a manner expected of a nursing student in the beginning-level clinical nursing course and the application of knowledge in meeting the nursing needs of an adult postoperative patient was demonstrated.

**OBJECTIVE:** Student demonstrates use of the nursing process in the delivery of nursing care (cognitive domain of learning).

| Behavior | Yes | No | Comment |
|---|---|---|---|

1. Collects relevant objective data
   a) biological/physiological data
   b) psychological/emotional data
   c) social data
   d) spiritual data
   e) cultural data
   f) pathophysiological data
   g) data on prescribed medications
   h) laboratory data
2. Collects subjective data from the patient that is
   a) relevant to the patient situation
   b) Significant to the patient situation

3. Determines nursing diagnoses
   a) based on interpretation of data collected
   b) based on diagnoses originating from the
      Fifth National Conference on the Classifi-
      cation of Nursing Diagnoses
4. Develops goals of care that are
   a) relevant based on patient needs
   b) specific to the patient situation
   c) realistic for the patient situation
   d) short term/long term
   e) clearly stated
5. Prioritizes the goals of care in terms of significance to the present patient condition.
6. States rationale for the priorities of care that are
   a) accurate based on patient needs
   b) clearly specified
7. Develops plan of care based on the nursing
   diagnoses and goals of care that is
   a) accurate
   b) specific
8. Demonstrates during the implementation of
   plan of care
   a) organizational ability
   b) flexibility based on patient's preferences
      and needs
   c) accuracy in carrying out nursing
      interventions
   d) proficiency in carrying out nursing
      interventions
   e) thoroughness in completion of care
   f) safety in carrying out nursing interventions
9. Evaluates effectiveness of care given by
   describing clearly and specifically
   a) achievement of goals
   b) response of patient to care given
   c) modifications for the plan of care


**OBJECTIVE:** Student demonstrates use of oral and written communication
            skills (cognitive domain of learning).

| Behavior | Yes | No | Comment |
| --- | --- | --- | --- |

Oral Communication:
1. Initiates interaction by introducing self
2. Identifies the patient
3. Listens attentively to patient's comments
4. Maintains appropriate eye contact

5. Speaks to the patient
   a) clearly
   b) audibly
   c) directly
6. Speaks using language that is understandable to the patient
7. Elicits additional data during the interaction
8. Elicits patient's perception of the situation
9. Explains care to be given with correct information
10. Responds to patient's questions/comments using accepted therapeutic communication techniques.
11. Teaches patient based on need using teaching-learning principles
12. Observes for and responds to patient's nonverbal communication
13. Uses nonverbal communication techniques appropriately
14. Gives report of the patient's situation on an audiocassette tape being
    a) accurate as to needs, progress, changes, and/or additional data
    b) concise

Written Communication:
15. Uses the problem-oriented method of charting
16. Documents care given on the treatment form
17. Charts data related to identified problems
18. Includes objective and/or subjective data describing patient's situation
19. Uses descriptive terms to record data
20. Records assessment based on data
21. Writes the assessment in terms of interpretation of the data
22. Writes the plan including specific times and directions for providing the care
23. Reflects progress made relative to goal(s)
24. Uses standard abbreviations
25. Writes legibly
26. Includes signature

**OBJECTIVE:** Student demonstrates use of a helping relationship with the patient (affective domain of learning).

| Behavior | Yes | No | Comment |
| --- | --- | --- | --- |

1. Gives complete attention to the patient
2. Approaches patient in an accepting (nonjudgmental) manner
3. Demonstrates willingness to provide care
4. Demonstrates empathy during provision of care
5. Demonstrates patience during provision of care
6. Attends to feelings and concerns expressed or implied by the patient
7. Responds to feelings and concerns expressed or implied by the patient
8. Responds to patient in supportive manner
9. Responds to the spiritual needs of the patient
10. Respects the individuality of the patient by
    a)  offering appropriate choices in care
    b)  considering age of the patient
11. Accepts the strengths and limitations of the patient
    a)  considering patient's coping ability
    b)  considering patient's age

**OBJECTIVE:** Student performs the psychomotor skills according to accepted principles and procedure using the proper supplies (psychomotor and cognitive domains of learning).

| Behavior | Yes | No | Comment |
| --- | --- | --- | --- |

1. Gives the oral medications
   a)  Washes hands prior to giving the medications
   b)  Selects correct medication checking the standard 3 times
   c)  Measures correct dosage
   d)  Identifies patient by name and identification band
   e)  Gives medications at the correct time
   f)  Explains, giving correct information regarding the
       1) action
       2) dosage
       3) frequency
       4) significant side effects
   g)  Charts medications given immediately

2. Carries out a simple dressing change
   a) Washes hands prior to changing the dressing
   b) Provides privacy
   c) Explains procedure to be done accurately
   d) Places patient in proper position
   e) Removes soiled dressing without contaminating the wound or self
   f) Places soiled dressing in refuse bag
   g) Applies sterile dressing aseptically onto the wound
   h) Secures the new dressing properly with tape
3. Transfers patient from the bed to a chair using the pivot method
   a) Involves the patient actively in the procedure by encouraging independence as appropriate
   b) Prepares chair for usage, i.e., places pillows in chair to prevent flexion beyond 90° for a total hip replacement patient
   c) Assists patient to sit up on edge of bed using accepted methods
   d) Assists with putting on robe
   e) Puts walking shoes on
   f) Instructs patient about
      1) avoiding internal rotation of the leg with a hip replacement
      2) keeping the legs abducted with a hip replacement
   g) Assists patient to pivot on unaffected leg toward the chair
   h) Instructs patient in preparation to sitting
      1) to feel the chair back of the knees
      2) to reach for the arm of the chair
   i) Uses appropriate body mechanics
4. Ambulates patient using a 3- or 4-point gait with crutches
   a) Involves the patient actively in the procedure by encouraging independence as appropriate
   b) Checks proper fitting of crutches to the patient
   c) Gives correct information about usage of proper gait
   d) Checks for
      1) erect posture
      2) steadiness
      3) amount of weight bearing per doctor's order

**OBJECTIVE:** Student demonstrates application of knowledge essential in meeting the nursing needs of an adult postoperative patient (cognitive domain of learning).

| Knowledge essential based on simulated patient needs and the behavior | Yes | No | Comment |
|---|---|---|---|

A.  Alteration in comfort
    1.  Assess the pain for
        a) location
        b) duration
        c) intensity
        d) quality
        e) onset
    2.  Intervenes by
        a) checking time of last analgesic administration
        b) selection of appropriate pain medication
        c) use of comfort measures (positioning, rest, relaxing environment)
B.  Alteration in urinary system function
    1.  Assess for signs of cystitis
        a) dysuria
        b) frequency
        c) urgency
        d) inspection of urine
    2.  Intervenes by
        a) encouraging increased oral fluid intake
        b) recording intake and output
        c) giving correct information on preventive measures (cleansing, undergarments, irritants)
C.  Function of gastrointestinal system
    1.  Assess bowel status by checking for
        a) date of last movement
        b) characteristics of the bowel movement
    2.  Intervenes by
        a) allowing a choice by the patient of taking a medication or not
        b) giving correct information on diet, fluid intake, activity
D.  Function on musculoskeletal system
    1.  Assess movement and sensation of the toes
    2.  Intervenes by observing for accuracy when the patient does the
        a) isometric exercises (quadricap, hamstring, gluteal)
        b) range of motion of the ankle exercises

E. Function of the respiratory system
   1. Assesses the color/warmth of the toes or the pedal pulses
   2. Intervenes by informing the patient about the findings
F. Function of the respiratory system
   1. Assesses patient's method of deep breathing exercises
   2. Intervenes by giving correct information about deep breathing
G. Integrity of the skin
   1. Assesses the surgical incision for
      a) intactness
      b) drainage
      c) redness
      d) warmth
      e) swelling
   2. Intervenes by informing the patient about the healing of the incision

## Scoring Key*

Pass – performs 85% of the behaviors.
Fail – does not perform 85% of the behaviors.
Total number of behaviors – 140; 85%=119 behaviors.

*Guidelines are available for evaluators to use in determining if the behaviors were performed or not.

# 15

# Measuring Baccalaureate Students' Nursing Process Competencies: A Nursing Diagnosis Framework

## Ursel Krumme

*This chapter discusses four tools – Critical Elements for Clinical Performance for Oriented Adult Clients with Acute Pain, ...with Chronic Pain, ...with Altered Sleep-Wakefulness Patterns, and ...Requiring Health Teaching – measures of nursing process competencies.*

The purpose of this study was to measure baccalaureate students' nursing process competencies using valid and reliable instruments developed around nursing diagnoses. The specific objectives were (1) to describe students' nursing assessment behaviors: the identification of subjective data, objective data, nursing diagnoses and "related to" statements; and (2) to describe students' nursing management behaviors: the identification of client-family outcomes, deadlines, client-family/nurse actions and the extent to which outcomes are met.

## OUTCOME VARIABLE SELECTED FOR MEASUREMENT

Nursing process competencies of baccalaureate students in clinical practice were selected as the study outcome variable for measurement. The faculty's commitment to the assessment of student learning outcomes at Seattle University's School of Nursing (1981a) is stated in its philosophy:

This study was supported in part by the Measurement of Clinical and Educational Nursing Outcomes Project, University of Maryland School of Nursing; a Seattle University Fall 1984 sabbatic; and a Seattle University 1981 Summer Fellowship. The author gratefully acknowledges the support of student participation by School of Nursing faculty, especially that of Rose DeGracia. Inquiries can be sent to the author at Seattle University School of Nursing, Seattle, WA 98122.

"We believe the teacher must evaluate learning outcomes"; "We believe the teacher is responsible for evaluation of the learner's progress toward objectives" (p. 7). Nursing process competencies comprise major educational outcomes of students working with client-families. These competencies are reiterated in the school's program, level, and clinical course objectives (Seattle University School of Nursing 1981a, 1981b). To cite an example, students enrolled in Basic Nursing II, who work with adult client-families in medical-surgical hospital settings, are expected to demonstrate the following nursing process competencies (see Table 15.1 for detailed behaviors):

   I. Applies process of systematically collecting a nursing data base.
  II. A. Articulates client-family problems.
     B. Establishes expected client-family outcomes and deadlines.
     C. Determines client-family/nurse actions.
     D. Discusses extent to which outcomes are met.

The school's expected student nursing process competencies are appropriately modeled after the nursing process components found in the profession's *Standards of Nursing Practice* [American Nurses' Association (ANA), 1973]:

     I. The collection of data about the health status of the client/patient is systematic and continuous.
    II. Nursing diagnoses are derived from health status data.
   III. The plan of nursing care includes goals derived from the nursing diagnoses.
 IV, V, VI. The plan of nursing includes. . . client-patient/nurse. . . measures to achieve the goals derived from the nursing diagnoses.
 VII, VIII. The client/patient's progress or lack of progress. . . toward goal achievement directs reassessment. . . and revision of the plan of nursing care. (pp. 2-5)

This study attempted to describe baccalaureate students' nursing process competencies, specifically students' nursing assessment and management behaviors with client-families in clinical practice (see Table 15.1). Selected nursing diagnoses were used as the framework around which to develop valid and objective test items. Students' nursing assessment behaviors were defined as the identification of subjective data, objective data, nursing diagnoses, and "related to" statements. Students' nursing management behaviors were defined as the identification of client-family outcomes, deadlines, client-family/nurse actions, and the extent to which outcomes are met.

**TABLE 15.1 Nursing Process Competencies Expected of Basic Nursing II Students**[a]

| | | |
|---|---|---|
| C3 | I. | Applies process of systematically collecting a nursing data base of one client-family assigned weekly by clinical instructor |
| C3 | A. | Takes a nursing history that includes sociocultural and religious assessments |
| C3 | B. | Records physical assessment data |
| C3 | C. | Records diagnostic, laboratory, medication, and treatment data |
| C3 | II. | Applies the nursing process to one client-family assigned weekly |
| C3 | A. | Articulates client-family problems (physiological and psychosocial) |
| C2 | 1. | Classifies problems according to actual, potential, and possible categories |
| C3 | 2. | Established priorities among identified problems |
| C3 | 3. | Relates subjective data from client-family for each identified problem |
| C3 | 4. | Relates objective data from client-family record for each identified problem: e.g., diagnostic, laboratory test, operating room, pathology, and PT/OT reports |
| C2 | 5. | Cites psychosocial and cultural factors underlying problems |
| C2 | 6. | Estimates possible cause(s) of problem(s) |
| C2 | 7. | Explains pathophysiological alteration underlying problem(s) |
| C3 | B. | Establishes expected client-family outcomes and deadlines for both short- and long-term goals |
| C3 | 1. | Articulates optimal health outcomes and deadlines referenced in the literature for identified client-family problems |
| C2 | 2. | Cites health outcomes and deadlines selected by client-family for identified problems |
| C3 | C. | Determines client-family/nurse actions |
| C3 | 1. | Articulates actions client-family selected to achieve health outcomes including nursing actions |
| C2 | 2. | Explains rationale behind contracted client-family/nurse actions |
| A3 | 3. | Appreciates roles played by members of the health team |
| C2 | 4. | Explains rationale behind therapeutic regimens initiated by other health team members (physician, physical/occupational therapist, social worker, nutritionist, etc.) |
| C2 | 5. | Discusses results of nursing research findings when planning and/or carrying out client-family/nurse actions |
| C2 | D. | Discusses extent to which outcomes are met. |
| C2 | 1. | Cites client-family behaviors that meet/do not meet each health outcome |
| C2 | 2. | Cites alternative actions possible to assure each health outcome is attained |

[a] Classified according to the taxonomies of educational objectives accepted by faculty.

## REVIEW AND ANALYSIS OF LITERATURE RELATED TO NURSING PROCESS COMPETENCIES

In 1973 the nursing profession, by publishing its *Standards of Nursing Practice* identified the nursing process as a specific activity that distinguished it from other health care disciplines (ANA, 1973, pp. 2-5). In a recent survey of National League for Nursing (NLN)-accredited baccalaureate programs, Gaines and McFarland (1984) reported that nearly all (98.6%) of such programs hold students accountable for nursing process competencies according to these practice standards. The *Standards,* reaffirmed by the American Nurses' Association in its 1980 *Social Policy Statement* (pp. 15-16), were originally conceived as a means "to provide measures to judge the competency of its members" as well as "to evaluate the quality of its services" (ANA, 1973, p. 1).

Fredette and O'Connor's (1979) belief that "knowledge and skill in the utilization of the nursing process is one of the most significant and relevant areas of expertise that the student of nursing must acquire" (p. 541) led their baccalaureate faculty to search for ways to operationalize this belief in their program's theory and clinical nursing courses. They describe student/faculty efforts to devise course-specific patient collection tools to serve as guides for the identification of subjective and objective data to support each nursing diagnosis and for subsequent student writing of weekly clinical papers, with instructor feedback to provide the needed repetition for the development of patient care planning skills. The authors state that a majority of the accepted nursing diagnoses have been integrated into their junior year theoretic content and that it is essential for professional nursing programs to evaluate the competency of students' abilities in these areas in actual practice. Yet, no mention is made of tested instruments developed by faculty around which to evaluate students' nursing process competencies with the identified nursing diagnoses.

The aforementioned findings regarding the lack of faculty-developed, tested, and reliable instruments around which to evaluate student's nursing process competencies using a nursing diagnosis framework is not surprising. Kritek, in 1978, argued that nursing is in a dilemma because its *Standards of Practice* exceed the tools that it possesses to measure that practice. Mallick (1983), however, in countering this argument as it relates to student evaluation of nursing process competencies, states: "Tools are available even though they may be primitive instruments" (p. 459). She supports Gordon's (1982) case for the use of the approved nursing diagnoses as the "ideal tool for writing nursing-specific process and outcome standards" (p. 276). Gordon also points out that "nursing diagnoses describe the independent domain of nursing practice. Thus nurses assume accountability for health problems described by these diagnostic labels. It follows logically that nursing diagnoses should be used to define client populations for care review" (p. 276). Indeed, in an attempt to tie in such an approach to the evaluation of a practicing nurse's clinical performance, Warren (1983) concludes:

Given the patient data base, . . the diagnosis, . . the expected patient outcomes, . . and appropriate nursing interventions, . . peers could determine
whether or not a nurse was demonstrating competent practice. It would also
facilitate in identifying areas for growth and development. . . . This is an
exciting concept: can staff consistently and accurately diagnose and treat
(actual or potential problems)? . . . and . . . what can staff development do to
assist their mastery of these diagnoses? (p. 36)

To date, however, no instrument has been reported in the literature
that uses nursing diagnoses as the framework around which to measure
the nursing process competencies outlined in the profession's standards.
Indeed, the research that has been conducted to date has focused primarily on making the nursing diagnosis itself. Guided by the belief that without such problem identification there is no need to continue with the
other components of the process, researchers have found that nurses are
neither comfortable nor highly competent with the activities related to
this strategic aspect of the nursing process.

For example, Aspinall (1976) designed a study to examine the nursing
diagnostic skills of graduate nurses from associate, diploma, and baccalaureate programs through use of written case studies. Although the
information given about the patient's history and clinical follow-up
pointed to 12 possible nursing diagnoses (as validated by a group of nurse
experts), results revealed that none of the graduates could identify all 12;
only 1 to 9 problems, with a mean of 3.44, were listed by the graduates.
Still, an interesting finding reported here was that the diagnostic skills of
baccalaureate graduate nurses were significantly better than those of the
graduates of the other two programs, leading the author to conclude that
nursing diagnostic skills may prove to be a truly distinguishing characteristic between technical and professional nursing practice.

In one other study reported in the literature, DeBack (1981) analyzed
nursing care plans of senior nursing students in baccalaureate schools by
applying predetermined criteria to the nursing diagnosis step of the nursing
process (which she also felt was not only an assumed outcome of their educational preparation but also the most crucial aspect of the nursing process to
be evaluated). These findings were not the resounding success anticipated:
of 200 care plans analyzed, only 28% met all three predetermined criteria,
and 35% of them met none of the three outlined criteria (with no significant
effect noted for a school's particular curricular model). Nevertheless, 56%
of the care plans met Criterion 1, the statement of an actual or potential
health concern of the client; 34% met Criterion 2, a client concern
expressed according to level of dysfunction; and 49% met Criterion 3, a
statement of a client concern that nurses could resolve.

From these data, DeBack (1981) concluded that senior students in baccalaureate nursing programs are seriously deficient in their ability to
carry out the most strategic step of the nursing process – the formulation
of nursing diagnoses. She conjectures that this deficit may be due to the
lack of attention given to the needed detail in this step of the problem-

solving methodology of the nursing process. She further feels that untilthe extent to which nursing diagnosis is used, understood, and taught by nursing faculty is investigated and curricula altered accordingly, students' abilities in this crucial step of the nursing process are likely not to improve. She makes a case for the assessment of nursing students' abilities to include types of testing that can determine whether needed skills for formulating nursing diagnosis have been learned: "In the absence of a problem identification there is no need to continue with the other components of the [nursing] process because there would exist no objective basis for planning, for interventions, or for evaluative judgments about the client's problems" (p. 52).

In a survey conducted by McLane (1982) in 1980, it was reported that 81% of NLN-accredited baccalaureate programs integrated nursing diagnosis concepts and skills in most or all of their program's clinical courses. Gaines and McFarland subsequently report in a 1984 survey that this number has increased to 94.7%, with 89.2% of baccalaureate programs including nursing diagnosis content in both theory and clinical medical-surgical courses (81.5% of the schools reported that they taught the diagnostic categories developed by the National Conference Group, since 1982 known as the North American Nursing Diagnosis Association). They further stated:

> Documentation of nursing diagnoses in the patient's permanent record is a way of demonstrating the extent to which the ANA standards of nursing practice are being met . . . as more nursing students who use nursing diagnosis as a natural part of their care graduate, adequate tests of its clinical usefulness can be conducted . . . . The continued interest in nursing diagnosis in the practice setting provides an exciting challenge to nurse educators and clinicians alike. (pp. 42, 49)

There continues to be consensus, as reported by nurse educators and administrators in the literature since the dissemination of the 1973 standards, that nursing process competencies are expected performance behaviors of graduates of nursing programs (see, for example, ANA, 1981; National League for Nursing, 1982; New Mexico SNAP Project, 1979; Orange County/Long Beach Nursing Consortium, 1981; Williams & Scott-Warner, 1985). However, the measurement of nursing process competencies with client families in actual practice as reported in the literature, seems to continue to raise more questions than answers. For example, Benner (1982) in discussing the issues involved in assessing nursing process abilities of students in a competency-based testing program, states: "While the nursing process works well for teaching the beginning student how to approach a patient care situation, it does not work well as a means of identifying required competencies . . . . The competency statements it generates are too global (pp. 303-304). In citing a typical competency test item as an example – "Defines complex problems utilizing multiple resources including the client, family, community, etc." – Benner

(1982) justifiably points out that the content and practices inherent in the performance behavior item are omitted, thereby limiting its usefulness in a competency-based testing program for assessing nursing process competencies; "The skills included in this 'assessment competency' are legion and the possible variations are infinite" (p. 304).

Mallick, in 1977, stated that even when nursing knowledge is presented according to a nursing diagnosis framework, such as the care of a patient with pain, there is a similar lack of attention paid to the content and practices of expected nursing performance behaviors. For example, she cites the following:

> Students are given no guidance as to what data need to be collected in order to make an assessment that pain is indeed present, no description of systematic methods by which reliable data can be collected, no criteria by which levels of pain may be differentiated, and so on. . . . Students are overwhelmed by the task. . . that they must reorganize their knowledge into an action-oriented framework appropriate to the clinical setting. (p. 246)

In chiding nurse educators for their neglect of providing such explicit guidance for the application of nursing process skills with client-families during practice, Mallick (1977) concludes with the statement that "application is something that can be taught; it need not be left for the student to discover for herself" (p. 247).

Citing the challenge presented for the 1980s as the improvement of the quality of nursing care delivered to client-families, Van Maanen (1981) states that the majority of quality monitoring instruments developed to date have "focussed on nursing tasks and procedures rather than on more comprehensive aspects of nursing and patient care. . . comprehensive care. . . includes how the patient feels about his anxiety/pain" (p. 33). Conceding that the objective measurement of comprehensive patient care will be hard to accomplish, Van Maanen nevertheless identifies that one optimum feasible approach at present is to quantify the process of care in detail. The study reported here used such an approach in the measurement of baccalaureate students' nursing process competencies: Detailed nursing assessment and management behaviors were identified for selected nursing diagnoses. Nursing process competencies were determined by an instructor's evaluation of a student's application of the expected behaviors with client-families in clinical practice.

## REVIEW AND ANALYSIS OF EXISTING CRITERION-REFERENCED MEASUREMENT TOOLS AND PROCEDURES FOR MEASURING NURSING PROCESS COMPETENCIES

Relatively few attempts to measure nursing process competencies of baccalaureate students or practicing nurses against objective and valid criteria, using criterion-referenced measurement tools, have been reported in the literature. These efforts nevertheless point out the importance that some faculty and administrators have placed on the measurement of nursing process competencies as expected outcomes of their program's educational experience(s) and/or nursing practice.

Pearson (1977), for example, described faculty work undertaken at the University of Wisconsin – Milwaukee to design five evaluation videotapes for a response television system that tests the "complete nursing process competencies of baccalaureate students" (p. 1). The videotapes describe "common episodes" encountered in "real practice" that test each component of the nursing process via a different simulated patient situation. Content-validated by nursing faculty, "the competency testing is seen as an integral part of the clinical aspects of the nursing curriculum" (p. 14). The tapes are stated to be also used as evaluation tools for determining placement of the RN student in the baccalaureate curriculum. Reliability data for the predetermined criteria, however, are not reported. Interestingly, moreover, the identification of nursing diagnoses is not included as one of the phases comprising nursing process (in this study noted to be data collection, validation, interpretation, formulation of hypotheses, formulation of plan of care, implementation, and evaluation of nursing care).

In yet another study that used videotapes with simulated patient situations to assess baccalaureate students' nursing process competencies, Loustau and her faculty (1980) at the University of Washington describe the difficulties encountered in establishing interrater reliability for items related to nursing process. In no instance of a paired faculty observation of a student's videotaped performance was the desired 80% agreement attained. In this study, however, students' identification of nursing diagnoses was included as a component of nursing process competencies.

As part of the bachelor of science in nursing requirements for the University of the State of New York Regents External Degree Program at Albany (1976, 1978), students take a specially designed Clinical Performance Nursing Examination (CPNE). Originally designed for the associate-degree evaluation program and administered in a hospital setting, this 2½-day examination tests students' application of nursing process in caring for several child and adult patients (University of the State of New York, 1976, pp. 7-9). Critical elements are listed for required and selected areas as well as for areas of overriding concern (see Table 15.2 for tested areas). The rigorous validity and reliability testing procedures undertaken for this examination included generation and validation of nursing process domain items by a panel of experts representing respective clinical areas, a comparison of performance by qualified and unqualified student groups, and determination of interrater agreement by faculty clinical evaluators following an intensive orientation program (University of the State of New York, 1976; Lenburg, 1976, 1979).

Subsequently added to the evaluation program for the bachelor of science in nursing degree were three simulated tests: (1) the Health Assessment Examination, which measures students' ability to collect and analyze data from a client's health assessment; (2) the Teaching Examination, which measures students' ability to assess, plan, and implement a brief teaching episode; and (3) the Professional Performance Examination, which uses videotaped vignettes to assess students' competencies in the management of client care, leadership, research, collaboration, and clinical decision making (University of the State of New York, 1978, p. 6). Despite the rigor and comprehensive nature of this competency program, it should be noted, however, that an integrative system incorporating nursing diagnoses as a framework for the development of test items to assess baccalaureate students' nursing process competencies was not used.

As part of the University of Washington School of Nursing's baccalaureate curriculum revision project, Krumme (1977) described a model and methodology for evaluating students' nursing process competencies around patient population health/wellness outcomes. It was also suggested at the time that "Patient Problems (Actual and Potential)" could be substituted without changing the essence of the model. As in the aforecited studies, criterion-referenced measurement was used because "objectivity in evaluation and validity and reliability in measurement of performance, can best be secured using criterion-referenced rather than norm-referenced tools" (Krumme, 1975, p. 764; see also Ward & Lindeman, 1978, pp. 257-530).

Krumme's (1977) suggested process for constructing and validating nursing assessment and management performance evaluation items was subsequently refined at Seattle University's School of Nursing around a nursing diagnosis framework (Krumme, 1981; see also Table 15.2). Instruments were developed to measure students' nursing process competencies for the nursing diagnoses "alterations in comfort (acute or chronic)," "sleep pattern disturbance," and "knowledge deficit." As part of the University of Maryland Outcome Measurement Project, of which Krumme was an ongoing participant, these instruments underwent additional validity and reliability testing and revision. Also, work was initiated in the construction of new instruments to measure students' nursing process competencies for other high-priority nursing diagnoses identified by faculty: "ineffective breathing pattern/airway clearance," "potential impairment of skin integrity," and "impaired physical mobility."

A review of published instruments to date reveals that criterion- referenced tools that measure an individual's nursing process competencies around nursing diagnoses do not exist outside this author's developmental efforts (see, for example, Ward & Fetler, 1979, Ward & Lindeman, 1978). An analysis of existing criterion-referenced instruments reveals instead that performance items are organized around Abdellah's 21 nursing problems (Abdellah, 1960; Carter, Hilliard, Castles, Stoll, & Cowan, 1976); the phases of assessment, planning, implementation, and evaluation (Haussmann, Hegyvary, & Newman, 1976); outcome criteria for patient populations with medical diagnoses (ANA, 1977; McBride, Mohr,

Smith, Swanson, & Kelly, 1975); and outcome criteria organized around universal and health deviation self-care demand categories adapted from Orem (Horn & Swain, 1977a, b). A brief discussion of the methodology and field testing undertaken in the development of these instruments, although not developed specifically for assessing baccalaureate students' nursing process competencies but rather practicing nurses' competencies, still seems appropriate to include in this review. Particular emphases will be placed on an instrument's evidence of reliability and validity.

Two early 1970 evaluation tools rigorously field-tested for their reliability and validity focus on expected nurse actions with client-family populations (Carter et al., 1976; Haussmann et al., 1976). Carter's process criteria, delineated in the Medical-Surgical and Obstetrical Standards, include items for the "Nursing Care Plan," the "Nursing Record," and "The Patient and His Environment." Conceptually organized around Abdellah's 21 nursing problems into four groups, (Abdellah, 1960; Carter et al., 1976, pp. 8-9), the items specify the following, see also Table 15.2):

1. Nursing measures necessary to maintain hygiene, physical comfort, activity, rest and sleep, safety, and body mechanics.
2. Nursing measures necessary to maintain oxygen supply, nutrition, elimination, fluid and electrolyte balance, regulatory mechanisms, and sensory functions.
3. Nursing measures that should be helpful to the patient and family during their emotional reactions to the patient's illness.
4. Nursing measures that will assist the patient and his family to cope with the illness and the necessary life adjustment.

Evaluators conduct a review of patient records and nursing care plans for baseline data against which to judge whether the indicated measures have indeed been carried out by the nurse. Items are either asked of the patient and/or the family during an interview or answered through observation. Independent scoring of 1,572 items for eight clients by two evaluators revealed disagreement on only eight items; coder agreement on four patient situations was 100%.

Building on the work of Carter et al. (1976) and others, the Medicus Systems Corporation and Rush-Prebyterian-St. Luke's Medical Center (Haussmann & Hegyvary, 1976; Haussmann et al., 1976; Hegyvary, Gortner, & Haussmann, 1976), under a contract awarded by the Division of Nursing in 1972, constructed and validated patient-specific criteria for medical, surgical, pediatric, nursery, and recovery room units. The resulting "Criteria Master List" includes 257 items organized around the following nursing process framework for patients requiring self-, partial, complete, or intensive care (Haussmann, et al., 1976, pp. 71-101):

1. A plan of nursing care is formulated,

2. Physical needs are attended,
3. Nonphysical needs are attended,
4. Nursing care objectives are evaluated.

Data are collected from patient records, interviews, and observations or from nursing personnel interviews and observations. Field-tested in 19 hospitals across the nation, it has been found that with an orientation session two observers achieve better than 90% agreement using an identical 50-item worksheet in a patient situation (Haussmann et al.,1976, p. 17). The Medicus-Rush process tool reportedly continues to fill the need for objective measurement of a hospital's nursing process activities (see, for example, Medicus System Corp., 1985; Smeltzer, Feltman, & Rajki, 1983).

In contrast to Carter and associates' (1976) and Rush-Medicus Corporation's focus on item development around client-family/nurse actions, the Joint Commission on Accreditation of Hospitals' (JCAH) Performance Evaluation Procedures (McBride et al., 1975) and the American Nurses' Association's Guidelines for Review of Nursing Care (1977) focus on the assessment of outcomes, that is, the end results achieved by client-family/nurse actions (see Table 15.2). Organized around medical diagnoses, measurement is done after actions have been taken and recorded. Content-validated by nurse experts in the respective clinical area, high interrater agreement for the items has been reported following detailed orientation sessions to the instruments (Deets, 1976; JCAH, 1974).

One last performance evaluation instrument rigorously tested for its reliability and validity also focuses on the end results of client-family/nurse actions, or "the assessment of outcomes of nursing care process as reflected by patients' physical and emotional status, extent of their knowledge, and their ability to perform self-care" (Horn & Swain, 1977a, p. 1). Discarding medical diagnoses, as well as body systems, around which to develop items, Horn and Swain (1977a, b) used 7 "Universal" and 10 "Health Deviation Demand" categories adapted from Orem's Theory of Self-Care for the instrument's "Health Care Measures of Nursing Care for Adult Medical-Surgical Hospitalized Patients" (see Table 15.2):

1. *Universal Self-Care Demand Measures* necessary for maintaining activities for daily living – 329 items,
2. *Health Deviation Self-Care Demand Measures* necessitated as a result of illness, injury, or disease – 211 items.

In contrast to the retrospective review methodology used in the JCAH Procedures (McBride et al., 1975) and the ANA Guidelines (1977) outcome measurement instruments, data for this tool are collected through direct patient observation and interview while care is administered. All 539 items of Horn and Swain's (1977a) instrument were content-validated by three groups of experts: the nursing project research staff, practicing clinical specialists, and a national advisory panel. A large proportion of 414 items subjected to reliability testing (70 are informational and do not need such testing) achieved 80% or higher interrater agreement.

A synthesis of criterion-referenced measurement instruments that have been used to assess nursing process competencies is presented in Table 15.2.

**TABLE 15.2 Synthesis of Criterion-Referenced Measurement Instruments Used to Assess Nursing Process Competencies**

| Instrument/Framework | Methodology | Field testing |
|---|---|---|
| Carter et al., 1976 Process Criteria Organized Around Abdellah's 21 problems Gp. I Comfort, activity, rest sleep, safety Gp. II Oxygen, nutrition, elimination, fluid-electrolytes, regulatory-sensory functions Gp. III Emotional reaction to illness Gp. IV Coping with illness and life adjustment | Item Forms Nursing care plan Patient record Patient and environment Care sampled on Units: Med-Surg and OB Two observers go to bedside: One interviews patient Other observes patient and environment 80% score considered safe care (25% penalty if safe-level care item not passed) | Validity: content validity by experts Reliability: Independently scored 1,572 items on 8 patients showed disagreement on only 8 items; coder agreement on 4 patient audits, 100% |
| Medicus-Rush: Haussmann et al., 1976 Process criteria organized around nursing process for self-care, partial care, complete care, intensive care | 257 items grouped within 28 subobjectives of nursing care for med-surg, peds/newborn, RR units (50 items relate to environment) Computer generates 50-item worksheet Care sampled on unit Sources of information Patient record, observation, interview Nursing personnel interview Observation Patient environment observation Observer inference Unit management observation | Validity: content validity by experts Reliability Tested in 19 hospitals across nation .9 interrater agreement with orientation session |
| JCAH, 1974; McBride et al., 1975 | Item forms Audit criteria | Validity: Nursing audit commit- |

*(continued)*

**TABLE 15.2** (*Continued*)

| Instrument/Framework | Methodology | Field testing |
|---|---|---|
| Outcome criteria organized around patient population with medical diagnoses | worksheets<br>Records pulled that meet patient population criteria<br>Medical records personnel prepare audit report<br>Outcomes categorized:<br>Those desired to be present 100%<br>Complications 0% of time present | tees content validate items<br>Criteria compared to literature e.g., *Quality Review Bulletin*<br>Reliability: interrater agreement reported high with orientation workshops |
| ANA, 1977<br>Outcome criteria organized around patient populations with medical diagnoses | Item forms<br>Essential HTN, well-population-family, osteoarthritis, nutritional deficiencies, bedridden, maintenance habilitation, respiratory distress, first stage labor, adolescent nutrition, pregnancy, colostomy, acute MI, cholecystectomy, depression – nonpsychotic, alcoholic, psychotic withdrawal | Validity:<br>Content validity by National Task Force experts in Community Health Nursing (CHN) Maternal Child Nursing (MCN), Med-surg, Psych.<br>Reliability:<br>.9 interrater agreement with orientation |
| Horn & Swain, 1977a, 1977b<br>Outcome criteria organized around 8 universal and 10 health deviation self-care demand categories adapted from Orem (1971) | 539 items<br>Universal: 328<br>Demands for air, 70; water, 29; food, 22; elimination, 73; rest/activity/sleep, 110; normality, 23; solitude, 1<br>Health deviation: 211<br>IV and wound observation, 28; pt. knowledge of health deviation, 13; med/injection performance, 61; diet, 23; fluids, 11; exercises, 17; activity restrictions, 11; rest, 13; skin/wound care, 19; using appliances, 15<br>Categorized also according to<br>Evidence that requirement is met | Validity<br>Items content validated for domain representativeness/appropriateness/completeness by research staff members, National Advisory Panel, Clinical Nurse Specialists. Panel and specialists also ranked significance and devised measurements for the variables<br>Reliabiilty<br>Pair of observers used; items scoring .80 or better interrater agreement retained<br>414 items tested for reliability (70 are informational only): 230 (58% proved reliable. |

(*continued*)

**TABLE 15.2** (*Continued*)

| Instrument/Framework | Methodology | Field testing |
| --- | --- | --- |
| | Evidence that patient has necessary knowledge, skill, or motivation to meet requirement<br>Data collected through direct patient observation and interview | |
| CPNE: Univ. of the State of New York, 1976, 1978; Lenburg, 1976, 1979.<br>Process criteria organized around<br>  Required areas: usually readily available and provide uniformity to exam (e.g., vital signs (VS), fluids, mobility)<br>  Selected areas: pre-established array from which to select (e.g., meds, oxygen, dressing change<br>  Overriding areas: continuously monitored: asepsis, physical and emotional jeopardy | Item forms<br>  Critical elements listed for required, selected and overriding areas of care<br>  Planning, implementation, and evaluation phase of nursing process judged; 5 patient care situations–2 children, 3 adults–must be passed<br>  Two nursing laboratory experiences; oral meds, IM & IV meds/sterile dressing change must be passed<br>  Standard to pass: 100% of critical elements met and no failure of overriding areas | Validity<br>  Item generation of domain examined<br>  Panel of experts representing clinical areas content validate items<br>  Qualified and unqualified groups compared<br>Reliability: High interrater agreement achieved with orientation to instrument |
| Krumme, 1977; 1981<br>Process criteria organizes around nursing process<br>  Client-family problems/ nursing diagnosis<br>  Subjective data<br>  Objective data<br>  "Due to" statement<br>  Expected outcomes with deadlines<br>  Client-family/nurse actions<br>  Extent to which outcomes are met | Item forms<br>  Acute pain<br>  Chronic pain<br>  Sleep pattern disturbance<br>  Knowledge deficit<br>  Ineffective breathing pattern/airway clearance<br>  Potential impairement of skin integrity<br>  Impaired physical mobility<br>Data collected through:<br>  Nursing database form<br>  Nursing care plan<br>  Progress note recording<br>Critical elements must be met; however, 80% pass considered mastery | Validity<br>  Tables of specifications for content/objectives<br>  Criterion-referenced test specifications<br>  Interrater agreement of relevance and importance of items by nurse educators, clinical specialists<br>Reliability<br>  Interrater agreement of item scoring<br>  Stability of ratings over time |

## STEPS UNDERTAKEN IN THE DEVELOPMENT, REFINEMENT, AND TESTING OF INSTRUMENTS

### Construction of Tools Measuring Students' Nursing Process Competencies With Client-Families

Students' expected nursing assessment and management behaviors are outlined in Table 15.1. A student's nursing process competencies are determined by the instructor's evaluation of the application of the expected behaviors with client-families in clinical practice. Prior experience indicated that the clinical objectives were clearly vulnerable to instructor bias and subjectivity in rating. The specific problem that remained was how to develop test items that would be referenced to the expected nursing process behaviors. The decision was made to use the framework of nursing diagnosis. In the context, nursing assessment behaviors were defined as the identification of subjective data, objective data, nursing diagnosis, and "related to" statements. Nursing management behaviors were defined as the identification of client-family expected outcomes, deadlines, client-family/nurse actions, and the extent to which outcomes are met.

Using the list of the Task Force of the National Group for the Classification of Nursing Diagnoses (Kim, McFarland, & McLane, 1984), faculty selected "Alteration in comfort: acute and chronic pain," and "Sleep pattern disturbance" as diagnoses around which initial test items would be developed that could serve as representative samples of the domain of students' nursing process behaviors. Test items measuring students' nursing process behaviors with adult clients with "Knowledge deficit(s)" were subsequently added. As part of this Measurement Outcomes Project, additional work was undertaken in the development of test items for three other nursing diagnoses identified as high priority by faculty: "Ineffective breathing pattern/airway clearance," "Potential impairment for skin integrity," and "Impaired physical mobility" (these tools are still being refined and are not included in this presentation).

There were basically four steps involved in the construction of test items referenced to students' expected nursing assessent and management behaviors for the selected nursing diagnoses. (For further elaboration see Gronlund, 1973; Krumme, 1977; Popham, 1972.)

1. Identification of criteria that must be met by the client-family for the identified nursing diagnoses (for example, for "Alterations in comfort: acute or chronic pain" the adult must be oriented and have an analgesic prescribed, as needed or time-contingent; for "Sleep pattern disturbance" the adult must be oriented and have a hypnotic prescribed, as needed, etc.).
2. Development of a table of specifications outlining the essential item-content areas for the selected nursing diagnoses on one axis and the nursing assessment and management objectives on the other axis. (See sample in Table 15.3.)

3. Identification of the specific student behaviors for each cell of the resulting two-dimensional table of specifications that would provide evidence for the attainment of the objectives for the essential item-content areas outlined for the selected nursing diagnoses. (See sample in Table 15.3.)
4. Writing, pilot-testing, and rewriting test items in objective, measurable terms. (See instruments at end of chapter.)

**TABLE 15.3 Sample Table of Specifications: Critical Student Nursing Assessment and Management Behaviors for Adult Clients with Acute Pain**

| Content areas/objectives | Collects data in specific client situation Cognitive: application | Implements client-family/ nurse actions Cognitive: application-evaluation |
|---|---|---|
| Subjective data | | |
| Location | States location of client's pain | |
| Intensity | Describes intensity of client's pain on scale of 1 to 10 | |
| Type | Describes type of client's pain e.g., burning, cramping, bloating | |
| Duration | States how long client's pain has been present | |
| Chronology | Describes precipitating events/aggravating factors | |
| Coping methods | Describes ways client controls pain (past/current) | Implements individual ized pain relief measures |
| Beliefs | States client's beliefs about pain (culture/ religion) | |
| | | |
| Objective data | | |
| Behavioral responses | States behavioral responses, e.g., body position, facial expression, splinting activity | |
| Physiological responses | States physiological responses, e.g., alterations in pulse/ respiration/blood pressure, persp., nausea/vomiting, pallor, distention | |
| Contributing factors | State contributing factors e.g., fatigue, concerns, worries | Encourages/listens to expressions of fears/ concerns/worries |

*(continued)*

**TABLE 15.3** (*Continued*)

| Content areas/objectives | Collects data in specific client situation Cognitive: application | Implements client-family/ nurse actions Cognitive: application-evaluation |
|---|---|---|
| Possible cause of pain "Due to" statement Underlying patho-psychosocial alteration | Gives "due to" statement Explain underlying pathophysiological/ psychosocial alteration | |
| Comfort measures Bedpan/bath/ pericare/change of linen, dressing rein-forcement Positioning/ambulating Hot/cold applications | | Offers/gives bed pan, bath, oral, pericare, change of linen, rein-forcement of dressing Positions/ambulates Applies hot/cold measures |
| Other relief measures Distraction | | Provides distraction, e.g., radio, TV, visits |
| Relaxation techniques | States presence/location of muscle tension | Implements relaxation technique e.g., DB, mas-sage (unless contraindi-cated), centering |
| Medication administration Pattern of analgesic administration | Describes client's pat-terns of analgesic ad-ministration past 48 hr | Offers analgesic at pre-cribed intervals (if respi-ration 10-12 for narcotics) |
| Analgesic | | Administers analgesics within 15 min of request |
| Expected outcomes/ deadlines/evaluation No verbal or nonverbal expression of pain | States "no verbal or non-verbal expression of pain" | Checks client within 30 minutes following pain relief measure other than analgesic |
| Performs activities, e.g., deep breathing, cough-ing, ambulating | States "performs activi-ties, e.g., deep breathing, coughing, ambulating | Checks client within 30 minutes following pain administration of analgesic |
| Pulse and respiration within normal limits for client | States pulse and respira-tion within normal limits for client | Records response to pain management program |
| Checking interval of prescribed analgesic or other pain relief measure | States checking intervals of prescribed analgesic or other pain relief measure | Reports client's response to pain management program to primary RN/team leader/MD |

Developed Spring 1979 in collaboration with Brenda Geyer; revised fall 1985.

Criterion-referenced test specifications similar to the illustrative set presented by Waltz, Strickland, & Lenz (1984) were also developed to facilitate the construction of new test items (e.g., general description, sample item directions, stimulus attributes/item characteristics, and response attributes):

> . . . the purpose of test specifications is to communicate the specifics related to the construction of the measure. This includes explication of not only what the items on the measure will assess but also the rules that govern the creation and administration of the measure. The goals of the development of test specifications are to be sufficiently specific to communicate the scope and constraints to potential users of the measure; and to be sufficiently targeted and explicit to guide those who might be involved in the construction and development of the measure. (p. 171)

## Administration and Scoring

Student's written nursing data base forms, care plans and SCAP recordings of subjective and objective observations as well as their assessments and management behaviors for the identified nursing diagnosis were met. Specific guides, incorporated in the nursing data base form, allowed students to gather the relevant subjective and objective data. For example, for the nursing diagnosis "Alterations in comfort: acute or chronic pain," the following Pain Assessment guides were listed:

Acute pain? Chronic pain? (please circle)
What is location, intensity (1 lowest to 10 highest), type, duration, chronology/precipitating events?
What cultural/religious beliefs of control, past/current ways/drugs to control pain?
Interfere with activities of daily living or family/work responsibilities?
Currently ordered meds: dates/times prescribed; when prn's given last 48 hr

For the nursing diagnosis "Sleep pattern disturbance" the following Sleep-Wakefulness Assessment guides were listed for patterns "usual at home" and "during hospitalization":

What beliefs of duration; usual bedtime/arising hours (also naps); how long to fall asleep; number/reason of awakenings (what helps to fall asleep again); what dream recall? if snoring/waking patterns present in sleep; awake feeling state (refreshed)?
What environmental controls: temp/ventilation; number of pillows/ blankets; noise level; lighting?
What physical activity during day; snack/drink, physical care, quiet recreation prior to bedtime/on arising?
Use of caffeine (coffee, tea, cola), alcohol, hypnotic/other drug?

For the nursing diagnosis "Knowledge deficit," the following health teaching needs assessment guides were listed:

What does the client-family know about his health status? (that is, cognitive, affective, and psychomotor)
What does the client-family want or need to know about his health status? (that is, cognitive, affective, and psychomotor)
Readiness to learn?
What cultural patterns may influence teaching-learning?

Students' nursing care plans and SCAP rescorings were additional data sources used to provide evidence that the expected nursing process behaviors were met. Contrary to Ciuca's (1972) findings that the "unit nursing care plan was primarily a place for the notation of functional duties such as medications, treatments, etc. (p. 710)," most care plan forms used in the Seattle area agencies in which students practice include designated areas for "Client-Family Problems," "Expected Outcomes" with "Deadlines," and "Client-Family/Nurse Actions." The Seattle University School of Nursing's (1981a) care plan, following an analysis of the components of nursing process in clinical courses, has similarly designated such areas since 1978.

Scoring consisted of placing a check mark in the Yes column for an item in the respective instrument if the performance behavior was met, in the No column if omitted, or in the NA column if the item did not apply. Percentage scores, that is the proportion of the maximum possible raw score points that were obtained by an individual or group of individuals, were determined using the formula described by Waltz and associates (1984), who note: "The percentage score represents the proportion of a content domain that an individual has mastered or responded to appropriately. hence, it indicates an individual's level of performance in relation to the possible minimum and maximum raw scores on a measure" (p. 177). A percentage score of 80 or higher of the possible maximum raw score on a measure was set by faculty as the standard of mastery against which to judge an individual's or group of individuals' performance.

## Reliability Testing

Since "reliability is a necessary prerequisite for validity" (Strickland, 1984), the steps undertaken to determine reliability of the instruments will be presented first. This process involved basically two steps:

1. *Interrater agreement of item scoring.* Two raters, using the same instrument, evaluated the identical individual on the specified test items; all items retained in the instruments were those where interrater agreement was .80 or higher.

2. *Stability of ratings over time.* Using the same instrument, a student's performance was evaluated approximately 2 weeks following the first administration (i.e., without formative evaluative feedback); all items retained in the instruments were those where .80 or higher agreement was achieved (both intrarater and interrater agreement).

## Validity of Test Items

According to Waltz and associates (1984), the "validity of the content of the measure is requisite to the validity of the total measure or test" (p. 194). The steps undertaken to assure validity of the content of the items in the instruments were as follows:

1. *Review of the research reported in the literature* as the primary source for the content of the test items, that is, the subjective and objectives assessments and management behaviors – independent and interdependent – considered essential for students' practice with clients with the identified nursing diagnoses.
2. *Development of tables of specifications* described earlier (see sample in Table 15.2). According to Cox (1972), "In general. . . criterion-referencing itself suggests that the validity must depend upon the correspondence of test items with the objectives to which the test is referenced. . . thus the test items must be constructed for, or matched to, the goals of instruction" (p. 74).

Criterion-referenced test specifications, also developed for each instrument, outlined the rules that governed the creation and administration of the measures (for further discussion, see Waltz et al., 1984, p. 171). Interrater agreement of relevance and importance of test items as measures of student assessment and management behaviors for clients with the relevant nursing diagnoses were rated by faculty and clinical nurse specialists as follows:

Using the designated scale(s) please rate each performance item for its relevance and importance as a nursing assessment or management behavior to be demonstrated by baccalaureate students when working with adult oriented clients with. . . acute pain on analgesics (sample client-family with nursing diagnosis inserted):

|  Relevance Scale | Importance Scale |
| --- | --- |
| 1. Not Relevant | 1. Not Important |
| 2. Somewhat Relevant | 2. Somewhat Important |
| 3. Quite Relevant | 3. Quite Important |
| 4. Very Relevant | 4. Very Important |

An index of content validity (CVI) of the proportion of items rated as Quite/Very Relevant (3 or 4) and Quite/Very Important (3 or 4) by two judges, was calculated for nurse faculty and clinical nurse specialists (see Waltz et al., 1984, p. 143). Acceptable levels for $P_o$ were .80 or greater; K values equal to or greater than .25 (Waltz et al., 1984, p. 198). All measures retained in the instruments met this minimum standard of acceptability.

## MAJOR FINDINGS AND RESULTS

As part of this Measurement Outcomes Project, a cross-validation study by clinical nurse specialists of the relevance and importance of test items measuring baccalaureate students' nursing process competencies was conducted for four tools: Critical Elements for Clinical Performance for Oriented Adult Clients with Acute Pain, . . .with Chronic Pain, . . .with Altered Sleep-Wakefulness Patterns, and . . .Requiring Health Teaching (validity of items had been previously established by faculty). Tables of specification delineating item content and nursing behaviors as well as criterion-referenced test specifications guiding the development and scoring of the measures were developed for three additional tools: (a) Critical Elements for Clinical Performance for Adult Clients with Ineffective Breathing Patterns/ Airway Clearance, (b) . . . Potential Impairment of Skin Integrity, and (c) . . . Impaired Physical Mobility. Faculty interrater agreement for relevance and importance of test items, item scoring, and test-retest reliability were accomplished for the instrument Critical Elements for Clinical Performance for Adult Clients with Ineffective Breathing Patterns/Airway Clearance. However, because additional validity and reliability testing is needed for the three new tools evolved during this measurement project, they are not included at this time as part of the remainder of the presentation.

Student participation was secured through informed, consent procedures, with opportunities for feedback of findings provided. Item analysis summaries of students' nursing assessment and management performance behaviors, using both the Difficulty Index (DI) (the number responding correctly) and the $p$-value (the percentage responding correctly for each item) were prepared for four instruments ($N = 66\text{-}175$). These summaries revealed that a large number of the expected performance items were met by the participating students at the mastery level. For example:

1. More than 80% stated the location, intensity, type duration, chronology, and behavioral response of clients with acute or chronic pain.
2. More than 80% stated client's usual bedtime/arising hours, time of nap hours, use of caffeine, and use of drugs to fall asleep prior to and during hospitalization.
3. More than 80% stated client's willingness/interest/availability for learning and learning needs in the cognitive, psychomotor, and affective domains.

However, results also indicated that several expected performance items did not meet the desired 80% level. For example:

1. Including relaxation techniques as a nursing management behavior for clients with acute pain.
2. Providing for adjustments/restrictions of intake of caffeine or other stimulants for clients with sleep pattern disturbance.
3. Using an evaluation tool at the end of teaching for clients with knowledge deficit(s).

Review of such findings allowed for a systematic evaluation of areas needing improvement.

A positive student response to the use of criterion-referenced measurement instruments around nursing diagnoses was found. Three classes of students, when asked how helpful the tools were for their evaluation of nursing process competencies, 64 to 74% indicated they were either "very" or "somewhat helpful" to them ($N = 42$, 53, and 61, respectively). A majority of students in the three classes agreed that other tools should be evolved around nursing diagnoses (69-71%).

## IMPLICATIONS FOR NURSING/CONCLUSIONS

In her presentation "The State of the Art of Measurement in Nursing Ourcomes," Waltz (1984) cited a paucity of studies that focus on the measurement of educational outcomes and made a strong case that "educators are just as accountable for their outcomes as are clinicians." This research, initiated in 1979 and refined and expanded through this project, focused on the measurement of nursing process competencies-major educational outcomes identified in Seattle University School of Nursing (1981a) objectives. A nursing diagnosis framework was used. Although the sample in this study was small and nonrandom and limited to a few nursing diagnoses, the findings process competency data. Recent studies support the need for continued work in the measurement of baccalaureate students' clinical competencies (Field, Gallman, Nicholson, & Dreher, 1984; Lee & Strong, 1985).

**TABLE 15.4 Item Analysis Summary of Students' Nursing Process Behaviors for Adult Clients with Acute Pain**

| | | DI[a] | p[a] | DI[b] | p[b] | DI[c] | p[c] |
|---|---|---|---|---|---|---|---|
| I. Assesses client's pain | | | | | | | |
| A. Collects subjective data | | | | | | | |
| 1. States location | 1. | 58 | .95 | 53 | 1.00 | 32 | 1.00 |
| 2. Describes intensity (on scale of 1, no pain, to 10, unbearable pain) | 2. | 56 | .92 | 51 | .96 | 31 | .97 |
| 3. Describes type (e.g. burning, cramping, bloating, radiating) | 3. | 54 | .89 | 49 | .92 | 29 | .91 |
| 4. States duration (how long pain has been present?) | 4. | 57 | .93 | 43 | .81 | 31 | .97 |
| 5. Describes chronology (precipitating events/ aggravating factors) | 5. | 56 | .92 | 46 | .87 | 26 | .81 |
| 6. Describes ways client controls pain (past/current) | 6. | 50 | .82 | 41 | .77 | 26 | .81 |
| 7. States beliefs about pain control (culture/religion) | 7. | 44 | .72 | 29 | .55 | 22 | .69 |
| B. Collects objective data | | | | | | | |
| 1. Describes behavioral responses, e.g., body position, facial expression, splinting, activity level | 1. | 58 | .95 | 50 | .94 | 27 | .84 |
| 2. States physiological responses, e.g., alterations in pulse/respiration/blood pressure, perspiration, nausea/vomiting, pallor, distention, muscle tension | 2. | 52 | .85 | 40 | .75 | 25 | .78 |
| 3. States contributing factors, e.g., fatigue, concerns/fears or worries | 3. | 54 | .89 | 34 | .64 | 24 | .75 |
| 4. States pattern of pain medication administration for past 48 hr | 4. | 33 | .54 | 41 | .77 | 27 | .84 |
| C. Identifies possible cause of client's pain | | | | | | | |
| 1. Gives "due to" statement | 1. | 59 | .92 | 44 | .86 | 26 | .81 |
| 2. Explains underlying pathophysiological/ psychosocial alteration | 2. | 59 | .97 | 48 | .91 | 32 | 1.00 |
| II. Identifies expected outcomes and deadline | | | | | | | |
| 1. States "No verbal or nonverbal expression of pain" | 1. | 56 | .92 | 44 | .86 | 26 | .81 |
| 2. States: "Performs activities, e.g., deep breathing (DB), C, ambulating" | 2. | 52 | .85 | 40 | .78 | 28 | .88 |
| 3. States: "P and R within NML for client" | 3. | 42 | .69 | 31 | .61 | 22 | .69 |
| 4. States checking interval of prescribed analgesic or other pain relief measures | 4. | 50 | .82 | 38 | .75 | 29 | .91 |
| III. Implements client-family/nurse actions | | | | | | | |
| A. Provides comfort measures | | | | | | | |
| 1. Implements individualized pain relief methods (see IA6) | 1. | 49 | .80 | 39 | .76 | 29 | .91 |
| 2. Offers/gives bed pan/bath/oral, pericare, change of linen, reinforcement of dresing(s) | 2. | 53 | .87 | 44 | .86 | 29 | .91 |
| 3. Positions/repositions client/ambulates as prescribed | 3. | 54 | .89 | 48 | .94 | 29 | .91 |
| 4. Applies hot/cold measures as prescribed | 4. | 25 | 1.00 | 10 | .91 | 17 | 1.00 |

(*continued*)

**TABLE 15.4** (*Continued*)

|  | DI[a] | p[a] | DI[b] | p[b] | DI[c] | p[c] |
|---|---|---|---|---|---|---|
| 5. Encourages/listens to expressions of fears/concerns/worries | 5. 43 | .70 | 45 | .88 | 29 | .91 |
| B. Implements pain relief measures other than comfort measures |  |  |  |  |  |  |
| 1. Provides distraction, e.g., radio, TV, visits | 1. 54 | .89 | 42 | .82 | 29 | .81 |
| 2. Includes relaxation technique, e.g., DB, massage (unless contraindicated), centering exercises | 2. 44 | .72 | 35 | .69 | 20 | .63 |
| C. Medicates appropriately if required |  |  |  |  |  |  |
| 1. Offers pain medications at prescribed intervals (if R⇑ 10-12 for narcotics) | 1. 57 | .93 | 42 | .82 | 29 | .91 |
| 2. Administers pain medications within 15 min of request | 2. 53 | .87 | 45 | .88 | 29 | .91 |
| IV. Evaluates extent to which outcomes are met |  |  |  |  |  |  |
| 1. Checks client within 30 min for effectiveness of pain relief, measures other than medications | 1. 54 | .89 | 44 | .86 | 28 | .88 |
| 2. Checks client within 30 min following administration of analgesic(s) | 2. 52 | .85 | 44 | .86 | 28 | .88 |
| 3. Records response to pain management program | 3. 54 | .89 | 44 | .86 | 29 | .91 |
| 4. Reports client's response to pain management program to primary nurse/team leader/MD | 4. 53 | .87 | 44 | .86 | 29 | .91 |

[a] Class of 1982, $N = 61$ for all items except IIIA4 (25).
[b] Class of 1983, $N = 53$ for all items in I; $N = 51$ for all items in II-IV except IIIA4 (11).
[c] Class of 1987, $N = 32$ for all items except IIIA4 (17).
DI (difficulty index), number of students responding correctly.
$p$-value, percentage of students responding correctly.

**TABLE 15.5 Item Analysis Summary of Students' Nursing Process Behaviors for Adult Clients with Acute Pain**

| I. Assesses client's pain | DI[a] | p[a] | DI[b] | p[b] |
|---|---|---|---|---|
| A. Collects subjective data |  |  |  |  |
| 1. States location | 1. 30 | .97 | 31 | 1.00 |
| 2. Dscribes intensity (on scale of 1, no pain, to 10, unbearable pain) | 2. 28 | .90 | 29 | .94 |
| 3. Describes type (e.g. burning, cramping, bloating) | 3. 27 | .87 | 25 | .81 |
| 4. States duration (how long pain has been present?) | 4. 29 | .94 | 29 | .94 |
| 5. Describes chronology (precipitating events/ aggravating factor) | 5. 26 | .84 | 27 | .87 |
| 6. Describes ways client controls pain (past/current) | 6. 24 | .77 | 27 | .87 |
| 7. States belief about pain control (culture/religion) | 7. 23 | .74 | 16 | .52 |
| 8. States if pain interferes with Activities of Daily Living (ADLs) | 8. 26 | .84 | 27 | .87 |
| 9. States if pain interferes with family role, social interaction/work | 9. 26 | .84 | 29 | .94 |
| B. Collects objective data |  |  |  |  |
| 1. Describes behavioral responses, e.g. body position, facial expression, splinting/muscle tension | 1. 31 | 1.00 | 25 | .81 |
| 2. States contributing factors, e.g. concerns/fears/worries | 2. 30 | .97 | 20 | .65 |

(*continued*)

**TABLE 15.5** (*Continued*)

| | DIᵃ | pᵃ | DIᵇ | pᵇ |
|---|---|---|---|---|
| 3. States level of activity (how much time per day in bed/chair/active?) | 3. 31 | 1.00 | 25 | .81 |
| 4. States pattern of pain medication administration for past 48 hr | 4. 26 | .84 | 25 | .81 |
| C. Identifies possible cause of client's pain | | | | |
|   1. Gives "due to" statement (original injury/surgery when pain started) | 1. 29 | .93 | 30 | .97 |
|   2. Explains underlying pathophysiological/ psychosocial alteration | 2. 25 | .81 | 27 | .87 |
| II. Identifies expected outcomes and deadlines | | | | |
|   1. States: "Able to cope with pain" | 1. 28 | .90 | 27 | .87 |
|   2. States: "Pain doesn't interfere with necessary activities" | 2. 25 | .81 | 23 | .74 |
|   3. States alternate ways of dealing with pain other than medication. | 3. 25 | .81 | 20 | .65 |
|   4. States checking interval of prescribed analgesic or other pain relief measures | 4. 25 | .81 | 25 | .81 |
| III. Implements client-family/nurse actions | | | | |
|   A. Provides comfort measures | | | | |
|     1. Implements individualized pain relief methods (see IA6) | 1. 23 | .74 | 23 | .74 |
|     2. Offers/gives bed pan/bath/oral, pericare, change of linen | 2. 29 | .94 | 26 | .84 |
|     3. Positions/repositions client/ambulates as prescribed | 3. 31 | 1.00 | 27 | .87 |
|     4. Applies hot/cold measures as prescribed | 4. 25 | .96 | 9 | 1.00 |
|     5. Listens to expressions of fears/concerns/worries | 5. 31 | 1.00 | 27 | .87 |
|     6. Responds to c/o pain factually, not sympathetically | 6. 29 | .94 | 22 | .71 |
|   B. Implements pain relief measures other than comfort measures | | | | |
|     1. Encourages conversation not related to pain | 1. 30 | .97 | 27 | .87 |
|     2. Gives positive feedback for activities that do not focus on pain | 2. 27 | .87 | 25 | .81 |
|     3. Provides distraction, e.g. radio, T.V, visits, reading | 3. 29 | .94 | 27 | .87 |
|     4. Includes relaxation techniques, e.g. DB, massage (unless contraindicated) | 4. 26 | .84 | 23 | .74 |
|     5. Provides alternative methods of pain relief, e.g. biofeedback, TENS | 5. 15 | .48 | 13 | .42 |
|   C. Medicates appropriately | | | | |
|     1. Administers medications at prescribed intervals | 1. 31 | 1.00 | 28 | .90 |
| IV. Evaluates extent to which outcomes are met | | | | |
|   1. Checks client within 30 min for effectiveness of pain relief measures other than medications | 1. 29 | .94 | 23 | .74 |
|   2. Checks client within 30 min following administration of analgesic(s) | 2. 29 | .94 | 20 | .65 |
|   3. Records client's level of activity | 3. 29 | .94 | 23 | .74 |
|   4. Reports client's level of activity to primary nurse/ team leader/MD | 4. 30 | .97 | 25 | .81 |
|   5. Records client's response to pain management program | 5. 30 | .97 | 23 | .74 |
|   6. Reports client's response to pain management program to primary nurse/team leader/MD. | 6. 30 | .97 | 21 | .68 |

[a]Class of 1982, $N = 31$ for all items except III A4 (26).
[b]Class of 1983, $N = 31$ for all items except III A4 (9).
*DI* (difficulty index), number of students responding correctly.
*p* value, percentage of students responding correctly.

**TABLE 15.6 Item Analysis Summary of Students' Nursing Process Behaviors for Adult Clients with Sleep Pattern Disturbance**

| | Prior to hospital | | | | During hospital | | | |
|---|---|---|---|---|---|---|---|---|
| I. Assesses Client's sleep/wakefulness pattern/ environmental controls/other influencing factors<br>A. Collects subjective data | | | | | | | | |
| Sleep-wakefulness pattern | $DI^a$ | $p^a$ | $DI^b$ | $p^b$ | $DI^a$ | $p^a$ | $DI^b$ | $p^b$ |
| 1. States client's beliefs of number of hours of sleep/naps to stay healthy | 1. | 43 | .90 | 34 | .87 | 38 | .79 | 27 | .73 |
| 2. States client's usual bedtime/arising/hours | 2. | 44 | .92 | 37 | .95 | 41 | .85 | 35 | .90 |
| 3. States time of naps hours | 3. | 43 | .90 | 24 | .62 | 43 | .90 | 22 | .56 |
| 4. States how long it usually takes client to fall asleep | 4. | 32 | .67 | 26 | .67 | 32 | .67 | 22 | .56 |
| 5. States number of awakenings during sleep | 5. | 28 | .58 | 30 | .77 | 33 | .69 | 35 | .90 |
| 6. States what wakes client up once asleep | 6. | 28 | .58 | 27 | .69 | 31 | .65 | 34 | .87 |
| 7. States what helps client get back to sleep if awoken | 7. | 23 | .48 | 28 | .72 | 26 | .54 | 30 | .77 |
| 8. Describes client's dream patterns (no recall/pleasant/frightening) | 8. | 18 | .38 | 20 | .51 | 22 | .46 | 16 | .41 |
| 9. Describes patterns of waking behavior that may appear during sleep (e.g. sleepwalking/grinding of teeth/ jerking movements) | 9. | 14 | .29 | 12 | .31 | 16 | .33 | 10 | .26 |
| 10. States if snoring is present during sleep | 10. | 15 | .31 | 17 | .44 | 17 | .35 | 18 | .46 |
| 11. Describes awake state following sleep (refreshed/fatigued) | 11. | 36 | .75 | 34 | .87 | 39 | .81 | 33 | .85 |
| Environmental controls | | | | | | | | |
| 1. Describes temperature/ventilation used (thermostat setting/windows open or closed) | 1. | 37 | .77 | 34 | .87 | 39 | .81 | 38 | .97 |
| 2. Describes bedding used (number of blankets/pillows) | 2. | 35 | .73 | 34 | .87 | 34 | .71 | 38 | .97 |
| 3. States lighting used (none/dim/night/ full light) | 3. | 32 | .67 | 29 | .74 | 37 | .77 | 32 | .82 |
| 4. States noise level present (quiet/loud) | 4. | 35 | .73 | 33 | .85 | 39 | .81 | 33 | .85 |
| Physical activity/care/recreation | | | | | | | | |
| 1. Describes pattern of physical activity during waking hours/prescribed activity level | 1. | 34 | .71 | 36 | .92 | 39 | .81 | 31 | .79 |
| 2. Describes snack/drink taken prior to retiring | 2. | 33 | .69 | 28 | .72 | 34 | .71 | 28 | .72 |
| 3. States physical care routine followed prior to bedtime (bath/shower/teeth brushing) | 3. | 35 | .73 | 26 | .67 | 35 | .73 | 25 | .64 |
| 4. Describes quiet recreation followed prior to bedtime (reading/TV/radio/handwork) | 4. | 36 | .75 | 29 | .74 | 36 | .75 | 26 | .67 |
| 5. Describes waking routine followed (drink/food/bath/shower) | 5. | 34 | .71 | 23 | .59 | 33 | .69 | 23 | .59 |

(*continued*)

**TABLE 15.6** (*Continued*)

| | Prior to hospital | | | | During hospital | | | |
|---|---|---|---|---|---|---|---|---|
| | DI[a] | p[a] | DI[b] | p[b] | DI[a] | p[a] | DI[b] | p[b] |
| Other influencing factors | | | | | | | | |
| 1. Describes client's concerns/worries at home/work/hospitalization | 1. 38 | .79 | 28 | .72 | 45 | .94 | 29 | .74 |
| 2. Describes use of caffeine (coffee/tea/ carbonated drinks) | 2. 40 | .83 | 38 | .97 | 40 | .83 | 35 | .90 |
| 3. Describes use of other stimulants (e.g. alcohol) | 3. 34 | .71 | 30 | .77 | 35 | .73 | 26 | .67 |
| 4. Describes use of drugs to assist sleep | 4. 42 | .88 | 28 | .72 | 40 | .83 | 32 | .82 |
| B. Collects objective data | | | | | | | | |
| 1. Describes behavioral responses, e.g., full concentration/decreased attention span; easygoing/irritable; active/inactive | | | | | 1. 43 | .90 | 30 | .77 |
| 2. States physiological responses, e.g., muscle weakness (droopy eyelids); yawning; oriented/disoriented | | | | | 2. 42 | .88 | 29 | .74 |
| 3. Describes contributing factors, e.g., presence of pain, IVs bandages/casts, incontinence. | | | | | 3. 45 | .94 | 30 | .77 |
| 4. Reviews record of several days sleep-activity cycle (notes/graphs/diary) | | | | | 4. 35 | .73 | 11 | .28 |
| C. Identifies client problem and possible cause of altered sleep-wakefulness pattern | | | | | | | | |
| 1. States problem (e.g., sleep deprivation; primary sleep disorder; insomnia/hypersomnia/narcolepsy, secondary sleep disorder: depression/alcoholism/ chronic renal insufficiency/hypothyroidism/ schizophrenia/anorexia nervosa) | | | | | 1. 48 | 1.00 | 39 | 1.00 |
| 2. Gives "due to" statement, e.g., situational stress/ crises, medical pathophysiology, psychosocial illness, drug-related disorder, aging process | | | | | 2. 48 | 1.00 | 39 | 1.00 |
| II. Identifies expected outcomes and deadline | | | | | | | | |
| 1. States: "Falls asleep within 15-30 min | | | | | 1. 42 | .88 | 20 | .56 |
| 2. States: "Sleeps 6½-8 hr uninterrupted" | | | | | 2. 43 | .90 | 24 | .67 |
| 3. States: "Feels refreshed/rested/slept out" | | | | | 3. 46 | .96 | 30 | .83 |
| 4. States: "Slept through the night" | | | | | 4. 47 | .98 | 33 | .92 |
| 5. States checking interval of prescribed hypnotic/other sleep management action (Q.D.) | | | | | 5. 44 | .92 | 26 | .72 |
| III. Implements client-family/nurse actions | | | | | | | | |
| A. Establishes sleep environment | | | | | | | | |
| 1. Implements client's usual temperature/ventilation used | | | | | 1. 41 | .85 | 19 | .53 |
| 2. Provides number of blankets/pillows usually used by client | | | | | 2. 41 | .85 | 19 | .53 |
| 3. Adjusts lighting to level preferred by client | | | | | 3. 41 | .85 | 17 | .47 |
| 4. Adjusts noise to level of client's usual setting | | | | | 4. 41 | .85 | 13 | .36 |
| 5. Provides for privacy (e.g., curtains pulled/doors closed) | | | | | 5. 41 | .85 | 18 | .50 |
| B. Provides for physical activity/care/recreation reflective of client's usual pattern | | | | | | | | |
| 1. Encourages usual pattern of physical activity during waking hours/implements prescribed activity level (OOB, wheelchair, ambulation) | | | | | 1. 44 | .92 | 26 | .72 |
| 2. Provides usual snack/drink taken by client prior to retiring (as permitted) | | | | | 2. 40 | .83 | 9 | .25 |

(*continued*)

**TABLE 15.6** (*Continued*)

| | DI[a] | *p*[a] | DI[b] | *p*[b] |
|---|---|---|---|---|
| 3. Provides for/assists with physical care routine followed by client prior to bedtime (elimination/bath/shower/teeth brushing) | 3. 36 | .75 | 9 | .25 |
| 4. Provides for clean/unwrinkled bed linen | 4. 39 | .81 | 24 | .67 |
| 5. Positions/repositions as permitted for comfort | 5. 38 | .79 | 23 | .64 |
| 6. Adjusts binders/bandages/tubes | 6. 38 | .79 | 12 | .33 |
| 7. Encourages/provides for usual quiet recreation prior to bedtime | 7. 37 | .77 | 10 | .28 |
| 8. Provides for usual waking routine of client | 8. 41 | .85 | 15 | .42 |
| C. Promotes relaxation | | | | |
| 1. Encourages/provides opportunity to talk about concerns/worries | 1. 47 | .98 | 29 | .81 |
| 2. Provides information regarding hospital care activities | 2. 45 | .94 | 26 | .72 |
| 3. Offers/gives back massage | 3. 45 | .94 | 26 | .72 |
| 4. Encourages/provides for centering | 4. 38 | .79 | 17 | .47 |
| D. Implements other influencing actions | | | | |
| 1. Adjusts/restricts intake of caffeine/other stimulants | 1. 25 | .52 | 10 | .28 |
| 2. Medicates appropriately for pain if present | 2. 28 | .58 | 21 | .58 |
| 3. Medicates appropriately for sleep disorder if other measures fail | 3. 27 | .56 | 11 | .31 |
| 4. Plans uninterrupted sleep cycles of 60-90 min when giving care during sleep period | 4. 26 | .54 | 11 | .31 |
| 5. Encourages/provides for recording of sleep-activity patterns by client | 5. 27 | .56 | 6 | .17 |
| IV. Evaluates extent to which outcomes are met | | | | |
| 1. Checks client within 15-30 min following implementation of sleep-assisting measures other than hypnotic | 1. 23 | .48 | 17 | .47 |
| 2. Checks client within 15-30 min following administration of hypnotic | 2. 23 | .48 | 16 | .44 |
| 3. Checks client from $6^1/_2$-8 hr to ascertain if uninterrupted sleep | 3. 40 | .83 | 24 | .67 |
| 4. Describes client's expressions of wake state following sleep hours/interventions | 4. 41 | .85 | 29 | .81 |
| 5. Records response to sleep management program | 5. 40 | .83 | 30 | .83 |
| 6. Reports response to sleep management program to primary nurse/team leader/MD | 6. 39 | .81 | 30 | .83 |

[a]Class of 1982, $N = 48$ for all items.
[b]Class of 1983, $N = 39$ for all items in I; $N = 36$ for all items in II-IV.
*DI* (Difficulty index), number of students responding correctly.
*p*-value, percentage of students responding correctly.

**TABLE 15.7** Item Analysis Summary of Students' Nursing Process Behaviors for Adult Clients with Knowledge Deficit

| | $DI^a$ | $p^a$ | $DI^b$ | $p^b$ |
|---|---|---|---|---|
| I   Assesses client-family's health teaching needs | | | | |
| A. Collects subjective data | | | | |
|    Client-faily readiness for learning | | | | |
|    1. States client-family's willingness/interest/availability for learning | 1. 51 | .94 | 40 | .95 |
|    2. States client-family's psychological/physical readiness | 2. 44 | .81 | 36 | .86 |
|    3. States client-family's learning needs in the cognitive domain (knowledge of facts/concepts) | 3. 49 | .91 | 41 | .98 |
|    4. States client-family's learning needs in the psycho-motor domain (technical skills) | 4 44 | .81 | 41 | .98 |
|    5. States client-family's learning needs in the affective domain (attitudes/feelings) | 5. 46 | .85 | 36 | .86 |
|    6. States client-family's educational level/experience(s) | 6. 45 | .83 | 31 | .74 |
| B. Collects objective data | | | | |
|    Client-family experiential readiness | | | | |
|    1. Describes client-family's background knowledge in the cognitive domain | 1. 45 | .83 | 35 | .83 |
|    2. Describes client-family's proficiency of psychomotor skills | 2. 43 | .80 | 34 | .81 |
|    3. Describes client-family's nonverbal behaviors indicating learning needs in affective domain (e.g. smoking/drinking/overeating) | 3. 42 | .78 | 31 | .74 |
|    4. Evaluates cultural patterns influencing teaching-learning | 4. 40 | .74 | 29 | .69 |
| II. Identifies client-family problem related to health teaching needs and possible cause | | | | |
|    1. States specific problem (e.g., lack of knowledge, lack of readiness to learn, unavailable for learning) | 1. 52 | .96 | 37 | .88 |
|    2. Gives "due to" statement (e.g., never having been informed, misinformed, decreased perceptual field resulting from anxiety) | 2. 51 | .94 | 41 | .98 |
| III. Identifies client-family expected outcomes and dealine(s) | | | | |
|    1. Client-family verbalizes the expected outcomes of teaching-learning | 1. 44 | .81 | 40 | .95 |
|    2. Client-family state-deadline date(s) for expected outcomes to be met | 2. 40 | .74 | 31 | .74 |
|    3. Client-family demonstrates that learning has occurred | 3. 44 | .81 | 34 | .81 |
| IV. Implements client-family/nurse actions | | | | |
| A. Prior to teaching | | | | |
|    1. Validates with client-family the main objective(s) goal(s) purpose(s) of teaching-learning | 1. 44 | .81 | 40 | .95 |
|    2. Formulates with client family expected outcomes of teaching-learning | 2. 44 | .81 | 40 | .95 |
|    3. Formulates with client family deadline date(s) | 3. 40 | .74 | 31 | .74 |
|    4. Contracts with client-family for time and date(s) available for teaching-learning | 4. 45 | .83 | 22 | .52 |
|    5. Formulates a written teaching plan with teacher objective(s), outcome criteria, deadline date(s), content outline, teaching-learning actions | 5. 32 | .59 | 25 | .60 |

*(continued)*

**TABLE 15.7** (*Continued*)

| | DI[a] | p[a] | DI[b] | p[b] |
|---|---|---|---|---|
| 6. Controls the environment for teaching-learning effectiveness (necessary equipment available and in working order; privacy and freedom from noise/distractions provided) | 6. 48 | .89 | 24 | .57 |
| B. During teaching | | | | |
| 1. Uses patient education materials suited for client-family educational experiental level: pamphlets, written hand-outs, AV aids | 1. 45 | .83 | 21 | .50 |
| 2. Provides for discussion/role playing | 2. 46 | .85 | 20 | .48 |
| 3. Demonstrates skill(s) to be learned | 3. 43 | .80 | 18 | .43 |
| 4. Provides for return demonstration of skills (a minimum of 3 times) | 4. 43 | .80 | 18 | .43 |
| 5. Elicits feedback at least twice during teaching | 5. 44 | .81 | 23 | .55 |
| 6. Modifies content and/or approach based on feedback | 6. 44 | .81 | 19 | .45 |
| 7. Gives positive feedback during return demonstration of knowledge/skills/attitudes (a minimum of 3 times during teaching) | 7. 49 | .91 | 18 | .43 |
| 8. Summarizes content/teaching-learning activities | 8. 51 | .94 | 23 | .55 |
| C. At the end of teaching | | | | |
| 1. Uses an evaluation tool (e.g., test questions, behavioral skills checklist) | 1. 10 | .19 | 3 | .07 |
| 2. Summarizes client-family learning that occurred | 2. 51 | .94 | 19 | .45 |
| 3. Stays within agreed on time frame | 3. 45 | .83 | 15 | .36 |
| 4. States possible follow-up of learning-teaching activities by staff | 4. 49 | .91 | 15 | .36 |
| V. Determines extent to which client-family outcomes are met | | | | |
| 1. States if client-family expected outcomes of teaching-learning are met | 1. 50 | .93 | 28 | .67 |
| 2. If not, states follow-up of teaching and learning actions | 2. 44 | .88 | 15 | .41 |
| 3. Documents teaching and learning to assure continuity | 3. 50 | .93 | 37 | .88 |
| 4. Reports teaching and learning to primary nurse/team leader/MD | 4. 52 | .96 | 38 | .90 |

[a]Class of 1982, $N = 54$ except v2 (50).
[b]Class of 1983, $N = 42$ except v2 (37).
*DI* (dificulty index) = number of students responding correctly.
*p*-value, percentage of students responding correctly.

# REFERENCES

Abdellah, F. G., et al. (1960). *Patient-centered approaches to nursing.* New York: McMillian.

American Nurses' Association. (1973). *Standards of nursing practice.* Kansas City, MO: Author.

American Nurses' Association. (1977). *Guidelines for review of nursing care at the local level: Emphasis given to PSRO and use of outcome criteria in the review of nursing care.* Kansas City, MO: Author.

American Nurses' Association. (1980). *Nursing: A social policy statement.* Kansas City, MO: Author

American Nurses' Association. (1981). *Educational preparation for nursing.* Kansas City, MO: Author

Aspinall, M. J. (1976). Nursing diagnosis-the weak link. *Nursing Outlook, 24,* 433 – 437.

Benner, P. (1982). Issues in competency-based testing. *Nursing Outlook, 30*(5), 303 – 309.

Carter, J. H., Hilliard, M., Castles, M. R., Stoll, L., & Cowan, A. (1976). *Standards of nursing care: A guide for evaluation* (2nd ed.). New York: Springer Publishing Co.

Ciuca, R. L. (1972). Over the years with the nursing care plan. *Nursing Outlook, 20*(11), 706 – 711.

Cox, R. C. (1972). Evaluative aspects of criterion-referenced measures. In W. J. Popham (Ed.), *Criterion-refernced measurement: An introduction* (pp. 67 – 75). Englewood Cliffs, NJ: Educational Technology Publications.

DeBack, V. (1981). The relationship between senior nursing students' ability to formulate nursing diagnosis and the curriculum model. *Advances in Nursing Science, 3*(3), 51 – 66.

Deets, C. (1976). Criterion referenced measurement and quality of care criteria: The ANA PSRO study. In American Nurses' Association (Ed.). *Issues of evaluation research* (pp. 83 – 91). Kansas City, MO: American Nurses' Association.

Field, W. E., Gallman, L., Nicholson, R., & Dreher, M. (1984). Clinical competencies of baccalaureate students. *Journal of Nursing Education, 23*(7), 284 – 293.

Fredette, S., & O'Connor, K. (1979). Nursing diagnosis in teaching and curriculum planning. *Nursing Clinics of North America, 14*(3), 541 – 552.

Gaines, B. C., & McFarland, M. B. (1984). Nursing diagnosis: Its relationship and use in nursing education. *Topics in Clinical Nursing, 5*(4), 39 – 49.

Gordon, M. (1982). *Nursing diagnosis: Process and application.* New York: McGraw-Hill.

Gronlund, N. E. (1973). *Preparing criterion-referenced tests for classroom instruction.* New York: McMillian.

Haussmann, R. K. D., & Hegyvary, S. T. (1976). Field testing the nursing quality monitoring methodology: Phase II. *Nursing Research, 25,* 324 – 331.

Haussmann, R. K. D., Hegyvary, S. T., & Newman, J. F. (1976). *Monitoring quality of nursing care: Part II. Assessment and study of correlates* (DHEW Pub. No. HRA 76-77). Bethesda; MD: U.S. Department of Health, Education and Welfare.

Hegyvary, S. T., Gortner, S., & Haussmann, R. K. D. (1976). The development of criterion measures for quality of care: The Rush-Medicus experience. In *Issues in evaluation research* (pp. 106 – 127). Kansas City, MO: American Nurses' Association.

Horn, B. J., & Swain, M. A. (1977a). *Development of criterion measures in nursing care: Reliability test results; Instrument of health status measures* (vol. 1) (PB-267 004). Springfield, VA: National Technical Information Service.

Horn, B. J. , & Swain, M. A. (1977b). *Development of criterion measures in nursing care: Manual for instrument of health status measures* (vol. 2) (PB-267 005). Springfield, VA: National Technical Information Service.

Joint Commission on Accreditation of Hospitals (1974, January). *Staff communication: Workshop on evaluation & documentation of nursing care.* Seattle, WA.

Kim, M. J., McFarland, G. K., & McLane, A. M. (Eds.). (1984). *Pocket guide to nursing diagnosis.* St. Louis: C. V. Mosby.

Kritek, P. B. (1978). The generation and classification of nursing diagnosis: Toward a theory of nursing. *Image, 10,* 30 – 43.

Krumme, U. (1975). The case for criterion-referenced measurement. *Nursing Outlook, 23*(12), 764 – 770.

Krumme, U. (1977). Criterion-referenced measurement for student evaluation. Council on BAC and Higher Degrees program, National League of Nursing, In *Evaluation of students in baccalaureate nursing programs* (pp. 25 – 61) (Publication No. 15-1684). New York: National League for Nursing.

Krumme, U, (1981). *Criterion-referenced measurement of student clinical performance* (Summer Fellowship Follow-Up Report). Seattle: Seattle University.

Lee, H. A., & Strong, K. A. (1985). Using nursing diagnosis to describe the clinical competence of baccalaureate and associate degree graduating students: A comparative study. *Image, 17*(3), 82 – 85.

Lenburg, C. (1976). *Criteria for developing clinical performance evaluation* (Publication No. 23-1634). New York: National League for Nursing.

Lenburg, C. (1979). *The development and implementation of clinical performance examinations: Transition to accountabililty in education and service.* New York: Appleton-Century-Crofts.

Loustau, A., Lenz, M., Lee, K., McKenna, M., Hirako, S., Walker, W. F., & Goldsmith, J. W. (1980). Evaluating students' clinical performance: Using videotapes to establish rater reliability. *Journal of Nursing Education, 19*(7), 10 – 17.

Mallick, M. J. (1977). Do nursing educators preach what they want practiced? *Nursing Outlook, 25*(4), 244 – 247.

Mallick, M. J. (1983). Nursing diagnosis and the novice student. *Nursing and Health Care, 4,* 445 – 459.

McBride, J. L., Mohr, J. L., Smith, A. P., Swanson, D. J., & Kelly, P. (1975). *PEP workbook for nurses: Advanced.* Chicago: Joint Commission on Accreditation of Hospitals.

McLane, A. M. (1982). Nursing diagnosis in baccalaureate and graduate education. In M. J. Kim & D. A. Moritz (Eds.), *Classification of nursing diagnosis: Proceedings of the third and fourth national conferences (pp. 105 – 113). New York: McGraw- Hill.*

Medicus Systems Corp. (1985). *Nursing productivity and quality system: Group health cooperative-Eastside Hospital* (Final Report). Evanston, IL: Author.

National League for Nursing. (1982). *Competencies of graduates of nursing programs* (Publication No. 14-1905). New York: Author.

New Mexico SNAP Project: System for a Nursing Articulation Program. (1979). *Minimum behavioral expectations of new graduates from Mew Mexico schools of nursing.* Albuquerque, NM: University of Albuquerque.

Orange County/Long Beach Nursing Consortium. (1981). *Expected educational competencies of nursing graduates.* Orange County, CA: Orange County/Long Beach Nursing Consortium.

Pearson, B. D. (1977). *Clinical simulations for teaching the nursing process: Final progress report* (PHS Special Project Grant 05D00531-01 NUD10). Milwaukee, WI: University of Wisconsin.

Popham, W. J. (1972). *An evaluation guidebook: A set of practical guidelines for the educational evaluator.* Los Angeles: The Instructional Objectives Exchange.

Seattle University School of Nursing. (1981a). *Self-report for National League for Nursing accreditation: Curriculum* (vol. 1). Seattle: Author.

Seattle University School of Nursing. (1981b). *Self-report for National League for Nursing: Course descriptions* (vol. 2). Seattle: Author.

Smeltzer, C. H., Feltman, B., & Rajki, K. (1983). Nursing quality assurance: A process, not a tool. *Journal of Nursing Administration, 13*(1), 5 – 9.

Strickland, O. (1984, February). *Classical and non-classical approach to measurement.* Paper presented at the Measurement of Clinical and Educational Nursing Outcomes Workshop I, Baltimore.

University of the State of New York – Regents External Degree Program at Albany. (1976). *The New York regents external degrees in nursing: Historical developments and program study guides for the associate degree.* Albany, NY: Author.

University of the State of New York – Regents External Degree Program at Albany. (1978). *New York regents external degree, bachelor of science (nursing) degree description.* Albany, NY: Author.

Van Maanen, H. M. (1981). Improvement of quality of nursing care: A goal to challenge in the eighties. *Journal of Advanced Nursing, 6*(1), 31 – 37.

Waltz, C. (1984, January). *State of the art of measurement in nursing outcomes.* Paper presented at the Measurement of Clinical and Educational Nursing Outcomes Workshop I, Baltimore.

Waltz, C., Strickland, O. L., & Lenz, E. R. (1984). *Measurement in nursing research.* Philadelphia: F. A. Davis.

Ward, M. J., & Fetler, M. E. (Eds.). (1979). *Instruments for use in nursing education research.* Boulder, CO: Western Interstate Commission for Higher Education.

Ward, M. F., & Lineman, C. A. (Eds.). (1978). *Instruments for measuring practice and other health care variables* (vol. 2) (Publication No. HRA 78 – 54). Bethesda, MD: U.S. Department of Health, Education and Welfare.

Warren, J. J. (1983). Accountability and nursing diagnosis. *Journal of Nursing Administration, 13*(10), 34 – 37.

Williams, E. M., & Scott-Warner, M. (1985). *The preparation and utilization of new nursing graduates.* Boulder, CO: Western Interstate Commission for Higher Education.

# Clinical Performance Evaluation Tool for Measuring the Ability to Apply

Patient's initials _____Med. diagnosis/date \_\_\_\_ Prescribed analgesic \_\_\_\_
Student name _____Surg. prodedures/date \_\_ Activity _____
Date(s) of clinical _____ Hot/cold application \_\_\_\_

## CRITICAL ELEMENTS FOR CLINICAL PERFORMANCE FOR ORIENTED ADULT CLIENTS WITH ACUTE PAIN ON ANALGESIC MEDICATIONS

The items marked with a box ☐ may be asked of the client/nursing staff; those items that are circled must be observed; remaining items may be validated with a student. Place a check mark in Yes column when performance behavior met, in No column if omitted, or in NA column if item does not apply.

Yes No NA

I. Assesses client's pain
   A. Collects subjective data
      1. States location    1.
      2. Describes intensity (on scale of 1, no pain, to 10, unbearable pain).    2.
      3. Describes type (e.g., burning, cramping, bloating, radiating).    3.
      4. States duration (how long pain has been present).    4.
      5. Describes chronology (precipitating events/ aggravating factors).    5.
      6. Describes ways client controls pain (past/current).    6.
      7. States beliefs about pain control (culture/religion).    7.
   B. Collects objective data
      ☐1.☐ Describes behavioral responses, e.g., body position, facial expression, splinting, activity level.    1.
      ☐2.☐ States physiological responses, e.g., alterations in P/R/BP, perspiration, N/V, pallor, distention/ muscle tension.    2.
      ☐3.☐ States contributing factors, e.g., fatigue, concerns/ fears or worries.    3.
      ☐4.☐ States pattern of pain medication administration for past 48 hours.    4.
   C. Identifies possible cause of client's pain.
      1. Gives "due to" statement.    1.
      2. Explains underlying pathophysiological/ psychosocial alteration.    2.

II. Identifies expected outcomes and deadline.                    Yes No NA
   1. States: "No verbal or nonverbal expression of pain".   1.
   2. States: "Performs activities, e.g., DB, C, ambulating".   2.
   3. States: "P and R within NML for client".   3.
   4. States checking interval of prescribed analgesic or
      other pain relief measures.   4.

III. Implements client-family/nurse actions.
   A. Provides comfort measures.
     [1.] Implements individualized pain relief methods (see
       IA6).   1.
     [2.] Offers/gives bedpan/bath/oral, pericare, change of
       linen, reinforcement of dressing(s).   2.
     [3.] Positions/repositions client/ambulates as prescribed. 3.
     [4.] Applies hot/cold measures as prescribed.   4.
     [5.] Encourages/listens to expressions of fears/
       concerns/worries.   5.
   B. Implements pain relief measures other than comfort
     measures.
     1. Provides distraction, e.g., radio, TV, visits.   1.
     2. Includes relaxation technique, e.g. DB, massage
       (unless contraindicated), centering exercises.   2.
   C. Medicates appropriately if required.
     1. Offers pain medications at prescribed intervals. (If
       Rt above 10-12 for narcotics)   1.
     2. Administers pain medications within 15 minutes of
       request.   2.

IV. Evaluates extent to which outcomes are met.
   [1.] Checks client within 30 minutes for effectiveness of
     pain relief measures other than medications.   1.
   [2.] Checks client within 30 minutes following administration
     of analgesic(s).   2.
   (3.) Records response to pain management program.   3.
   4. Reports client's response to pain management program
     to primary nurse/team leader/MD.   4.

## CRITICAL ELEMENTS FOR CLINICAL PERFORMANCE FOR ORIENTED ADULT CLIENTS WITH CHRONIC PAIN

The items marked with a box ☐ may be asked of the client/ nursing staff; those items that are circled must be observed; remaining items may be validated with student. Place a check mark in Yes column when performance behavior met; in No column if omitted, or in NA column if item does not apply.

I. Assesses client's pain.                                    Yes No NA
   A. Collects subjective data
     1. States location   1.
     2. Describes intensity (on scale of 1, no pain, to 10,
       unbearabe pain).   2.

      3.  Describes type (e.g., burning, cramping, bloating,   Yes  No  NA
          radiating).    3.
      4.  States duration (how long pain has been present).  4.
      5.  Describes chronology (precipitating events/
          aggravating factors).    5.
      6.  Describes ways client controls pain (past/current).  6.
      7.  States beliefs about pain control (culture/religion).  7.
      8.  States if pain interferes with ADL's.  8.
      9.  States if pain interferes with family role, social
          interaction/work.    9.

  B.  Collects objective data
      1.  Describes behavioral responses, e.g., body position,
          facial expression, splinting/muscle tension.  1.
      2.  States contributing factors, e.g., concerns/fears/
          worries.    2.
      3.  States level of activity (how much time per day in
          bed/chair/active).    3.
      4.  States pattern of pain medication administration
          for past 48 hours.    4.

  C.  Identifies possible cause of client's pain.
      1.  Gives "due to" statement (original injury/surgery
          when pain started).    1.
      2.  Explains underlying pathophysiological/
          psychosocial alteration.    2.
      3.  Identifies expected outcomes and deadline.

II.  Identifies expected outcomes and deadlines
    1.  States: "Able to cope with pain."  1.
    2.  States: "Pain doesn't interfere with necessary activities."  2.
    3.  States Alternative ways of dealing with pain other than
       medication.    3.
    4.  States checking interval of prescribed analgesic or
       other pain relief measures.    4.

III.  Implements client-family/nurse actions.
  A.  Provides comfort measures.
      1.  Implements individualized pain relief methods (see
          IA6).    1.
      2.  Offers/gives bedpan/bath/oral, pericare, change of
          linen.    2.
      3.  Positions/repositions client/*ambulates as prescribed.*  3.
      4.  Applies hot/cold measures as prescribed.  4.
      5.  Listens to expressions of fears/concerns/worries.  5.
      6.  Responds to c/o pain factually, not sympathetically.  6.

  B.  Implements pain relief measures other than comfort
      measures.
      1.  Encourages conversation not related to pain.  1.
      2.  Gives positive feedback for activities that do not
          focus on pain.    2.
      3.  Provides distraction, e.g., radio, TV, visits.  3.
      4.  Includes relaxation technique, e.g. DB, massage
          (unless contraindicated), centering exercises.    4.

     5.   Provides alternative methods of pain relief, e.g.     Yes No NA
         biofeedback, TENS, opportunity for self-hypnosis.  5.

  C.  Medicates appropriately.

     1.   Administers medications at prescribed intervals.   1.

IV.  Evaluates extent to which outcomes are met.

     $\boxed{1.}$  Checks client within 30 minutes for effectiveness of
         pain measures other than medications.         1.

     $\boxed{2.}$  Checks client within 30 minutes following administration
         of analgesic(s).                         2.

     ③  Records client's level of activity.           3.

     4.   Records client's level of activity to primary nurse/
         team leader/MD.                     4.

     ⑤  Records response to pain management program.   5.

     6.   Reports client's response to pain management program
         to primary nurse/team leader/MD.         6.

## CRITICAL ELEMENTS FOR CLINICAL PERFORMANCE FOR HOSPITALIZED ADULTS WITH ALTERED SLEEP PATTERN DISTURBANCE PATTERNS, ON HYPNOTIC MEDICATION

The items marked with a Box ☐ may be asked of the client/ nursing staff; those items that are circled must be observed; remaining items may be validated with student. Place a check mark in Yes column if performance behavior met; in No column if omitted, or in NA column if item does not apply.

I.  Assesses client's sleep/wakefulness pattern/environmental controls/other influencing factors.

|  |  | Prior to hospital | During hospital |
|---|---|---|---|
|  |  | Yes No NA | Yes No NA |
| A. | Collects subjective data Sleep-wakefulness pattern |  |  |
| 1. | States client's beliefs of number of hours of sleep/ naps to stay healthy. | 1. | 1. |
| 2. | States client's usual bedtime/arising/hours. | 2. | 2. |
| 3. | States time of naps hours. | 3. | 3. |
| 4. | States how long it usually takes client to fall asleep. | 4. | 4. |
| 5. | States number of awakenings during sleep. | 5. | 5. |
| 6. | States what wakes client up once asleep. | 6. | 6. |
| 7. | States what helps client get back to sleep if awoken. | 7. | 7. |
| 8. | Describes client's dream patterns (no recall/pleasant/ frightening). | 8. | 8. |
| 9. | Describes patterns of waking behavior that may appear during sleep (e.g. sleepwalking/grinding of teeth/jerking movements). | 9. | 9. |

|  | Prior to hospital | During hospital |
|---|---|---|
|  | Yes No NA | Yes No NA |

10. States if snoring is present during sleep.      10.      10.

11. Describes awake state following sleep (refreshed/ fatigued).      11.      11.

Environmental controls

1. Describes temperature/ventilation used (thermostat setting/windows open or closed.)      1.      1.

2. Describes bedding used (number of blankets/pillows).      2.      2.

3. States lighting used (none/dim/ night/full light).      3.      3.

4. State noise level present (quiet/loud).      4.      4.

Physical activity/care/recreation

1. Describes pattern of physical activity during waking hours/prescribed activity level.      1.      1.

2. Describes snack/drink taken prior to retiring.      2.      2.

3. States physical care routine followed prior to bedtime (bath/ shower/teeth brushing).      3.      3.

4. Describes quiet recreation followed prior to bedtime (reading/TV/radio/handwork).      4.      4.

5. Describes waking routine followed (drink/food/bath/ shower).      5.      5.

Other influencing factors

1. Describes client's concerns/worries at home/work/ hospitaization.      1.      1.

2. Describes use of caffeine (coffee/ tea/carbonated drinks).      2.      2.

3. Describes use of other stimulants (e.g., alcohol).      3.      3.

4. Describes use of drugs to assist sleep.      4.      4.

B. Collects objective data

   1. Describes behavioral responses, e.g., full concentration/decreased attention span; easygoing/irritable; active/inactive.      1.

   2. States physiological responses, e.g., muscle weakness (droopy eyelids); yawning; oriented/disoriented.      2.

   3. Describes contributing factors, e.g., presence of pain, IVs, bandages/ casts, incontinence.      3.

       4.  Reviews record of several days          Yes No NA
           sleep-activity cycle
           (notes/graphs/diary).               4.

C.  Identifies client problem and possible
     cause of altered sleep-wakefulness
     pattern.
     1.  States problem (e.g., sleep depriva-
         tion; primary sleep disorder;
         insomnia/hyper-somnia/narcolepsy,
         secondary sleep disorder:
         depression/alcoholism/chronic
         renal insufficiency/ hypothyroidism/
         schizophrenia/anorexia nervosa).     1.
     2.  Gives "due to" statement, e.g., situ-
         ational stress/ crises, medical path-
         ophysiology, psychosocial illness,
         drug-related disorder, aging process.    2.

II.  Identifies expected outcomes and deadline.
     1.  States: "falls asleep within 15-30
         minutes."                       1.
     2.  States: "Sleeps 6-8 hours uninterupted."   2.
     3.  States: "Feels refreshed/rested/slept
         out."                         3.
     4.  States: "Slept through the night."     4.
     5.  States checking interval of prescribed
         hypnotic/other sleep management
         action (Q.D.)                 5.

III.  Implements client-family/nurse actions
    A.  Establishes sleep environment
       1.  Implements client's usual
           temperature/ventilation used.     1.
       2.  Provides number of blankets/
           pillows usually used by client.     2.
       3.  Adjusts lighting to level preferred
           by client.                 3.
       4.  Adjusts noise to level of client's
           usual setting.             4.
       5.  Provides for privacy (e.g., curtains
           pulled/doors closed).         5.
    B.  Provides for physical activity/care/
      recreation reflective of client's usual
      pattern.
       1.  Encourages usual pattern of physi-
           cal activity during waking hours/
           implements prescribed activity level
           (out of bed, wheelchair, ambulation).  1.
       2.  Provides usual snack/drink taken
           by client prior to retiring (as
           permitted).                 2.

        3.   Provides for/assists with physical        Yes No NA
            care routine followed by client prior
            to bedtime (elimination/bath/
            shower/teeth brushing).        3.
        4.   Provides for clean/unwrinkled bed
            linen.        4.
        5.   Positions/repositions as permitted
            for comfort.        5.
        6.   Adjusts binders/bandages/tubes.        6.
        7.   Encourages/provides for usual
            quiet recreation prior to bedtime.        7.
        8.   Provides for usual waking routine
            of client.        8.
  C.  Promotes relaxation.
        1.   Encourages/provides opportunity
            to talk about concerns/worries.        1.
        2.   Provides information regarding hos-
            pital care activities.        2.
        3.   Offers/gives back massage.        3.
        4.   Encourages/provides for centering.        4.
  D.  Implements other influencing actions.
        1.   Adjusts/restricts intake of caffeine/
            other stimulants.        1.
        2.   Medicates appropriately for pain if
            present.        2.
        3.   Medicates appropriately for sleep
            disorder if other measures fail.        3.
        4.   Plans uninterrupted sleep cycles of
            60-90 minutes when giving care
            during sleep period.        4.
        5.   Encourages/provides for recording
            of sleep-activity patterns by client.        5.
IV.  Evaluates extent to which outcomes are
    met.
    1.   Checks client within 15-30 minutes fol-
        lowing Implementation of sleep-assisting
        measures other than hypnotic.        1.
    2.   Checks client within 15-30 minutes fol-
        lowing administration of hypnotic.        2.
    3.   Checks client from 6–8 hours to ascer-
        tain if uninterrupted sleep.        3.
    4.   Describes client's expressions of wake
        state following sleep hours/interventions.        4.
    5.   Records response to sleep management
        program.        5.
    6.   Reports response to sleep management
        program to primary nurse/team
        leader/MD.        6.

## CRITICAL ELEMENTS FOR CLINICAL PERFORMANCE WITH CLENT-FAMILIES WITH KNOWLEDGE DEFICIT

Items marked with a box ☐ may be asked of the client-family/ nursing staff; those items that are circled must be observed; remaining items may be validated with student. Place a check mark in Yes column when performance behavior met, in No column if omitted, or in NA column if item does not apply.

I. Assesses client-family's health teaching needs
   A. Collects subjective data                          Yes No NA
       Client-family readiness for learning
         ☐1. States client-family's willingness/interest/ availability for learning.     1
         ☐2. States client-family's psychological/physical readiness.     2.
       Client-family/nursing staff's perception of teaching needs
         ☐3. States client-family's learning needs in the cognitive domain (knowledge of facts/concepts).     3.
         ☐4. States client-family's learning needs in the psychomotor domain (technical skills)     4.
         ☐5. States client-family's learning needs in the affective domain (attitudes/feelings)     5.
         ☐6. States client-family's educational level/ experience(s).     6.
   B. Collects objective data
       Client-family experiential readiness
         ☐1. Describes client-family's background knowledge in the cognitive domain.     1.
         ☐2. Describes client-family's proficiency of psychomotor skills.     2.
         ☐3. Describes client-family's nonverbal behaviors indicating learning needs in affective domain, (e.g., smoking/ drinking/overeating).     3.
         ☐4. Evaluates cultural patterns influencing teaching-learning.     4.
II. Identifies Client-family problem related to health teaching needs and possible cause.
   1. States specific problem (e.g., lack of knowledge, lack of readiness to learn, unavailable for learning).     1.
   2. Gives "due to" statement (e.g., never having been informed, misinformed, decreased perceptual field resulting from anxiety).     2.
III. Identifies client-family expected outcomes and deadline(s).
   1. Client-family verbalizes the expected outcomes of teaching-learning.     1.
   2. Client-family state deadline date(s) for expected outcomes to be met.     2.
   3. Client-family demonstrates that learning has occurred.     3.

IV. Implements Client-family/nurse actions          Yes No NA
    Prior to teaching
    1.  Validates with client-family the main objective(s) goal(s) purpose(s) of teaching-learning.     1.
    2.  Formulates with client-family expected outcomes of teaching-learning.     2.
    3.  Formulates with client-family deadline date(s).     3.
    [4.]  Contracts with client-family for time and date(s) available for teaching-learning.     4.
    ⑤  Formulates a written teaching plan with teacher objective(s), outcome criteria, deadline date(s), content outline, teaching-learning actions.     5.
    ⑥  Controls the environment for teaching-learning effectiveness (necessary equipment available and in working order; privacy and freedom from noise/distractions provided).     6.
    During teaching
    ①  Uses patient education materials suited for client-family educational/experiental level: pamphlets, written handouts, AV aids.     1.
    ②  Provides for discussion/role playing.     2.
    ③  Demonstrates skill(s) to be learned.     3.
    ④  Provides for return demonstration of skills (a minimum of three times).     4.
    ⑤  Elicits feedback at least twice during teaching.     5.
    ⑥  Modifies content and/or approach based upon feedback.   6.
    ⑦  Gives positive feedback during return demonstration of knowledge/skills/attitudes (a minimum of three times during teaching).     7.
    ⑧  Summarizes content/teaching-learning activities.     8.
    At the end of teaching
    ①  Uses an evaluation tool (e.g., test questions, behavioral skills checklist).     1.
    ②  Summarizes client-family learning that occurred.     2.
    [3.]  Stays within agreed upon time frame.     3.
    [4.]  States possible follow-up of learning-teaching activities by staff.     4.

V. Determines extent to which client-family outcomes are met.
    1.  States if client-family expected outcomes of teaching-learning are met.     1.
    2.  If not, states follow-up of teaching and learning actions.   2.
    ③  Documents teaching and learning to assure continuity.     3.
    [4.]  Reports teaching and learning to primary nurse/ team leader/MD.     4.

# 16
# Measuring the Validity of Computer-Assisted Instructional Media

*Sandra Millon Underwood*

*This chapter discusses the Software Evaluation Tool for Nursing, a measure for assessing computer-based instructional programs for nursing education.*

The primary responsibility of nurse educators who teach in generic programs is to prepare their learners as generalists, capable of functioning in any of the multiple roles of the profession. In order to do this, they must provide the learners with the necessary direct instruction, clinical experiences, and laboratory activities that will lead to the acquisition of a broad base of scientific nursing knowledge and to the development of a minimal level of clinical competence for safe and effective nursing practice. Jacobs, Fivars, Edwards, and Fitzpatrick (1978) utilized the critical incident technique developed by Flanagan (1954) to identify the critical requirements for safe and effective nursing practice. These incidents reflect not only the need for the practicing nurse to have acquired a wide base of knowledge that relates to the behavioral, social, and natural sciences but also the importance of synthesizing this knowledge base into specific demonstrable nursing behaviors. The incidents themselves are (1) measures of performance of specific nursing behaviors, (2) limited to patient-oriented components of nursing care, and (3) noted as emphasizing nurse/patient interaction and intervention. Therefore, the instructional settings utilized in the various schools of nursing should allow for the development of such learning outcomes. To ensure that the educational goal has been and is being fulfilled, it has often been suggested that educators and researchers further this investigation to determine if a relationship exists between the actual educational experiences provided by nursing schools and the specific incidents for safe and effective nursing practice, to ensure that such a relationship has been maintained.

McManus (1949) asserted that in order to teach to a high level of nursing competence the educational experiences and expected learning outcomes should not only include the lower-level processes of remembering, recalling, recognizing, conceiving, defining, and distinguishing *but also the higher-level processes* of generalizing, deducing, analyzing, understanding, knowing, reasoning, qualifying, formalizing and asserting propositions, inferring and demonstrating the ability to systematize knowledge deductively. It would be pretentious to state that schools of nursing are not in favor of creating an educational environment that fosters the development of such higher-level mental abilities. However, in doing so instructional strategies must be implemented that provide learning situations that challenge the student to think and test solutions on the spot. In the clinical setting, the immediate needs of the client provide the student with the opportunity to implement novel nursing interventions that will contribute to client well-being, comfort, and recovery. However, the development of higher mental abilities can be affectively achieved, only where instruction is provided to assist the learner to do so. The learner must be taught to pull together concepts, principles, skills, and implications pertinent to the problem at hand and to fuse them in planning, intervening, and evaluating a program of action for solving the problems identified.

The higher mental abilities of reasoning, judging, inferring, and evaluating are inherent aspects of professional nursing most often developed through experience. Yet it is the quality of those experiences provided to students that will determine if he or she develops proficiency and mastery of these mental abilities. Dewey (1938) reemphasized this notion when he stated the belief that all genuine education comes about through experience does not mean that all experiences are "genuinely" or "equally" educative. Likewise, Dale (1969) and Russel (1976) described a hierarchy of learning experiences and suggested that those experiences that were the most concrete were limiting in regard to student participation; for example, reading or hearing lectures of an experience are the least desirable and least educative alternative approaches to instruction. These experiences, documented as being the least desirable, are noted as being the most frequently used. The clinical settings of hospitals and health care agencies as we know them provide student nurses with the opportunity to administer direct patient care. Although these settings provide students access to actual clients whom they may collaborate with and minister to, it also limits them in that the hospital setting does not offer students the flexibility of experimenting with alternative nursing actions and nursing interventions. Such experiences would be necessary to develop skill in processing higher-order nursing problems. The integration of simulated nursing laboratories into the curriculum may be a remedy for this limitation.

Interactive computing systems have emerged as a primary component for simulating nursing experiences during the last two decades. While their use appeared to be primarily experimental in the late 1960s, interactive computing systems have proved to be effective for presenting nursing concepts, fostering the development of skills in problem solving and critical decision making, and testing applications and the utilization of the nursing process. Milner (1980) describes the benefits as being that of instructional enhancement and cost-effectiveness, but interactive computing capabilities have been observed to transcend their value for providing direct didactic instruction to include that of "assuring" the transference of knowledge, concepts, attitudes, and behaviors expected of a nurse within a professional setting. Their qualities are thought to be a function of their inherent pedagogical features, which resemble those of effective teaching as described by Bloom (1976). Within the conceptual model proposed by Bloom, four variables are described as essential for the development and implementation of quality instruction within any learning process:

1. Cues – instruction as to what is to be learned as well as directions as to what the learner is to do in the learning process.
2. Participation – the extent to which the learner actively participates or engages in the learning process.
3. Reinforcement – the extent to which the student is rewarded for learning.
4. Corrective feedback – the testing of learners comprehension.

These characteristics, which are inherent pedagogical features of simulated computer-assisted instruction, are, if effectively utilized, believed to provide nursing educators and learners with an excellent medium for individual and group instruction.

Given their educational potential, pedagogical capabilities, and marketability in the health care arena, there is a wealth of computer simulations for nursing education. The aim of most authors of computer software is to provide the profession with highly marketable instructional media that will ultimately enhance the aquisition of health-related concepts and health-related behaviors. However, little effort has been expressed regarding the development of specific evaluation tools that may be utilized by authors and consumers alike to assess computer media, before or after their development for quality, appropriateness, and usability within various curricula. The goal of this proposed endeavor was to develop and test an evaluation tool that may effectively evaluate the content of computer simulations developed for use in nursing education and also evaluate the cognitive skills employed by the learner within the framework of the simulation.

## REVIEW OF THE LITERATURE

Too little attention has been focused on the development of tools for evaluating the multitude of computer simulations being mass-produced today. The few reports of evaluation tools that are available and easily accessible tend to be so generalized that they merely reflect an overall interest in the subject matter and/or appeal of the general graphic displays. In addition, they are so pedagogically limited that they neglect to place an emphasis on establishing content validity, determining core objectives, or monitoring the author's/teacher's reference to cognitive, affective, and psychomotor behavioral outcomes, criteria that are deemed essential outcomes in nursing education.

Diane Billings (1984), in her recent report on the evaluation process of instructional computing, argues that the current and anticipated increased use of simulated computer-assisted instructional media in nursing education requires mechanisms for ongoing assessment. Given the limited resources for such an evaluation, she reports her recommendation for a naturalistic evaluation focus and implies that the data collected during the evaluation of simulated computer-assisted instructional programs should determine the "values," "needs," and "activities of the individual groups involved."

Because of the fact that very few educational software evaluation standards are presently available, many educators are said to be forced to quickly develop and use guidelines in the form of checklists, to provide an idea of what they can expect from select software programs. Wade (1980) described the characteristics of good learning situations and proposed the development of an evaluation tool utilizing a similar format. She reported that such a rating tool should utilize five criteria for identifying and rating computer-assisted instruction (CAI) for learning program characteristics. This tool would then attempt to assume that the following demands be met: (1) the learner must be right; (2) the learner must be ready; (3) learning needs must be managed or facilitated; (4) assimilation must be practicable; and (5) learning must be efficient. Hecht, Johnson, and Kansky (1981) developed a similarly structured tool; however, they utilized even more global descriptors, such as a passive/active program characterized on a present/absent scale.

The computer technology program of the Northwest Regional Educational Laboratory (Weaver & Johnson, 1984) was also prompted to develop an evaluator's guide for microcomputer-based instructional programs, given the fierce competition among program developers to increase the quality of courseware/software. They initially utilized an evaluation scale in the form of a 21-item checklist, which was further expanded in 1982 to include areas for more descriptive assessments by the evaluators. This tool emphasizes the evaluation of content characteristics as the key variables to be evaluated when assessing a computer program's worth.

Klopfer (1983) constructed a microcomputer software evaluation instrument to aid educators in examining and discussing the merits of a microcomputer software package. The primary intent was for the science instructional program; however, it provides a sensible process and basic criteria for assessing software packages of all kinds. Through a 7-point Likert-type scale their tool evaluates (1) "policy issues" (the degree of appropriateness, compatability, cost-effectiveness, and instructional effectiveness of the software); (2) "instructional quality" (the degree of effective pedagogy, application of good instructional design principles, adaptibility of the software to students' individual preference, assessment of student's learning, and the role envisioned for the student using the software package): (3) "subject matter standards" (accuracy of content, sound application of the scientific process, and the absence of stereotypes); (4) "technological quality" (how well the computer program runs, how carefully its operational features are designed, and how well designed the accompanying student/teacher materials are).

## THE INSTRUMENT DEVELOPMENT PROCESS

In an attempt to further identify the critical characteristics of computerized instructional media used in nursing that should be assessed through formal evaluation, more than 30 authors, editors, and distributors of software for nursing were contacted by this researcher and requested to complete a questionnaire that asked the following question: "Given your experience with the development and utilization of computerized instructional media, identify what you consider to be the most critical characteristics of computerized instructional media for nursing that should be assessed through formal evaluation."

An analysis of the data obtained revealed that nurse educators, administrators, and clinicians engaged in the utilization of computer-based media believed the following to be included among the most critical variables for evaluation of computer software for nursing:

Application to nursing
Program purpose
Program objectives
Program clarity
Effectiveness of the simulation
Instructional design
Adequacy of documentation
Content accuracy
Clinical correlates
Effective utilization of the technology
Hardware and software requirements

Their recommendations appeared to cluster around the four main themes expressed in the Software Evaluation Tool proposed by Klopfer (1983) which was cited previously. Specification of these qualitites is listed in Table 16.1.

**TABLE 16.1** Important Characteristics of Computerized Instructional Media as Identified by Authors, Editors, and Distributors of Nursing Software

Policy Issues
  Does the CAI demonstrate an appropriate use of the computer?
  Is there good branching?
  Is there an appropriate use of color, sound, animation and graphics?
  What are the hardware and, if applicable, software requirements?
  Does the mediated instruction utilize the technology being employed?
  Are the resources available for the implementation of the media (i.e.,
    faculty skilled in the development and/or integration of CAI
    into the current instructional program)?
  Can the end results of the user's efforts be saved on a disk or printer
    for later reference?

Instructional quality
  Is the content accurate?
  Is there adequate documentation?
  Is there integrity of instructional design?
  Is the CAI logical and well structured?
  Is the CAI innovative?
  Is the CAI educationally sound?
  Is the program effective?
  Is the CAI user "simple". . .not just "friendly"?
  Is there an obvious match between CAI and curriculum design?
  Is the CAI based on tightly defined learning outcomes?
  Does the program fulfill its purpose?
  Does the program fulfill the curriculum goals/objectives/behaviors?
  Is the CAI educational?
  Does the software meet the needs that have been defined for its par-
    ticular use?
  Does the program meet the learners' identified learning needs?
  Does the material meet the particular needs of the users?
  How true to life is the simulation, i.e. does it take into account all the
    essential variables and allow for their interaction with each other
    in determining the simulations results?
  Is there shaped feedback and remediation incorporated into the
    instructional design?
  Are the computers' responses meaningful?
  Does the program operate on varying levels of difficulty?
  Is modification of certain variables and their parameters permitted
    by the program (i.e., can you change a drug dose)?
  Does the software provide a form of instruction or experience that
    cannot be provided through another media?
  Does the CAI offer something more for learning than textbooks and
    traditional materials?

Subject matter standards
  Is the CAI clear/
  Is the content valid?

*(continued)*

**TABLE 16.1** *(Continued)*

Is the information accurate?
Is the simulation applicable to nursing?
Is the content applicable to professional practice?
Does the author specifically identify the objective(s) to be accom-
   plished within the CAI?

Technical quality
   Are the screen displays clear and crisp?
   Are the screens uncluttered?
   Does each display (screen) make one single point?
   Is this an effective simulation that applies theory?
   Is there freedom for the student to use this CAI with ease?
   Is there effective looping, branching, etc.?
   Is there effective use of graphics etc., as appropriate?
   Has the author created a sense of "fun" to understand the specified
      concepts as a means to "stimulate" self-directed learning?
   Is the CAI gentle to the user?

In addition it was suggested that within any program evaluation the
   following questions be asked:
   Is the simulation "friendly"?
   Does the program meet the needs of the defined population?
   Is the program "fun"?
   Does the program offer varying levels of difficulty?
   Does the program offer more than textbooks?
   Is/are the simulation/simulations true to life?
   Is modification of certain variables permitted within the simulation?

The data provided by the developers and reviewers of CAI software,
when compared to the many tools used today, suggest that many of the
critical characteristics related to the programs' content, teaching effectiveness, technical quality, and/or ability to develop higher-level cognitive, affective, and psychomotor behaviors are being assessed superfi-
cially. In addition, the most critical assessments are being left unasked.
We therefore suggest and support the development of a more complete
evaluation tool for nursing that addresses content analysis, contextual
variables pedagogical features, technical evaluations of the instructional
design for the content, and contextual, pedagogical, and technical features that reflect the integration of higher level cognitive, affective, and
psychomotor behaviors expected of the professional nurse. Such a
framework would not only provide for careful assessment of each
instructional situation for cognitive, affective, and, when appropriate,
psychomotor outcome behaviors but would also address the utilization
of the nursing process and higher-level cognitive skills throughout the
computer simulation. The proposed evaluation tool addresses those
objectives.

## Objectives

Utilization of the measurement tool will provide the user with a mechanism that will provide the opportunity to

1. Assess the instructional characteristics of selected computerized nursing simulations.
2. Critically evaluate the contextual design and constant presentation of selected computerized nursing simulations.
3. Describe the cognitive, affective, and psychomotor nursing behaviors required for the completion of selected computerized nursing simulations.
4. Identify the technical characteristics of select computerized nursing simulations that either aid or impede its utilization.

## Operational Definitions

*Contextual analysis*: description of the general content domain of the computer simulation, including evaluation of objective centrality, content analysis, and appropriateness of feedback.

*Instructional characteristics*: items that describe the instructional techniques and purposes employed in the package, including instructional strategies, stated objectives, and defined prerequisites.

*Instructional validity*: instructional programs within nursing that forster the utilization of higher-level cognitive skills and all aspects of the nursing process.

*Pedagogical characteristics*; the central variables of instruction, which include an analysis of the effective utilization of cues, participation, reinforcement, and feedback within the instructional program.

*Technical features*: user support materials and information displays that aid in the independent operation of the program.

## Conceptual Framework

Given the nature of this evaluation to measure the status of computer-assisted instructional materials for nursing within domains deemed essential for this type of media, a criterion-referenced framework was used as the basis of the tool development. Waltz, Strickland, and Lenz (1984) state that such should be the case given that criterion-referenced measures are used to assess for attainment of minimum requirements based on some predetermined criterion or performance standard.

## Tool Development

Following the critical review of the literature and the analysis of the data gathered from reviewers, developers, ,and users of computer-assisted instructional media, it appeared appropriate to structure the evaluation tool within four conceptual domains: nursing content, pedagogy, technical quality of the media, and policy issued, or the degree of appropriate use of the media itself. While using the *Evaluators Guide for Microcomputer-based Instructional Packages* (Weaver, 1982) as a model, items were specifically developed within each content area to assess the precision of the computer-assisted instructional program to meet expected standards for nursing media.

## ADMINISTRATION AND SCORING

Following the review of any computer-based instructional program for nursing, it was projected that evaluators may use the tool to critically assess the four content areas of any program designed for use within any nursing curriculum. Using multiple sets of bipolar descriptors, the evaluators are asked to rate the program being assessed using a 7-point Likert scale. After carefully considering the computer program being evaluated, the raters are requested to consider the descriptors at both ends of the scale and then assign a single value on the −3 to +3 scale according to how well the Right or Left descriptor applies to the software program being judged. Following the total evaluation, it is proposed that the scores would then be compiled and compared with an established profile of minimum standards for nursing educational media. As a consequence, decisions related to program acquisition, utilization, and recommendation could most and/or more efficiently be made.

The most critical component of the tool development appeared to be that of constructing appropriate and precise descriptors that would measure the content areas for nursing. Within-nursing concerns relate not only to the accuracy of content, effectiveness of the instructional design, and the appropriateness and ease with which media could be used but also to issues related to the three domains of learning and the higher levels of objective achievement. Therefore, much poise and creativity were warranted in the development of items (see instrument at end of chapter). These issues and concerns resulted in the initial development of a 45-item evaluation instrument. To ensure the integrity of each of the items, five content specialists were selected, each of whom agreed to serve as raters and evaluators of the items in the proposed software evaluation instrument. Included among the content specialists were a computer media specialist, a nurse educator and clinician who has authored multiple computer-assisted instructional programs, a nurse educator and administrator who has been involved in the evaluation of audiovisual media for patient and student education, a nurse educator who has frequently engaged in the selection and utilization of computer-assisted instructional materials in baccalaureate settings. Content validity assessment was done initially by each of the content specialists. Given that content validity measures are prerequisite to all other types of validity measures criterion-referenced frameworks, each content specialist was asked to examine the 45 items for format and content to determine if they were appropriate measures of the four specified content domains.

Using the procedure for determining item-objective congruence described in Waltz et al. (1984) to further establish the integrity of each item within its content domain, the content specialists were asked to evaluate each item for its congruence with the specified objective. Using a 3-point scale, they stated whether they were in agreement, disagreement, or undecided as to whether each individual item was indeed a representative measure of the stated content objective domain. Of the 45 items, 21 received perfect congruence ratings ($I = 1.00$); 15 received less than perfect yet satisfactory ratings of congruence ($I > .75$); and 9 received unsatisfactory ratings and were therefore removed from the evaluation instrument ($I < .75$).

Following the determination of item-objective congruence, attempts also were made to obtain an index of the relevance of each item to the content and to the objective domain. The technique described by Waltz et al. (1984) was used: Two content specialists rated the relevance of each item within a proposed criterion-referenced measurement tool as 1, not relevant; 2, somewhat relevant; 3, quite relevant; and 4, very relevant. $P_o$ and $K$ measures of interrater agreement and content validity (CVI) were obtained for the remaining 36 items in the instrument, using similar, yet not identical descriptors – 1, undesirable; 2, not essential; 3, desirable; and 4, essential for the assessment of computer-assisted instructional media for nursing. Much like the item-objective index of congruence, measures of interrater agreement are also rating scales frequently used to assess the validity of any group of items within a measure developed in a criterion-referenced framework. Following the proposed guidelines, a satisfactory degree of agreement related to content validity was established. $P_o$ and $K$ measures of interrater agreement and content validity are shown in Table 16.2.

**TABLE 16.2** $P_o$ **and** $K$ **Measures of Interrater Agreement and Content Validity**

| | Judge 1 | | |
| --- | --- | --- | --- |
| Judge 2 | Undesirable/ not essential | Essential/ desirable | Totals |
| Undesirable/ not essential | 2 | 2 | 4 |
| Essential/ desirable | 3 | 29 | 32 |
| Totals | 5 | 31 | 36 |

$P_o = 2 + 29/36 = .861.$
$P_c = (4/36)(5/36) + (32/36)(31/36) = 0.015 + 0.765 = 0.780.$
$K = P_o - P_c/1 - P_c = 0.861 - 0.780/1 - 0.780 = 0.368.$

In addition, a final test of validity was implemented. After again requesting the assistance of the content specialists, the CVI was obtained in attempts to quantify the extent of agreement between the judges relative to the relevance of the items and the objective domain. An index of .88 was obtained, and as a result, further evidence of the validity of the measurement tool was provided. Martuza (1977) and Waltz et al. (1984) suggest that assessments of content validity are indeed essential for all "measures" and/or "measurement tools." While focusing on determinations as to whether or not the items included within the sample adequately represent the domain of the content addressed by the instrument, the results of such indexing are largely a function and representation of how the instrument was developed. The anticipated result, often following item selection and deletion, is therefore a clearly defined domain from which items to measure the domain are construed.

In addition to assessing the extent to which a measure achieves the purpose for which it was intended, measures of the consistency with which the measuring device assesses the content domain are imperative in the development of any proposed tool. Test-retest, Cronbach's alpha, percent agreement, Cohen's (1960) $K$ and $K_{max}$ statistics were utilized as tests of this tool's reliability.

The test-retest procedure is most commonly used to determine the stability of any measurements obtained using this software evaluation tool, five nurse educators utilized the tool in the evaluation of two commercially produced computer-assisted instructional programs developed for nursing student populations. Evaluators were instructed to review the selected computer-assisted instructional programs at their own pace and then to complete the evaluation instruments. Two hours after completing the initial instrument, the evaluators were again asked to evaluate the computer-assisted instructional program, using an identically constructed evaluation instrument. Test-retest Pearson product-moment correlation coefficients were calculated. By correlating the scores obtained using the Software Evaluation Tool for Nursing, the resulting test-retest reliability observed was .8920. As a result, it may be inferred that there is an 89% consistency between measures from the first to the second occasion. This score provides statistical evidence of the short-term consistency of the measurement tool.

Likewise, the Cronbach's alpha, which statistically estimates the homogeneity of the subpoints of the tool was observed to be .8124. Therefore, it may be concluded that the test items are indeed homogeneous; or in other words, as suggested, the test is measuring one attribute.

To further ascertain the reliability of this instrument, many researchers suggest that percent agreement, Cohen's $K$ and $K_{max}$ evaluations be executed with test-retest data. Using the suggested formulas, the $P_o$ observed was .834. Therefore, 83.4% of the classifications made by the measurement tool on both testing occasions were in agreement. While recognizing that within the percent agreement are instances of item agreement due solely to chance, the Cohen's $K$ was calculated. The results revealed that 56% of the classifications on both measurement occasions were beyond that expected by mere chance. In addition, by using the $K_{max}$, it may be further inferred that there is a relatively high degree of consistency within the measures, since the $K$ versus $K_{max}$ are shown in Tables 16.3 and 16.4.

**TABLE 16.3** Classifications for Test-Retest Administrations of Tool

| Second Administration | First administration | | |
|---|---|---|---|
| | Positive | Negative | Totals |
| Positive | 24 (0.660) | 1 (0.027) | 25 (0.694) |
| Negative | 5 (0.138) | 6 (0.166) | 11 (0.306) |
| Totals | 29 (0.806) | 7 (0.194) | 36 (1.00) |

$P_o = 24/36 + 5/36 = 0.660 + 0.166 = .834$.
$P_c = (25/36)(29/36) + (11/36)(7/36) = 0.559 + 0.059 = 0.62$.
$K = P_c - (P_c/1 - P_c = 0.834 - 0.62/1 - 0.62 = 0.56$ (rounded).

**TABLE 16.4** Tabular Adjustments Required in Table 16.3 for Computation of $K_{max}$

| Second Administration | First administration | | |
|---|---|---|---|
| | Positive | Negative | Totals |
| Positive | 25 (0.694) | 0 (0.00) | 25 (0.694) |
| Negative | 4 (0.111) | 7 (0.194) | 11 (0.306) |
| Totals | 29 (0.806) | 7 (0.194) | 36 (1.00) |

$$K_{max} = \frac{0.694 + 0.194 - [(0.694)(0.806) + (0.306(0.194)]}{1 - [(0.694)(0.806) - (0.306)(0.194)]}$$

$= 0.888 - 0.618/1 - 0.618$
$= 0.207/0.382$
$= 0.71$ (rounded)
$K/K_{max} + 0.56/0.71 = 0.79$

## CONCLUSION AND RECOMMENDATIONS

While it is anticipated that there is much yet to learn regarding the use of automated media in the education and preparation of professional nurses, nurse educators recognize the challenge that awaits. And as the questions related to establishing the validity of teaching mechanisms are at the forefront, the greater question involves identifying those media that may most appropriately meet the needs of the professions populace and highlight those that will not.

The data obtained in this study provide evidence of the Software Evaluation Tool for Nursing's usefulness in the evaluation of computer-assisted instructional media for nursing education. Such evaluations are essential as educators consider alternative experiences for their learners, in hopes of meeting the ever-changing and widening demands of the profession and the needs of the learners. As a result, careful attention may then be focused on the selection, and more important, the development of quality instructional alternatives, especially when the selections are to be considered for use as a substitute for or in conjuction with the preferred clinical experience.

The concern related to establishing standards for computer-assisted instructional media and nontraditional educational techniques only emphasizes how far we have come in nursing education. However, given the expression of this concern, it also magnifies how far we have yet to travel. It is suggested that future research efforts focus on identifying further the pedagogic characteristics of computer-assisted instruction that result in enhanced student achievement. Among the research questions deemed critical to nursing education are (1) What is the most effective placement of computer-assisted instruction in nursing curricula? (2) Which subject areas are most suited for computerized instruction? (3) Is there a real advantage to putting instructional materials into a computerized format? (4) Does computer-assisted instruction achieve something that another more traditional medium could not, and if so, is it worth achieving?

## REFERENCES

Billings, D. M. (1984). Evaluating computer assisted instruction. *Nursing Outlook, 32*, 50-53.

Bloom, B. (1976). *Human characteristics and school learning.* New York: McGraw-Hill.

Cohen, J. (1960). A coefficient of agreement for nominal scales. *Educational and psychological measurement, 29*, 37-46.

Dale, E. (1969). *Audiovisual methods in teaching.* New York: Wiley.

Dewey, J. (1938). *Experience in education.* New York: Macmillian.

Flanagan, J. C. (1954). The critical incident technique.
*Psychological Bulletin, 51*, 327-350.

Hecht, W. P., Johnson, J., & Kansky, R. (1981). *Guidelines for evaluation of computerized instructional materials.* Reston, VA: Council for Teachers of Mathematics.

Jacobs, A. M., Fivars, G., Edwards, D. S., & Fitzpatrick, K. (1978). *Critical requirements for safe/effective nursing practice.* Kansas City; MO: American Nurses Association.

Klopfer, L. (1983). *Microcomputer software evaluation instrument.* Washington, DC: National Science Teachers' Association.

Martuza, V. R. (1977). *Applying norm-referenced and criterion- referenced measurement in education.* Boston: Allyn & Bacon.

McManus, R. (1949). *The effect of experience on nursing achievement.* New York: Teachers College of Columbia University.

Milner, S. (1980). How to make the right decision about microcomputers. *Instructional Innovations, 25,* 12-19.

Russel, J. (1976). *Modular instruction.* Burgess, MN.

Wade, T. E. Jr. (1980). Evaluation of computer-assisted instruction programs and other technical units. *Educational Technology, 20,* 32-35.

Waltz, C., Strickland, O., & Lenz, E. (1984). *Measurement in nursing research,* Philadelphia: F. A. Davis.

Weaver, P. (1982). *The evaluator's guide for microcomputer-based instructional packages.* Eugene, OR: International Council for Computers in Education.

Weaver, C. G., & Johnson, J. E. (1984). Nursing participation in computer vendor selection. *Computers in Nursing, 2,* 31-34.

# Software Evaluation Tool for Nursing (SET-N, 1985)
## Software Evaluation Tool for Evaluation of Computer-Based Instructional Media for Nursing Education (SET-N)

Given the apparent lack of valid and reliable means for evaluating computer-based instructional media for use within nursing education, the following software evaluation tool (SET-N) has been developed. Adapted from the 1983 Micro-Software Evaluation Instrument (Task force on Assessing Computer Augmented Science Instructional Materials – National Science Teachers Association), this SET-N purports to evaluate computer-based instructional materials for nursing.

Following the preview/review of any computer-based instructional program for nursing, evaluators may use this tool to assess the software package in four specific areas: Nursing Content, Pedagogy, Technical Quality, and Policy Issues – appropriateness of use of the media.

This program allows the evaluator to numerically describe any software program related to nursing. Using multiple sets of bipolar descriptors, the evaluators rate the program using a 7-point Likert scale. Following the evaluation, the scores may then be compiled and compared with an established profile of minimal standards for nursing educational media.

Each section of this tool contains a set of bipolar descriptors. Carefully consider the descriptors at both ends of each scale and then assign a value on the −3 to +3 scale according to how well the left or right descriptor applies to the software package you are judging.

| Definitely True | Partly True | Slightly True | Neither Description Applies | Slightly True | Partly True | Definitely True |
|---|---|---|---|---|---|---|
| −3 | −2 | −1 | 0 | +1 | +2 | +3 |

_____ _____ _____ _____ _____ _____ _____

Consider for a moment the following bipolar descriptor:

| | |
|---|---|
| The program makes the computer act as little more than a page turner or workbook. | The program exploits the computer's special capabilities (e.g., graphic animation, simulation) to provide a learning experience not easily possible through other media. |

If you believe that the left descriptor is definitely true about the program you just reviewed, you should rate that item as −3.

| Definitely<br>True<br>−3 | Partly<br>True<br>−2 | Slightly<br>True<br>−1 | Neither<br>Description<br>Applies<br>0 | Slightly<br>True<br>+1 | Partly<br>True<br>+2 | Definitely<br>True<br>+3 |
|---|---|---|---|---|---|---|
| X | | | | | | |

If you believe that the right descriptor is definitely true about the program you have just reviewed, you should rate the item +3.

| Definitely<br>True<br>−3 | Partly<br>True<br>−2 | Slightly<br>True<br>−1 | Neither<br>Description<br>Applies<br>0 | Slightly<br>True<br>+1 | Partly<br>True<br>+2 | Definitely<br>True<br>+3 |
|---|---|---|---|---|---|---|
| | | | | | | X |

If you cannot make a decision about a particular scale, mark the zero (0) point for the item.

| Definitely<br>True<br>−3 | Partly<br>True<br>−2 | Slightly<br>True<br>−1 | Neither<br>Description<br>Applies<br>0 | Slightly<br>True<br>+1 | Partly<br>True<br>+2 | Definitely<br>True<br>+3 |
|---|---|---|---|---|---|---|
| | | | X | | | |

To obtain the rating for each section, find the arithmetic sum of the values you assigned to all the scales in the section. A comparison of the obtained ratings within each category (Nursing Content, Pedagogy, Technical Quality, and Policy Issues) with the "established" minimums can lead to a recommendation concerning the suitability of the software package. (Please note that established minimums may be set by yourself, your faculty, or through peer review.)

## Characteristics of the Computer Assisted Instruction Software

Title

Author

Topics/subjects

Level of the learner

Instructional purpose and techniques

Remediation/development _____
Standard instruction _____
Enrichment _____
Data analysis _____
Drill and practice _____
Word processing _____
Tutorial _____
Information retrieval _____
Programming _____
Educational game _____
Laboratory device _____
Simulation _____
Teaching aid _____
Problem solving _____
Testing _____
Computer-managed instruction _____
Test construction _____
Program development _____

## Nursing Content Standards

The package presents topics which are irrelevant to the educational needs of the intended student users.

The topics included in the package are very significant in the education of the intended student/user population.

| Definitely True −3 | Partly True −2 | Slightly True −1 | Neither Description Applies 0 | Slightly True +1 | Partly True +2 | Definitely True +3 |
|---|---|---|---|---|---|---|
| _____ | _____ | _____ | _____ | _____ | _____ | _____ |

The nursing content is very inaccurate.

The nursing content is free from errors.

| Definitely True −3 | Partly True −2 | Slightly True −1 | Neither Description Applies 0 | Slightly True +1 | Partly True +2 | Definitely True +3 |
|---|---|---|---|---|---|---|
| _____ | _____ | _____ | _____ | _____ | _____ | _____ |

Racial, ethnic, or sex-role stereotypes are displayed.

The presentation is free from any objectionable stereotyping.

| Definitely True -3 | Partly True -2 | Slightly True -1 | Neither Description Applies 0 | Slightly True +1 | Partly True +2 | Definitely True +3 |
|---|---|---|---|---|---|---|

Biased or distorted information is paraded as factual information.

Well-balanced and representative information is presented.

| Definitely True -3 | Partly True -2 | Slightly True -1 | Neither Description Applies 0 | Slightly True +1 | Partly True +2 | Definitely True +3 |
|---|---|---|---|---|---|---|

The package includes nursing information which is greatly outdated.

The nursing content presented in the package represents current nursing theory and knowledge.

| Definitely True -3 | Partly True -2 | Slightly True -1 | Neither Description Applies 0 | Slightly True +1 | Partly True +2 | Definitely True +3 |
|---|---|---|---|---|---|---|

The presentation of the nursing content is confusing.

The nursing content is very clearly presented.

| Definitely True -3 | Partly True -2 | Slightly True -1 | Neither Description Applies 0 | Slightly True +1 | Partly True +2 | Definitely True +3 |
|---|---|---|---|---|---|---|

The package gives no attention to the utilization of the nursing process.

The application of the nursing process is well integrated into this software package.

| Definitely True -3 | Partly True -2 | Slightly True -1 | Neither Description Applies 0 | Slightly True +1 | Partly True +2 | Definitely True +3 |
|---|---|---|---|---|---|---|

Attention is primarily given to the utilization of lower-level cognitive processes.

Utilization of higher level cognitive processes are encouraged throughout the software program.

| Definitely True | Partly True | Slightly True | Neither Description Applies | Slightly True | Partly True | Definitely True |
|---|---|---|---|---|---|---|
| −3 | −2 | −1 | 0 | +1 | +2 | +3 |

_____   _____   _____   _____   _____   _____   _____

The software offers limited exposure to the development of affective behaviors related to the subject matter.

Multiple opportunities are provided for the application of higher-order processes within the affective domain.

| Definitely True | Partly True | Slightly True | Neither Description Applies | Slightly True | Partly True | Definitely True |
|---|---|---|---|---|---|---|
| −3 | −2 | −1 | 0 | +1 | +2 | +3 |

_____   _____   _____   _____   _____   _____   _____

No attempt is made to integrate processes related to psychomotor skills within the software package.

The program challenges the student to "demonstrate" proficiency in the psychomotor domain throughout the program.

| Definitely True | Partly True | Slightly True | Neither Description Applies | Slightly True | Partly True | Definitely True |
|---|---|---|---|---|---|---|
| −3 | −2 | −1 | 0 | +1 | +2 | +3 |

_____   _____   _____   _____   _____   _____   _____

There is limited opportunity for the user to become actively involved in the process of making clinical nursing decisions.

Clinical decision making by the student/user is encouraged throughout the software package.

| Definitely True | Partly True | Slightly True | Neither Description Applies | Slightly True | Partly True | Definitely True |
|---|---|---|---|---|---|---|
| −3 | −2 | −1 | 0 | +1 | +2 | +3 |

_____   _____   _____   _____   _____   _____   _____

## Comments (Nursing Content Standards):

## Software Program Profile

|  | Policy | Nursing Content | Pedagogy | Technical Quality |
|---|---|---|---|---|
| Ratings |  |  |  |  |
| Minimal Standards |  |  |  |  |

# 17

# Refinement and Validation of a Tool Measuring Leadership Characteristics of Baccalaureate Nursing Students

*Bonnie Ketchum Smola*

*This chapter discusses the Self-Assessment Leadership Instrument, a measure of leadership characteristics in nurses.*

## PURPOSE

The purpose of this study was to provide nurse educators with a valid and reliable instrument for the measurement of leadership characteristics in baccalaureate nursing students or practicing nurses. Using Copi (1961) as a guide for an operational definition, the term *leadership* in this study refers to the process of influencing the behavior of other persons in their efforts toward goal setting and goal achievement; this implies defining and planning for nursing in an interactional setting.

## CONCEPTUAL BASIS OF MEASUREMENT TOOL

Since this study utilized the leadership instrument originally developed by Yura (1970), it is important to refer to the theories identified by Yura (1970) as bearing upon her study. Tannenbaum, Weschler, and Massarik (1961) gave consideration to the psychological attributes of the follower, the group, the situation, interpersonal relationships, and communication. Argyris (1962) provided a theoretical framework relevant to the leader's interactions with others and position within an organizational structure. Stogdill's, (1958) theory related to the individual's behavior within the group structure, and Griffiths (1958) theory concerned decision making.

In addition, the present study utilizes the contributions of Cartwright and Zander (1960), the behavioral theorists who studied the general effects of the behavior of the individual in a particular situation. Wenrich and Wenrich (1974) are recognized for their work that identified and measured specific leadership behaviors and the effect of those behaviors on members of the group.

Criterion-referenced measurement theory is apparent in the nature of Yura's (1970) tool and in the instrument derived from it. Criterion-referenced measures are used to determine whether or not a subject has acquired a predetermined set of target behaviors. A subject's performance is compared to the criterion, not to the performance of others (Martuza, 1977). During the process of establishing the validity and reliability of the research tool, both the model of parallel measures and the domain-sampling model were used.

## METHODOLOGY

The discussion of methodology follows the chronological order of steps required for the project. First, a review of the literature was completed. Second, data collected by Yura (1970) in the development of the Leadership Behavior Tool was analyzed, using a chi-square statistic to test for relationships between selected categories of frequency data. Third, the tool was administered to senior-level baccalaureate nursing students. Data from this administration were used for (a) a comparison of responses between the faculty surveyed in the original study and the students to determine if the two groups shared the concept of leadership and (b) an item analysis. Fourth, using the results of these analyses, the instrument was refined; that is, the irrelevant or ambiguous items were eliminated or clarified. Items not eliminated were reworded into a self-report format. Content and construct validity of the new self-assessment tool were established as follows: content validity through a panel of judges; construct validity through the use of contrast groups. The judges used a modified semantic differential scale to rate each item on clarity and relevance, and an item-objective congruence index to verify the congruence of the item to the domain of leadership. Interrater and intrarater reliability were established by using the interclass correlation statistic. Fifth, a pilot test-retest procedure provided data for the Cohen's coefficient K statistic to reflect the reliability of the criterion-referenced instrument (Martuza, 1977).

## REVIEW OF THE LITERATURE

The review of the literature focused on the following: (a) leadership theory, (b) measurement theory, (c) documentation of the evolution of research tools to determine leader behavior, (d) nursing studies utilizing those instruments, and (e) self-assessment as formative and summative evaluation.

## Leadership Theory

No one all-inclusive theory exists to explain the leadership phenomenon. Some of the prevailing theories – trait, situational, or behavioral – still contain remnants of the two basic theories of leadership. These two basic theories are the great man theory and the time theory. Each of the five named theories; great man, time, trait, situational, and behavioral – offers a contribution to the explanation of the phenomenon of leadership, but no one of these theories is adequate when taken separately.

### Great Man Theory

In the more prominent civilizations of Europe and the Americas the great man theory has been most popular. Davenport (1976) states: "The great man theory emphasizes that certain individuals are hereditarily endowed with unique characteristics and abilities. . . .The doctrine of the divine right of kings gave birth to this idea and helped to sustain its perpetuity" (p. 27).

### Time Theory

The time theory has the social situation as its central focus. Leadership is thought to be a function of a variety of factors in a relatively small period of time. In the time theory, the personal characteristics or traits of the leader are secondary to the needs of the group. Chance plays an important part in determining leadership in this theory. A leader in one instance may not have the uniqueness needed for leadership in another period in time (Cooper & McGaugh, 1963). The rise of a powerful leader during a crisis may be cited as an example of the time theory of leadership. However, careful analysis of the time theory will show that it embraces a portion of the great man theory. The concept of individual differences is blended into the time theory. The unique qualities of the emergent leader meet the special needs of a given period of time (Burns, 1976).

### Trait Theory

The trait theory of leadership has been the topic of much research in education and business. Traits or qualities believed necessary for leadership were suggested in a rather dated work by Tead (1935), which listed 10 qualities necessary for the educational leader: physical and nervous energy, a sense of purpose and direction, enthusiasm, friendliness and affection, integrity, technical mastery, decisiveness, intelligence, teaching skill, faith and confidence. Barnard (1948), termed the father of modern organizational theory, concurred with the suggested list of traits. The qualities of friendliness, affection, and faith were also mentioned by Halpin (1956) in a publication that concluded by saying that all leaders needed to show more consideration toward their subordinates. Faber and Shearron (1970) listed the following from various investigations of leadership traits:

. . .age, height, weight, physique, energy, health, appearance, fluency of speech, intelligence, scholarship, . .knowledge, judgments, decision insight, originality, adaptability, introversion and extroversion, dominance, initiative, . .integrity and conviction, self-confidence, mood control, emotional control, . .social activity, mobility, and cooperation. (p. 310)

Three assumptions basic to the trait theory were identified by Pierce and Merril (1957):

(1) one has to assume that specific elements of behavior can be isolated and examined as entities in themselves;
(2) that such factors act independently of one another so they can be measured and analyzed;
(3) that the influence of a particular trait on leadership behavior is relatively constant and therefore somewhat predictable. (p. 321)

Ramseyer (1960) stated that personality traits were the ones most significantly related to leader behavior. However, an individual having possession of these traits has no guarantee of becoming a successful leader, and the same combination of traits is not found in all leaders.

Franseth (1961) categorized personality traits of a leader as follows: (1) democratic, (2) people-oriented, (3) perceives situations as others do, (4) proponent of group-centered leadership, (5) well informed, (6) scientific attitude, and (7) committed to helping others use energy creatively.

Organizational researchers such as Cooper and McGaugh (1963) and Stogdill (1970) concluded that trait identification alone is not sufficient for identification of leadership.

Adair (1968) offered hope to those not possessing leadership traits when he concluded that training for effective leadership is based on the belief that leadership potential can be developed.

## Situational Theory

The situational theory of leadership has been identified as an outgrowth of the time theory. It is more difficult to define situational leadership because the variables are not easy to observe, confine, and qualify.

Fiedler (1967) maintained that different situations require different leadership. In other words, the same leadership style or behavior will not be effective in all situations. Three major situational factors that may decide if a leader will have difficulty or ease in influencing the group are as follows:

(1) the degree to which the group accepts and trusts its leader;
(2) the leader's position power – that is, the power which the organization rests in the leadership position;
(3) the degree to which the task of the group is structured, unstructured. (p. 56)

Thus, to the proponents of situational leadership theory, a leader is not a person with skills inherent to leading that may be successfully transferred from one setting to another. Rather, an individual may emerge as the leader in a particular situation yet may not do so in another situation in which the social considerations are changed and other circumstances differ (Gross & Herriott, 1964; Lucio & McNeil, 1969).

The situational approach does not ignore or belittle the importance of traits or individual qualities. It embraces them while insisting that they are significant only in terms of a particular social or group situation (Stogdill, 1974).

The relationship between increased constraint and task-oriented leader behavior, and between job-mature faculty and decreased task and/or relationship behavior, were investigated by Goldenberg (1980). The results of the study were consistent with situational leadership theory but inconsistent with constraint theory. The study was limited to Ontario diploma nursing education programs.

The situational leadership theory was investigated by Gray (1983) in a study that examined leadership styles and leadership adaptability of nursing team leaders as perceived by nursing team members. The researcher suggested that a third dimension, the level of sophistication of tasks being performed in a situation, needs to be considered if situational leadership is to be useful in nursing practice.

## Behavioral Theory

The behavioral theory attempts to identify leader performance or behavior. Wenrich and Wenrich (1974) state that the behavior theory appears to be one of the more useful approaches to research on leadership. Cartwright and Zander (1960) focused on the behavioral theory of leadership in a study completed at the Research Center for Group Dynamics at the University of Michigan:

> Most group objectives may be accomplished through behaviors which can be classified as either "goal achievement behaviors" or "group maintenance behaviors." The kinds of leadership behavior directed toward goal achievement are those in which the leader initiates action. . .keeps members' attention on the goal. . .clarifies the issues. . .develops a procedural plan. . . evaluates the quality of work done and makes expert information available. The types of leadership behavior which serve the function of group maintenance are those through which the leader "keeps" interpersonal relations pleasant. . .arbitrates disputes. . .provides encouragement. . .gives the minority a chance to be heard. . .stimulates self-direction and increases the interdependence among members. (p. 496)

The main thrust of the behavioral theory is the interpersonal contribution a person makes in a particular situation. The traits of the individual are of lesser significance than the behavior that is exhibited.

A major study of the behavioral theory was done by the Personnel Research Board at The Ohio State University. Halpin (1956) explained that the leadership phenomenon could be more readily recognized by an examination of the leader behavior rather than the leader traits or leader-eliciting situations. The focus on leader behavior instead of leadership as such has made major contributions to the study of leadership.

Wallcnborn (1960) studied the behavior of the instructional leader; the results are similar to a study by Clark (1972). Both studies' view of leader behavior centers on interpersonal and group relationships, communication, problem solving, coordinating, planning, and guiding.

Kelley (1970) studied 505 registered nurses and senior nursing students from 8 hospitals and 13 schools of nursing in Alabama to determine the perception of registered nurses and nursing students concerning leadership behaviors believed to be important in the practice of nursing supervision in a general hospital. The Nursing Leadership Behavior Questionnaire was developed to measure leadership behaviors. Of the five goal oriented leadership behaviors – goal-setting, group-centered, individual-centered, leader-centered, and goal-achieving – the majority of the subjects perceived group-centered behaviors as the most important in the practice nursing supervision.

Johnson (1976) conducted a comparative study of self-concept, leadership style, and leadership effectiveness. The study used a self-report format. The results indicated that if head nurses wish to be viewed as effective by both superiors and subordinates, they should exhibit both structure and consideration behaviors to a high degree.

South (1981) designed the Nursing Questionnaire to determine what behaviors nurses perceive as nursing leadership behaviors. The Nursing Questionnair contains 15 vignettes designed to support a 6-point graphic rating scale for each of the three dimensions of the study: leadership, managerial skills, job competency. South (1981) concluded that a homogeneous definition of these three dimensions did not exist among the respondents.

Chang (1981) tested for differences in perceived leadership styles among graduates from diploma, associate degree, generic baccalaureate, and upper division nursing programs. No significant differences were found.

Lenz (1982) conducted a study to determine the relationships existing among the selected variables of age, education, and experience and the leadership behavior of initiation of structure and consideration for nursing education administrators. Two hundred participants, nursing education administrators from each level of nursing education programs, showed no difference among the variables.

A study to determine whether organizational factors, personal attributes, conflicts in expectations, and leader behaviors were related to job satisfaction of nurses was completed by Payne (1982). The major conclusion concerning leader behavior was that the only relationship among leader hierarchical influence, subordinate role ambiguity, and leader behavior of initiating structure is in the area of staff nurse satisfaction with supervision.

Ethnicity and perception of leadership behavior were studied by Castillo (1983) and Yearwood (1984). Castillo (1983) compared Anglo-American and Mexican-American baccalaureate nursing students' perceptions of ideal leadership and followership styles with the goal of finding a procedure for the development of a multivariate model to predict students' leadership and followership styles. A "best" model for followership was found that included ethnicity and Grade Point Average. However, a "best" model was not found for leadership. Yearwood's (1983) study focused on the self-reported effective and ineffective role behaviors of black and white nurse leaders. The critical-incident technique was used to identify 10 leader behaviors. The behaviors were operating politically, facilitating, negotiating, managing conflict, confronting, communicating, problem solving, group leadership, supervising, and risk taking.

## Measurement Theory

Measurement is a process that involves using rules to assign numbers to phenomena. The phenomenon is an attribute of an object, not the object itself. Because the attribute can vary in amount or type, the attribute is called a variable. The rules for assigning numbers to phenomena have been categorized hierarchically as either nominal, ordinal, interval, or ratio (Stevens, 1946). The numbers or values that result from measurement are referred to as scores (Waltz & Bausell, 1981). Statistical procedures are used to facilitate a better understanding of groups of numbers by providing numerical summaries of scores or data.

### *Criterion-Referenced Measurement Theory*

Criterion-referenced measurement theory states that measurements are used to determine whether or not a subject has acquired a predetermined set of target behaviors. A subject's performance is compared to the criterion, not to the performance of others (Martuza, 1977).

Even though the goal of measurement is to achieve accurate results, the goal is not completely possible because of measurement error (Waltz & Bausell, 1981). Random error, which primarily affects the reliability of measurement is always present (Stanley, 1971). According to Martuza (1977), these errors do not directly influence the meaning of the measurement; however, they do affect the precision of the measurement. Further, the validity of a specific measuring device is influenced by the degree to which systematic error is introduced into the measurement procedure. The greater the systematic error, the less valid the measure (Carmines & Zeller, 1979).

### Classical Measurement Theory

Classical measurement theory is a model for assessing random measurement error. According to Waltz, Strickland, and Lenz (1984):

> The basic tenet of classical measurement theory evolved from the assumption that random error is an element that must be considered in all measurement. The underlying principle of this theory is that every observed score is composed of a true score and an error score. The true score is the true or precise amount of the attribute possessed by the object or event being measured. The error score reflects the influence that random error has on the observed score. (p. 68)

Two conceptual models from classical measurement theory are used in the consideration of measurement error. These are the model of parallel measures and the domain-sampling model. Both are models for the computation of reliability coefficients.

### Model of Parallel Measures

This model purports to establish a measure's reliability by correlating parallel measurements. The model states that the correlation between any two tests of a domain is a precise determination of the reliability coefficient rather than an estimate (Nunnally, 1978).

### Domain-Sampling Model

This model states any measure is composed of a random sample of items from a hypothetical domain that it purports to measure. According to the domain-sampling model, "The extent to which any sample of items from the domain is correlated with the true score is an indication of its reliability" (Waltz et al. 1984, p. 74).

## Documentation of the Evolution of Research Tools

The major instruments developed to measure leadership include the Leader Behavior Description Questionnaire (Halpin, 1957) and the Leader Opinion Questionnaire (Fleishman, 1953).

### Leader Behavior Description Questionnaire (LBDQ)

A tool, the LBDQ, was developed by the Ohio State University Personnel Research Board staff in 1957 (Halpin, 1957). The original research for the questionnaire was done with approximately 30 different groups and group situations.

Halpin (1957) developed an adaptation of the instrument for an Air Force study. The Air Force study identified two dimensions of leader behavior termed "initiating structure" and "consideration." Initiating structure indicates the leader's ability to organize and define group activities, to establish patterns of organization and ways of getting a job done. Consideration refers to behavior indicating mutual trust, respect, and warmth in the leader-group member relationship.

In 1962, the LBDQ, Form XII, was developed by Stogdill (1963). Reliability of the instrument was established with a modified Kuder-Richardson formula. In the modified procedure, all items of a given subscale were correlated with the remainder of the statements in that subscale, instead of the subscale score including that item. The reliability coefficients ranged from 0.38 to 0.91 for nine different groups of leaders.

## *Leader Opinion Questionnaire*

Using the LBDQ-XII as a basis, Fleishman (1953) developed a short scale, the Leader Opinion Questionnaire (LOQ), for industrial use, Weissenberg and Gruenfeld (1966) concluded, from a study of civil service supervisors, that the LOQ is transparent and susceptible to faking unless used anonymously. However, Dagenais (1979) repudiated the criticism against the instrument with the results of a study of the relationship between the Consideration and Initiating Structure scales of the LOQ and the Response Bias scale of the Omnibus Personality Inventory (OPI).

The Response Bias scale purports to measure a "need to make a good impression" and was designed to differentiate between those who tend to fake "good" and those who fake "bad" responses for one reason or another. The Response Bias scale has a reliability index of 0.84 for a sample of college women and has been shown to be correlated with the Edwards Social Desirability Scale at the $r = 0.55$ level (Heist & Yonge, 1968).

## Nursing Studies Utilizing the Instruments

Following is a discussion of nursing leadership studies that utilized the LBDQ-XII and the LOQ.

## *LBDQ-XII*

The LBDQ-XII and an Activity Preference Questionnaire were used in a study by Anderson (1964) of leadership behavior of head nurses. The results indicated a difference in the perception of the head nurse as a leader between the ratings of subordinates and supervisors, as well as those of the nurses themselves. There was a positive correlation between the supervisors' and subordinates' ratings on initiating structure but no significant correlation on their rating of consideration or total leader acts.

Moloney (1967) used the LBDQ-XII and a rating scale to study the leadership behavior of deans of university schools of nursing. The conclusion was that leadership evaluation is closely related to the degree to which the leader conforms to the observers' norms. The Anderson (1964) and Moloney (1967) studies demonstrate that whether in nursing service or nursing education, three sets of perceptions must be taken into account: those of the leader, those of the supervisors, and those of the subordinates.

Yura (1970) developed a 70-item instrument to study the perceptions of faculty members relative to behavior indicating leadership potential of baccalaureate nursing students. The statements of leader behavior, taken from nursing leadership literature and the LBDQ-XII, were classified as relating to the self, critical thinking and decision making, interpersonal relationships (including communication), group relations, and job relations. A rating scale was formulated to score the perceived importances of items listed in an inventory of leadership behaviors. The 300 returned rating scales were tabulated for each behavioral statement for the total sample and for each segment of the sample in the study, namely: geographic area, level of student taught, educational background, and area of specialization. The range, mode, and percentage were calculated for each behavioral statement for the total sample and for all segments or categories of the sample.

According to Ward and Fetler (1979), the instrument developed by Yura is in need of item analysis, logical analysis of item content, and/or factor analysis to locate irrelevant or ambiguous items. Additionally, reliability studies and studies of both internal consistency and stability coefficients should be conducted by researchers considering using the instrument. Further, although the data in Yura's (1970) study are reported in categories of geographic location, educational level of the respondents, level of student taught, and specialty area taught, there are no statistical procedures to give an indication of the degree of the relationship between or among the categories.

Thornberry (1974) used the LBDQ to study the effects of organizational level on leadership behavior among nurses. He found there were no significant differences in leadership behavior as a result of differences in organizational level.

## LOQ

Oaklander and Fleishman (1964) used the LOQ and a six-item index of intraunit stress to study patterns of leadership related to organizational stress in hospital settings. Results indicated that the nursing supervisor's perception of her/his role is related to the amount of organizational stress perceived within that department and between that department and other organizational units.

DeBiase (1983) used the LOQ to investigate the relationship of head nurse initiating-structure and consideration leadership behaviors to the quality of patient care. It was concluded that head nurse initiating-structure and consideration behaviors, acting together, were not significantly related to quality or patient care.

## SELF-ASSESSMENT AS FORMATIVE AND SUMMATIVE EVALUATION

An issue that nurses confront is the knowledge that nursing professionals must be able to evaluate their own behavior objectively because as professionals they are accountable for their own actions. Professional nurses must understand the implications of their actions, accept the consequences of their decisions, describe their present abilities accurately, and identify areas that need further development (King, 1984).

Self-assessment has been found to be valid when compared to (1) test performance (Berdie, 1971; Gilmore, 1973), (2) academic success (Gaier, 1966), (3) peer rating (Amatora, 1956), and (4) instructor assessment (Geissler, 1973).

Self-assessment has been shown to result in superior work and better critical judgment (Abrams & Kelly, 1974; Geissler, 1973). Individuals experienced with self-assessment techniques tend to be more self-challenging, questioning, analytical, self-motivated, and curious (Wittich & Schuller, 1973).

As a formative evaluation procedure, self-assessment has been demonstrated to be a powerful and useful strategy. Abrams and Kelly (1974) reported that self-assessment resulted in quality clinical performance and was effective in promoting a positive attitude toward self-evaluation. Marriner's (1974) research supported the idea that self-evaluation has a strong influence on self-esteem and psychological health.

According to King (1984), "Many instructor-centered evaluation instruments such as the checklist can be converted to a self-evaluation format" (p. 182). The conversion of Yura's (1970) Leadership Behavior Tool into a self-assessment format can be of value to nursing in that it can serve as an evaluation as well as a teaching tool.

### Chi-Square Analysis

Yura (1970) reported the findings of her study in frequency data. With frequency data it is possible to compare the effects of two variables when there are more than two groups on either of the variables (Kleinbaum & Kupper, 1978).

Data in relation to subdefinitions of leadership identified by Yura (1970) – (a) self, (b) critical thinking and decision making, (c) interpersonal relationships, (d) group relations, and (e) job relations – were subjected to a chi-square analysis. In each category of items, a relationship was demonstrated. Results are given in Table 17.1.

**TABLE 17.1** Results of Chi-Square Analysis of Yura's (1970) Original Data

| Category | Degrees of Freedom | Chi-square | Decision |
|---|---|---|---|
| Self | 26 ($N-14$) | 7.579 $p > .05$ | Relationship |
| Critical thinking and decision making | 20 ($N=11$) | 6.294 $p > .05$ | Relationship |
| Interpersonal relationships | 32 ($N=17$) | 13.894 $p > .06$ | Relationship |
| Group relations | 28 ($N=15$) | 7.179 $p > .05$ | Relationship |
| Job relations | 24 ($N=13$) | 7.880 $p > .05$ | Relationship |

Based on the results of the chi-square analysis of data reported in Yura's 1970 study, whether subjects are from the eastern, central, or western geographical region of the United States, they will answer the same on each item of the tool. Further, regardless of geographical location, the subjects answer the same to the subdefinitions of leadership identified by Yura (1970). Therefore, a researcher using Yura's (1970) instrument may have some degree of confidence in generalizing to a larger group of nursing faculty from a random selection of a sample of nursing faculty in any one of the three geographical locations.

## Administration of Yura's Instrument

The 1970 study was repeated with 90 senior baccalaureate nursing students from three colleges as respondents to compare their perception of nursing leadership behavior with that of the faculty studied by Yura (1970). An analysis of variance of the mode of scores for each group was computed. The mean score for faculty was 3.514; the mean score for students was 3.542. The analysis of variance indicated no significant difference between the groups, $F(1,138) = 0.056$, $p > .05$.

This finding is significant because it gives credibility to the claim that nursing faculty and nursing students are in agreement about the characteristics of leadership. Also, the characteristics of leadership identified by the 1970 study defined the domain of leadership that formed the basis for the derivation of the self-assessment instrument.

### Item Analysis of Student's Response

An item analysis of the student's responses to Yura's (1970) tool was computed. The item analysis included an item $p$, or difficulty level, and an item $D$, or discriminatory power.

An item $p$-value can range from 0 to 1.00 and is the proportion of persons in a group of respondents who answered the item appropriately – in this case, at the higher level. The item $p$-level should be high for the items believed to be necessary attributes of leadership.

The focus of item discrimination indices was identification of ambiguous or irrelevant items. The $D$ assesses an item's ability to discriminate; that is, if performance on a given item is a good predictor of performance on the overall measure, the item is said to be a good discriminator. To determine the $D$-value for a given item, the procedure suggested by Waltz and Bausell (1981) was used.

$D$ ranges from $-1.00$ to $+1.00$. A negative $D$-value suggests that the item is not discriminating and is probably faulty. Possible explanations for a negative $D$-value are that the item provides a clue to the lower-scoring subjects that encourages them to score the item higher, while at the same time the item is misinterpreted by the higher scorers.

Items shown to be not difficult (i.e., a mean of more than .50) but poor discriminators (a discrimination rating of less than .50) were eliminated or rewritten. Items shown to be difficult (a mean of less than .50) and poor discriminators, a combination that indicates that the items are probably confusing, were also eliminated or rewritten. Forty-six items were retained for future use.

The internal consistency of the instrument was calculated using the Kuder-Richardson formula. The Kuder-Richardson was 0.93, indicating a very high internal reliability of the instrument. The high reliability coefficient means that the test was accurately measuring some characteristic of the people taking it. Further, it indicates that the individual items on the test were producing similar patterns of responding in different people.

## INSTRUMENT REFINEMENT

### Administration and Scoring

Next, the 46-item instrument was reworded into a self-report format. Two questions concerning the respondent were added: (1) Have you completed a course on leadership? and (2) Do you consider yourself to be a leader? The directions were altered in that the respondent was asked to consider the listed behaviors as they relate to his/her own leadership. A 5-point numerical scale was used. The respondent was asked to indicate his/her judgement of frequency of use of the particular behavior. The options ranged from 4 (Almost Always ) to 0 (Usually Not). A total score was derived by summating item scores. High scores represent high self- assessment of leadership characteristics.

### *Content Validity*

The instrument, Self-Assessment Leadership Instrument (SALI), was subjected to examination of content by a panel of five judges. Each judge was considered to have expertise in leadership as demonstrated by current, or in the recent past, teaching responsibility for leadership content at the graduate, undergraduate, or continuing education level. All judges were doctorally prepared. Each judge was asked to review the instrument for clarity, relevancy, and congruence. The scales for clarity and relevancy were modified semantic differentials (Rovinelli & Hambleton, 1977). For example, the items were rated as Very Unclear to Leadership – Very Clear to Leadership and Very Irrelevant to Leadership – Very Relevant to Leadership. Possible responses ranged from 0 (Very Unclear or Irrelevant) to 5 (Very Clear or Relevant).

Data from the modified semantic differential scale were analyzed to obtain a mean and a standard deviation per item. The cutoff score for retention of an item was a mean of greater than 3 and/or a standard deviation of less than 1. Six items were below the cutoff score of a mean of at least 3 and standard deviation of no greater than 1. The items were eliminated from the final draft of the SALI.

The matter of congruence was addressed in terms of item-objective congruence (Rovinelli & Hambleton, 1977). This procedure tested the individual item in relation to its subdefinition of leadership. The categories of subdefinitions established by Yura (1970) were used. The categories included (a) perception of leadership in relation to self, (b) critical thinking and decision making, (c) interpersonal relations, (d) group relations, and (e) job relations. Each item served as a unit of analysis. The categories were considered mutually exclusive; each item was assigned a value of +1, 0, or −1, depending on the item's congruence with the item's objective. Whenever an item was judged to be a definite measure of the objective, a value of +1 was assigned. A rating of 0 indicated that the judge was undecided about whether the item was a measure of the objective. The assignment of a −1 rating reflected a definite judgment that the item was not a measure of the objective. The data from the judge's ratings were used to compute the index of item-objective congruence. The index cutoff score was arbitrarily set at 0.75. Items with an index of item-objective congruence below 0.75 were deemed nonvalid as a measure of the objective; those with an index of 0.75 or above were considered valid.

Items were not eliminated on the basis of the item-objective congruence test. However, it was necessary to consider the items as covering the broad domain of leadership, not the specific category given.

Of the 14 items Yura listed as belonging to classification 1, Self, the judges agreed with 2 of the items. In other words, there was a 14% agreement between Yura and the judges as to which items belonged in the Self category. Yura listed 10 items as belonging in the Critical Thinking and Decision Making category. The judges agreed with three of the items, an agreement rate of 30% The highest agreement, 47%, between Yura and the judges was on the Interpersonal Relationships category. Of the 17 items identified by Yura as belonging in that category, the judges agreed with 8 items. There was a 20% agreement on the Group Relations category. Yura classified 15 items in that category; the judges agreed with 3 of the items. The Job Relations category showed no agreement. Yura had classified 13 items in that category, but the judges found no items appropriate to that classification.

## Interrater and Intrarater Reliability

An interrater agreement scale was used to determine agreement on clarity and relevancy. A measure of agreement among the judges was given by the interclass correlation. In both clarity and relevancy the reliability of the judges was very high: 94% and 91%, respectively. The results were reported as the reliability of average judges' ratings; the adjusted average reliability; the reliability of a single judge, or intrarater reliability; and the adjusted interclass reliability of a single judge. The adjusted average, or single-judge reliabilities, have been corrected for the variability that exists between the means of the judges. In estimating reliability, it is not always desirable to remove this source of unreliability because in actual practice it may be impossible to guarantee that judges would make equal average ratings (Kleinbaum & Kupper, 1978). Therefore, the unadjusted estimates of reliability were considered the most important. The results are presented in Table 17.2.

The intrarater reliability coefficients for clarity and relevancy were not as high, 77% and 68%, respectively. The reliability coefficients should reach at least 70%.

## Construct Validity

Construct validity was addressed through the use of contrasted groups. This type of validity is especially important for measures of affect (Waltz et al., 1984).

In the contrasted groups approach, two groups of individuals were identified to be extremely high or extremely low in the characteristics of leadership. This was done by asking peers, head nurses, or directors of nursing to name three to five of the top nurse leaders in the hospital or hospital unit. The individuals selected were identified as leaders by their actions, not by their positions in the facility. The same head nurses or peers were asked to identify nurses who are not leaders. Of these two groups of nurses, 20 identified as not leaders and 42 identified as leaders, were classified, one as the low group and the other as the high group. The instrument was administered to both the high and low groups; the difference in scores obtained by each group was assessed using an analysis of variance.

All 42 nurses identified by their peers as leaders answered yes to the question "Do you consider yourself to be a leader?" The 20 nurses identified by their peers as not leaders were placed in the group identified low in leadership characteristics. Fifteen of this group of nurses answered no to the question "Do you consider yourself to be a leader?" Five of the nurses identified by their peers as not leaders answered yes to the question "Do you consider yourself to be a leader?" If the instrument is sensitive to individual differences in leadership characteristics, the mean performances of these two groups should differ significantly.

A significant difference was found between the mean scores of the two groups for approximately two-thirds of the items. Since the two groups may differ in many ways in addition to varying on the characteristics of leadership, the mean differences in scores may be due to group noncomparability on some other variable that was not measured. Therefore, the claim for validity of the instrument must be offered in light of this possibility.

The results of the analysis of variance between the two groups is presented in Table 17.3.

One-third of the items did not discriminate between the groups. With 66% of the items discriminating between the groups, the SALI was thought to have both content and construct validity.

## Reliability and Pilot

The instrument was used in a pilot test-retest to establish reliability data. The focus of the test-retest procedure for criterion-referenced instruments is on the stability or reliability of the classification of persons on two separate occasions. In other words, the ability of the instrument to consistently classify the individual in the same category on two separate testing occasions. "The extent to which a criterion-referenced measure is able to reflect stability of results over time is an indication of the degree to which it is free from random measurement error" (Waltz et al., 1984, p. 188).

Twenty-four students volunteered to answer the questions on the instrument a second time 10 days after the first administration. Students were asked to identify their questionnaire with a four-digit number code that they could remember. For example, the last four numbers of their social security number or numbers that would represent a significant date to them. The questionnaires were matched for a test-retest procedure to establish reliability. Cohen's coefficient K was computed to determine the reliability of the instrument. The results showed Cohen's K coefficient of 0.545 or a 55% agreement on the two testing occasions over that achieved by chance alone. In other words, the agreement between the two tests did not happen by chance alone.

The SALI has been validated and has undergone reliability studies. The instrument is now ready to be used in the classroom or for in-service education, to allow nurses to assess their own leadership characteristics. The instrument can serve as a guide or criterion for nurses to measure their leadership characteristics. The instrument can be used independently, or the results of the instrument can be shared with the faculty responsible for teaching the leadership component of the curriculum.

Once aware of which items are missed, the student and/or faculty can examine the missed item and determine which leadership behaviors are in need of development.

Rather than presenting a course that gives only information about leadership, faculty can develop exercises to assist each student to develop the behaviors needed to become a leader in nursing. Clearly, the focus of evaluation of leadership in nursing should be in the assessment of what a person is able to do rather than how the person compares with others.

## RECOMMENDATIONS FOR FURTHER STUDY

Several recommendations for further study are suggested. The suggestions concern the continued use of the instrument as well as further refinement.

The instrument should be retested several times and under differing circumstances to verify the data.

An attempt to identify the exact nature of the subdefinitions of leadership should be carried out. This could be done by a factor analysis, followed by a content analysis of the items located within each factor.

A cutoff score or standard should be established to classify the subject and reflect the level of proficiency obtained. The score obtained on the Self-Assessment Leadership Instrument does not classify the subject as a leader or not a leader. A cutoff score or standard is a point along the scale of test scores that is used to classify a subject to reflect the level of proficiency obtained. According to Waltz et al. (1984), when using criterion-referenced measurement, the cutoff score could be set by determining the critical behaviors that distinguish leaders from not leaders. The standard is set depending on the critical behaviors or attributes that must be obtained. Because the instrument assesses more than one objective or subdefinition, different standards should be set in relation to the sets of items that measure the different objectives.

**TABLE 17.2 Interclass Reliability of Judges Rating Clarity and Relevancy**

| Category | Clarity | Relevancy |
|---|---|---|
| Reliability of ratings | 0.94 | 0.91 |
| Reliability of ratings (adjusted) | 0.95 | 0.94 |
| Reliability of a single judge | 0.77 | 0.68 |
| Reliability of a single judge (adjusted) | 0.80 | 0.76 |

**TABLE 17.3** ANOVA of Contrasted-Groups Performance on Self-Assessment Leadership Instrument

| Item | $F(1,60)$ | $p$ | Item | $F(1,60)$ | $p$ |
|------|-----------|------|------|-----------|------|
| 1 | 21.707 | <.05 | 2 | 1.468 | >.05 |
| 3 | 14.361 | <.05 | 4 | 14.017 | <.05 |
| 5 | 2.203 | >.05 | 6 | 2.502 | >.05 |
| 7 | 3.242 | >.05 | 8 | 17.345 | <.05 |
| 9 | 7.560 | <.05 | 10 | 7.246 | <.05 |
| 11 | 4.489 | <.05 | 12 | 4.840 | <.05 |
| 13 | 8.228 | <.05 | 14 | 9.427 | <.05 |
| 15 | 4.307 | <.05 | 16 | 0.742 | >.05 |
| 17 | 1.634 | >.05 | 18 | 16.156 | <.05 |
| 19 | 6.084 | <.05 | 20 | 2.882 | >.05 |
| 21 | 1.468 | >.05 | 22 | 12.328 | <.05 |
| 23 | 8.288 | <.05 | 24 | 13.014 | <.05 |
| 25 | 13.774 | <.05 | 26 | 25.487 | <.05 |
| 27 | 11.922 | <.05 | 28 | 24.622 | <.05 |
| 29 | 1.889 | >.05 | 30 | 6.650 | <.05 |
| 31 | 5.239 | <.05 | 32 | 11.193 | <.05 |
| 33 | 10.244 | <.05 | 34 | 5.916 | <.05 |
| 35 | 2.324 | >.05 | 36 | 15.201 | <.05 |
| 37 | 14.471 | <.05 | 38 | 7.384 | <.05 |
| 39 | 0.785 | >.05 | 40 | 2.800 | >.05 |
| 41 | 18.935 | <.05 | 42 | 15.264 | <.05 |
| 43 | 2.072 | >.05 | 44 | 1.582 | >.05 |
| 45 | 2.857 | >.05 | 46 | 10.342 | <.05 |

# REFERENCES

Abrams, R., & Kelly, M. (1974). Student self-evaluation in a pediatric-operative technique course. *Journal of Dental Education, 38*(7), 385-391.

Adair, J. (1968). *Training for leadership.* New York: MacDonald.

Anderson, R. (1964). Activity preference and leadership behavior of head nurses. *Nursing Research, 13*(3), 239-243.

Argyris, C. (1962). *Interpersonal competences and organizational effectiveness.* Homewood, IL: Dorsey.

Barnard, C. (1948). *Organization and management.* Cambridge; MA: Harvard University Press.

Berdie, R. F. (1971). Self-claimed and test knowledge. *Educational and Psychological Measures, 31*, 629-636.

Burns, J. M. (1976). *Leadership.* New York: Harper Row.

Carmines, E., & Zeller, R. (1979). *Reliability and validity assessment.* Beverly Hills, CA: Sage Publications.

Cartwright, D., & Zander, A. (1960). *Group dynamics: Research and theory* (2nd ed.). Evanston, IL: Row, Peterson.

Castillo, M. M. (1983). Perceptions of Mexican-American and Anglo- American nursing students toward an ideal leadership and followership style. (Doctoral dissertation, New Mexico State University, 1983). *Dissertation Abstracts International, 42*, 1409B.

Chang, Y. (1981). Perceived leadership styles and assertive characteristics of graduates from four types of nursing programs in Eastern North Dakota and Western Minnesota. (Doctoral dissertation, University of North Dakota, 1980). *Dissertation Abstracts International, 41,* 4064-B.

Clark, K. (1972). *A possible reality.* New York: Emerson Hall.

Cooper J., & McGaugh, J. (1963). *Integrating principles of social psychology.* Cambridge; MA: Schonkman.

Copi, I. (1961). *Introduction to logic.* New York: Macmillan.

Dagenais, F. (1979). Response bias and the Leadership Opinion Questionnaire Scales. *Journal of General Psychology, 100*(1), 161-162.

Davenport, I. W. (1976). *Analysis of the perceived leader behavior of male and female elementary school principals.* Unpublished doctoral dissertation, University of Missouri, Columbia; MO.

DeBiase, C. (1983). The relationship between selected leadership behaviors of head nurses and quality of patient care. (Doctoral dissertation, Northern Illinois University, 1982). *Dissertation Abstracts International, 43,* 2563-A.

Faber, C., & Shearron, G. (1970). *Elementary school administration: Theory and practice.* New York: Holt, Rinehart, Winston.

Fiedler, F. (1967). *A theory of leadership effectiveness.* New York: McGraw-Hill.

Fleishman, E. A. (1953). A leadership behavior description for industry. In M. Stogdill & A. E. Coons (Eds.), *Leadership behavior description and measurement* (pp.210-231). Columbus; OH: Ohio State University, Bureau of Research.

Franseth, J. U. (1961). *Supervision as leadership.* Evanston; IL: Row, Peterson.

Gaier, E. (1966). Student self-estimates of final course grades. *Journal of Genetic Psychology, 98,* 63-67.

Geissler, P. R. (1973). Student self-assessment in dental technology. *Journal of Dental Education, 37*(9), 19-21.

Gilmore, J. B. (1973). Learning and student self-evaluation. *Journal of College Science Teaching, 3*(1), 54-57.

Goldenberg, D. (1980). Relation of constraint and situational theory to diploma nursing program leadership. (Doctoral dissertation, Wayne State University, 1980). *Dissertation Abstracts International, 41*(5-A), 1861.

Gray, P. A. (1983). Leadership in nursing teams: Its perception by team leaders and team members. (Doctoral dissertation, The University of North Carolina at Chapel Hill, 1982). *Dissertation Abstracts International, 44*(1-a), 28.

Griffith, D. (1958). Administration as decision-making. In A. Halpin (Ed.), *Administrative theory in education* (pp.119-149). Chicago: University of Chicago, Midwest Administrative Center.

Gross, N., & Herriott. R. (1964). *The professional leadership of elementary school principals.* Cambridge; MA: Harvard Graduate School of Education.

Halpin, A. W. (1956). The behavior of leaders. *Educational Leadership, 24,*(12), 172.

Halpin, A. W. (1957). *Manual for the Leader Behavior Description Questionnaire.* Columbus; OH: Ohio State University: Bureau of Business Research.

Heist, P., & Yonge, G. (9168). *Manual for Omnibus Personality Inventory, Form F.* New York: Psychological Corporation.

Johnson, K. R. (1976). Nursing leadership: A comparative study of self concept, leadership style and leadership effectiveness. (Doctoral dissertation, University of Massachusetts, 1976). *Dissertation Abstracts International, 37,* 1886A.

Kelley, J. A. (1970). Leadership behaviors of the supervisor of nursing in general hospitals in Alabama as perceived by registered nurses and nursing students. (Doctoral dissertation, University of Alabama, 1969). *Dissertation Abstracts International, 30,* 5113B.

King, E. C. (1984). *Affective education in nursing: A guide to teaching and assessment.* Rockville, MD: Aspen Systems.

Kleinbaum, D. G., & Kupper, L. L. (1978). *Applied regression analysis and other multivariable methods.* Belmont, CA: Duxbury Press.

Lenz, C. L. (1982). A study of leadership behaviors and establishment of a demographic profile of nursing education administrators. (Doctoral dissertation, Ohio University, 1982). *Dissertation Abstracts International, 43*(6-B), 1796.

Lucio, W. H., & McNeil, J. D. (1969). *Supervision: A synthesis of thought and action* (2nd ed.). New York: McGraw-Hill.

Marriner, A. (1974, Spring). Student self-evaluation and the contracted grade. *Nursing Forum,* p. 13.

Martuza, V. R. (1977). *Applying norm-referenced and criterion- referenced measurement in education.* Boston: Allyn & Bacon.

Moloney, M. A. (1967). *Leadership behavior of deans in university schools of nursing.* Unpublished doctoral dissertation, Catholic University of America; Washington, DC.

Nunnally, C. (1978). *Psychometric theory* (2nd ed.). New York: McGraw-Hill.

Oaklander, H., & Fleishman, E. (1964). Patterns of leadership related to organizational stress on hospital settings. *Administrative Science Quarterly, 8*(3), 520-532.

Payne, A. M. (1982). Factors relating to the job satisfaction of nurses: Role conflict, sex-role identity, leader hierarchical influence, role ambiguity, and leader behaviors. (Doctoral dissertation, University of Texas, 1982). *Dissertation Abstracts International, 43*(2-A),329.

Pierce, T. M., & Merril, E. C. (1957). *Administrative behavior in education.* New York: Harper & Row.

Ramseyer, J. A. (1960). *Leadership for improving instruction.* Washington, DC: Association for Supervision and Curriculum Development.

Rovinelli, R. J., & Hambleton, R. K. (1977). On the use of content specialists in the assessment of criterion referenced test item validity. *Dutch Journal of Educational Research, 2,* 49-60.

South, L. L. (1981). Nurses' perceptions of nursing leadership behaviors. (Doctoral dissertation, University of Pittsburg, 1980). *Dissertation Abstracts International, 41,* 500-5001A.

Stanley, J. C. (1971). Reliability. In R. L. Thorndike (Ed.), *Educational Measurements* (2nd ed.). (pp. 356-442) Washington, DC: American Council on Education.

Stevens, S. S. (1946). On the theory of scales of measurement. *Science, 103* 677-680.

Stogdill, R. M. (1958). *Individual behavior and group achievement.* New York: Oxford University Press.

Stogdill, R. M. (1963). *Manual for the Leader Behavior Description Questionnaire – Form XII: An experimental revision.* Columbus; OH: The Ohio State University.

Stogdill, R. M. (1970). *A review of research on Leader Behavior Description Questionnaire – Form XII: An experimental revision.* Columbus; OH: Ohio State University, Bureau of Business Research.

Stogdill, R. M. (1974). *Handbook of leadership.* New York: Free Press.

Tannenbaum, R., Weschler, I., & Massarik, F. (1961). *Leadership and organization.* New York: McGraw-Hill.

Tead, O. (1935). *The art of leadership.* New York: Whittlesay House.

Thornberry, N. (1974). An exploration of the effects of organizational level of leadership behavior among nurses. (Doctoral dissertation, Bowling Green State University, 1974). *Dissertation Abstracts International, 35,* 1101B.

Wallenborn, A. (1960). *Instructional leadership in schools of nursing: What it is and how to prepare for it.* Unpublished doctoral dissertation, Columbia University, Teachers College.

Waltz, C. F., & Bausell, R. B. (1981). *Nursing research: Design, statistics, and computer analysis.* Philadelphia: F. A. Davis.

Waltz C., Strickland, O., & Lenz, E. (1984). *Measurement in nursing research.* Philadelphia: F. A. Davis.

Ward, M. J., & Fetler, M. E. (1979). *Instruments for use in nursing education research* . Boulder, CO: *Western Interstate Commission for Higher Education.*

Weissenberg, P., & Gruenfeld, L. (1966). Relationship among leadership dimensions and cognitive style. *Journal of Applied Psychology, 1*(5), 392-395.

Wenrich, R. C., & Wenrich, J. W. (1974). *Leadership in administration of vocational and technical education.* Columbus; OH: Charles E. Merrill.

Wittich, W. A., & Schuller, C. F. (1973). *Instructional technology: Its nature and use* (5th ed.). New York: Harper Row.

Yearwood, A. C. (1984). The effective and ineffective behaviors of black and white nurse leaders: An executive development program (Doctoral dissertation, Columbia University, Teacher's College, 1984). *Dissertation Abstracts International, 45,* 434A.

Yura, H. (1970). *Faculty perceptions of behavior indicating leadership potential of baccalaureate nursing students.* Unpublished doctoral dissertation, Catholic University of America, Washington, DC.

# Self Assessment Leadership Instrument

About the Questionnaire:

Please consider the following behaviors as they relate to your leadership. You should consider your reaction to each behavior and mark the rating accordingly.

A 5-point numerical scale (4...3...2...1...0) is used to indicate the rating. The interpretation of the extreme points on the continuum ranges from:

4 – Almost always behave in this manner

0 – Usually not behave in this manner

Thus the ratings:

| 4 | 3 | 2 | 1 | 0 |
|---|---|---|---|---|
| Almost always | More than 1/2 time | About 1/2 time | Less than 1/2 time | Usually not |

*Directions*: 1. Read each statement of behavior.
2. Indicate your judgment of how often you use this behavior.
3. Place the number that most closely indicates your estimate (i.e., 4 or 3 or 2 or 1 or 0) in the space provided at the end of the statement.
4. Respond to *every* statement.

| Statement of Leadership Behavior | Rating |
|---|---|
| 1. Evaluate your own needs | (_____) |
| 2. Fully grasp the ideas of the problem | (_____) |
| 3. Are aware of how you communicate with others | (_____) |
| 4. Are able to persuade groups to agree on specific issues | (_____) |
| 5. Organize your thoughts clearly and logically | (_____) |
| 6. Listen attentively for meaning and feelings | (_____) |
| 7. Get others to work together effectively | (_____) |
| 8. Predict the consequences of your decisions | (_____) |
| 9. Aware of the perceptions of others | (_____) |
| 10. Encourage the understanding of points of view of other group members | (_____) |
| 11. Plan ahead for what should be done | (_____) |
| 12. Recognize and locate resources in order to solve a problem | (_____) |
| 13. Show a willingness to make changes | (_____) |
| 14. Influence a group in goal setting | (_____) |
| 15. Make decisions on a factual basis | (_____) |

16. Alter your own behavior in order to meet a situation ( _____ )

17. Strive to understand other people ( _____ )

18. Assume responsibility for action taken based on your own decisions ( _____ )

19. Try to learn what impact you make on others ( _____ )

20. Grasp essentials of a problem, see solutions, and choose a course of action ( _____ )

21. Hold the attention of others while presenting pertinent ideas ( _____ )

22. Try out new ideas on a group ( _____ )

23. Delegate responsibility appropriately ( _____ )

24. Feel good about face-to-face exchanges of ideas ( _____ )

25. Discriminate between relevant, irrelevant, essential, and accidental data ( _____ )

26. Get others to follow your advice and direction ( _____ )

27. Encourage group members to work as a team ( _____ )

28. Direct group members or instruct them on what to do ( _____ )

29. Originate new approaches to problems ( _____ )

30. Have group members share in the decision making ( _____ )

31. Look for ways to improve yourself ( _____ )

32. Initiate action for new and better procedures and policies ( _____ )

33. Know how to proceed to get something done ( _____ )

34. Are friendly and approachable ( _____ )

35. Stand up for a group even if it makes you unpopular ( _____ )

36. Can define your role in a situation ( _____ )

37. Explain the reason for criticism ( _____ )

38. Encourage group members to express their ideas and opinions ( _____ )

39. Encourage slow-working members to improve their effort ( _____ )

40. Give credit when credit is due ( _____ )

# 18

# Assessing Students in Relation to Curriculum Objectives

## *Joan M. Johnson*

*This chapter discusses the Evaluation of Learning According to Objectives tool, a student measure of his or her own competence as an outcome of learning.*

Curriculum evaluation is becoming more important than ever to schools and colleges in this time of tighter budgets and greater expectations of all professionals. It is always important to consumers and the public that graduates will be competent practioners. The University of Wisconsin Oshkosh has recently developed a detailed evaluation plan. One facet of the plan is to have students evaluate their achievements and abilities at various points in their program and at its completion. Although students have evaluated courses and their own performances each semester and have evaluated the program at its completion, having them evaluate their perceived competency has not been part of the plan. This study proposed to develop a tool that would be useful for this purpose. It was expected that if the tool was effective in measuring competence as perceived by students the outcomes would be as follows:

1. There would be a significant positive relationship between students' perceptions of competency and their National League for Nursing (NLN) test scores.
2. There would be a significant positive relationship between students' perceptions of competency and their state board exam scores.
3. There would be a significant positive relationship between students' perceptions of competency and their college grade point average (GPA), as well as with their nursing grade point average (NGPA).
4. There would be a significant positive relationship between students' perceptions of competency and ratings of their competency by the clinical instructor.

5. There would be no significant relationship between sex, age, previous education, or patient care experience factors and students' competence.

The following definitions of competence were used:

*Conceptual competence* is the student's perceived achievement of clearly specified behavioral objectives, established to characterize competency in nursing, based on the University of Wisconsin Oshkosh curriculum.

*Operational competence* is the capability for performing as nurses as perceived by graduating baccalaureate students in relation to terminal behaviors of the curriculum at the University of Wisconsin Oshkosh College of Nursing, as determined by scores on a 67-item, Likert-scaled tool based on the curriculum objectives.

## REVIEW OF THE LITERATURE

Webster defines competence as capability, sufficiency, and adequacy. Clayton (cited in Chaska, 1983) defined competence as "achievement of clearly specified objectives which characterize competence in a given field" (p. 121). Benner (1982) stated that competence is viewed by beginning nurses as the performance of basic skills demonstrable in a lab setting," whereas experienced nurses viewed competence in relation to performance in an actual setting" (p. 303). Benner further defined competence as the "ability to perform a task with the desirable outcomes under the varied circumstances of the real world" (p. 304). Pottinger (1975) wrote that competencies should have "general significance to a wide variety of career and life outcomes" (p. 7). He pointed out that an endless list of skills, tasks, and actions is not meaningful if such activities are not used in the practice of the competence under examination.

### Tools

A number of nursing studies and associated tools were reviewed to determine their construction, validity and reliability, and their usefulness in this study. Nelson (1978) used the word "competency" and had nursing students rate themselves on three different categories of skills: technical, administrative, and communicative. Graduates of nine baccalaureate, diploma, and associate-degree programs were surveyed. Competence was not specifically defined, nor was the reliability of the tool determined. The tool was developed through a review of the nursing literature and as a result of professional experience and was later revised to include terminal behaviors from the nine schools taking part in the study. The competencies delineated were not intended to reflect all nine programs' objectives but rather functions common to all programs. In addition, a faculty member from each of the nine schools rated the ability of its graduates to perform the functions on a scale of Above Average, Average, or Below Average. The final list contained the functions rated average and above. Some of these functions are reasonable for most programs, but some were too specific to a disease or situation to be generalizable. One strength of the tool was the five rating levels, ranging from Extremely Competent to Incompetent. The usefulness of the category Incompetent seems questionable, however. It might have been better to use "unable to judge" or "unsure of competency." The use of a word comparable to competence (as used in the definition) might also introduce less bias and possibly decrease "self-serving answers" (according to Ward and Felter, 1979, p. 292).

In a follow-up study of graduates of a master's program, Hayter (1971) presented 17 functions for graduates and their employers to rate, using a scale of Excellent to Poor. Results were examined in relation to GPA and GRE scores and year of graduation. However, these functions were not appropriate for a baccalaureate graduate, nor did the rating scale seem appropriate to describe competence.

Brandt, Hastie, & Schumann (1967) conducted a study related to the effectiveness of major curriculum revisions. Fifty-one statements describing observable behaviors related to the curriculum objectives were rated by graduates, using a 5-point scale of Always to Never. This type of scale did not adequately conceptualize competence. There was no indication that this tool was tested for reliability or validity, and results of the study were inconclusive.

Following the inception of an associate-degree program, LaBelle and Egan (1975) use the terminal goals/behaviors established for graduates to study their competence. Graduates and their employers rated performance of the graduates using a scale of Great Difficulty, Some Difficulty, and No Opportunity to perform the behavior. They found that the yield from no Opportunity was difficult to interpret because it might have meant no opportunity to perform the task or no opportunity on the part of supervisors to observe the graduate perform the task. It was apparent that this scale was not adequate, though the use of the terminal behaviors of the curriculum was a good idea.

Although each of these tools and scales had some merit as well as weaknesses, none was appropriate for use in the current study for the reasons stated. To evaluate the graduates of the program, it seemed appropriate to use the stated terminal objectives/behaviors of the curriculum and the scale suggested by Waltz, Strickland, and Lenz (1984) to describe how well the student could perform the behavior.

## THE UNIVERSITY OF WISCONSIN OSHKOSH NURSING CURRICULUM

The University of Wisconsin Oshkosh nursing curriculum is built on a base of the humanities, natural and social sciences, and prenursing courses. The purpose of the program is to prepare professional nurses for a beginning-level position in any of a variety of settings. the major concepts of individual, environment, health, and nursing are the bases for the integrated curriculum. Selected threads within the four major concepts provide the focus for content, which is developed through use of the health/illness continuum.

The terminal objectives for graduates of the program include the expectations that graduates can

1. Use the nursing process to maintain, promote, or improve health of individuals, groups, and communities.
2. Use teaching methods to improve nursing and other health care.
3. Make informed decisions concerning the delivery of comprehensive health care.
4. Establish effective interpersonal relationships based on knowledge of human behaviors.
5. Collaborate in independent, dependent, and interdependent role relations to promote, restore, and maintain the health of individuals, groups, and communities.
6. Assume professional responsibility for providing quality nursing care.
7. Assume responsibility for their own personal and professional growth.

Performance indicators for each of the terminal objectives have also been developed. These indicators were the basis for the items in the instrument used in this study.

## METHODOLOGY

The sample for this study was the Spring 1985 class of the University of Wisconsin Oshkosh College of Nursing ($N = 60$). This was the fifth group of students to graduate from the integrated nursing curriculum. The students had evaluated courses and themselves each semester, and faculty at least once a year, so evaluation was not new to them.

### The Instrument

The seven terminal curriculum objectives have a total of 57 performance indicators. Four indicators encompass two or more activities, however, and so were broken down into their components to avoid ambiguity about which activity the student was rating. Prior to administration of the tool to students, two content specialists from the faculty reviewed the items and rated the relevance of each to the curriculum and its objectives. They used a 4-point scale: 1, Not Relevant; 2, Somewhat Relevant; 3, Relevant; and 4, Very Relevant. All of the items received a rating of 3 or 4; thus, all 67 items were used for the final tool. The content validity index was .91.

## Administration and Scoring

The instrument is a questionnaire that instructs the respondent to score each item on a Likert scale from 5 (Very Well) to 1 (Not at All) in regard to how well one perceives one's own ability to perform each terminal behavior. Item scores may be summed to obtain a total score.

# PROCEDURE

Three weeks before the end of the semester the graduating seniors were asked to rate themselves on each performance indicator according to "how well you are able to perform the terminal behavior without assistance." The scale ranged from 1, Not at All, to 5, Very Well. A score was obtained for each objective and for the total instrument. Three weeks later the same group of students was asked to rate themselves again on the performance indicators. this interval was necessary to determine if their perceptions were reliable. It is unlikely that competence itself would change in such a short period of time and at the end of the semester and program. In addition, each of the seven clinical faculty members were asked to rate two of their clinical students, using the same terminal behaviors and the same scale. Though rating all of the students was desirable, given the time of the semester, faculty were not willing to do so.

# MAJOR FINDINGS

The internal consistency reliability coefficient of the instrument was .96 on the first administration. Even thought the conditions for the retest were not ideal, the test-retest reliability coefficient was stable. Pearson correlations of objectves with each other were all significant (Table 18.1), and the alpha coefficient for internal consistency for each objective was .79 and above for all objectives (Table 18.2).

The Pearson correlation of student ratings with their NLN achievement test score was .08; with college GPA, .062; and with nursing GPA, .259; none significant at the .05 level ($N = 50$). The 10 usable faculty ratings correlated with student ratings at $-.288$, $p = 2.09$. Since only two students in the group were male, and only two students had degrees in another field, no corroborations were attempted for these variables. Age correlated with student ratings at .652, $p = .00$. A $t$-test relating patient care experience as a nursing assistant with students' ratings was not significant, which was the finding postulated ($t = 1.04$, $p = .304$, $N = 14$). Finally, correlation of students' ratings with their state board exam scores was .749, $p = .00$; and the correlation of faculties' ratings with the state board exam scores with those students rated ($N = 10$) was .429, $p = .108$.

**TABLE 18.1** Correlation Matrix – Objectives of Curriculum Correlated with Each Other

| Objective | 1 | 2 | 3 | 4 | 5 | 6 | 7 |
|---|---|---|---|---|---|---|---|
| 1 | .00 | | | | | | |
| 2 | .707 | 1.00 | | | | | |
| 3 | .456 | .429 | 1.00 | | | | |
| 4 | .548 | .532 | .536 | 1.00 | | | |
| 5 | .668 | .585 | .748 | .689 | 1.00 | | |
| 6 | .648 | .526 | .439 | .546 | .656 | 1.00 | |
| 7 | .255* | .243 | .485 | .374 | .466 | .456 | 1.00 |

$*p = .05$; all others, $p = .01$.

**TABLE 18.2** Internal Consistency of Students' Self-Rating on Curriculum Objectives

| | Objective | Alpha |
|---|---|---|
| I | Use of nursing process | .7905 |
| II | Use of teaching | .9966 |
| III | Decision making | .9937 |
| IV | Interpersonal relationships | .9945 |
| V | Collaborative role | .9926 |
| VI | Professional responsibility | .9928 |
| VII | Personal & professional growth | .9793 |

## DISCUSSION AND CONCLUSIONS

Students' ratings of self on items within objectives was stable from the first administration of the tool to the second, even though the second administration came on the last day of classes in the last 15 min of class. Their ratings correlated significantly with their state board exam scores.

Less sastisfying was the lack of correlation between the ratings of faculty and students regarding their ability on objectives and performance indicators. The range of student ratings was 2 to 5, with a mean of 4, and faculty ratings ranged form 1 to 5, with a mean of 3.5. This may indicate a need for faculty throughout the program to assist students to evaluate their skills more realistically and help them plan how to improve during the next semester.

Although the instrument demonstrated reliability, its validity is questionable. As with the end-of-program evaluation, the results are student perceptions rather than facts about their preparation for nursing practice. Questions that might be asked include the following: Are students prepared to evaluate their abilities realistically? Is there consistency between faculty and the students definition of "very well" and "well"? Do students understand the feedback that faculty give them about their performance?

Limitations of the study include the fact that the $N$ is not large, especially in comparing student and faculty ratings (10). This, plus the fact that some statements could not be judged by faculty because of the clinical setting in which they judged the student, may have affected the correlation of student-faculty ratings. Concern about state board exam results of the previous graduating class may have affected the results as well. Finally, the items on the tool are based on this college's curriculum objectives and thus may not be generalizable to other curriculum objectives and thus may not be generalizable to other curricula.

## IMPLICATIONS

For a measurement tool to be useful in the evaluation of a curriculum, it must be geared to the purposes or objectives of the curriculum. The terms used to describe achievement, perceptions, or skill must be clear to the individual who is completing the instrument, or the interpretation of results will be difficult.

## SUMMARY

The purpose of this study was to determine if an instrument based on curriculum objectives and performance indicators would be effective in measuring competence of graduating seniors. Effectiveness was to be determined through the correlation of students' ratings of their competence and NLN test scores, state board exam scores, college and nursing GPAs, ratings of clinical instructors, sex, previous education, and patient care experience. The only significant correlation found was between students' ratings of themselves on objectives (and performance indicators) and their state board exam scores. Although the tool was found to be highly reliable (.96), the validity is questionable. Further study is needed before this method of evaluation can be used with confidence to evaluate the curriculum and/or predict scholastic performance.

## REFERENCES

Benner, P. (1982). Issues in competency-based testing. *Nursing Outlook, 30*(5), 303 – 309.

Brandt, E. M., Hastie, B., & Schumann, D. (1967). Comparison of on-the-job performance of graduates with school nursing objectives. *Nursing Research, 16*(1), 50 – 60.

Chaska, N. L. (1983). *The nursing profession: A time to speak.* New York: McGraw-Hill.

Hayter, J. (1971). Follow-up study of graduates of the University of Kentucky, 1964 – 1969. *Nursing Research, 20*(1), 55 – 60.

LaBelle, B. M., & Egan, E. C. (1975). Follow-up studies in nursing. *Journal of Nursing Education, 14*(3), 7 – 13.

Nelson, L. F. (1978). Competencies of nursing graduates in technical, communicative, and administrative skills. *Nursing Research, 27*(2), 121 – 125.

Pottinger, P. S. (1975). Comments and guidelines for research in competency identification, definition and measurement. Syracuse, NY: Syracuse University, Education Policy Research Center. (ERIC Document Reproduction Service No. ED 134541).

Waltz, C. F., Strickland, O. L., & Lenz, E. R. (1984). *Measurement in nursing research*. Philadelphia: F. A. Davis.

Ward, M. J., & Felter, M. E. (1979). *Instruments for use in nursing education research*. Boulder, CO: Western Instruments Commission for Higher Education.

# Evaluation of Learning According to Curriculum Objectives

We are interested in how well your program has prepared students to implement program goals. Indicate the extent to which you are able to perform each of the following terminal behaviors.

|  | Very Well | | | | Not At all |
|---|---|---|---|---|---|
| 1. Use research findings to improve nursing practice. | 5 | 4 | 3 | 2 | 1 |
| 2. Use theoretical and empirical knowledge in the application of the nursing process. | 5 | 4 | 3 | 2 | 1 |
| 3. Collect data about the health status of clients. | 5 | 4 | 3 | 2 | 1 |
| 4. Collect data about the health status of a group or community. | 5 | 4 | 3 | 2 | 1 |
| 5. Determine the need for nursing intervention based on data analysis. | 5 | 4 | 3 | 2 | 1 |
| 6. Develop nursing diagnoses. | 5 | 4 | 3 | 2 | 1 |
| 7. Develop objectives based on identified nursing diagnoses. | 5 | 4 | 3 | 2 | 1 |
| 8. Evaluate the goals of nursing care, using knowledge from physical and behavioral science and nursing theories. | 5 | 4 | 3 | 2 | 1 |
| 9. Encourage the client to select own goals. | 5 | 4 | 3 | 2 | 1 |
| 10. Encourage the client to participate in own care. | 5 | 4 | 3 | 2 | 1 |
| 11. Determine care activities which require the specialized skills of the professional nurse. | 5 | 4 | 3 | 2 | 1 |
| 12. Determine community resources for promotion of optimal level of wellness for client/family. | 5 | 4 | 3 | 2 | 1 |
| 13. Implement a plan of nursing intervention which is consistent with scientific rationales. | 5 | 4 | 3 | 2 | 1 |
| 14. Implement a plan which facilitates health seeking behaviors with a select population within a community. | 5 | 4 | 3 | 2 | 1 |
| 15. Evaluate the effectiveness of nursing practice. | 5 | 4 | 3 | 2 | 1 |
| 16. Revise the nursing care plan based on evaluation of outcomes. | 5 | 4 | 3 | 2 | 1 |

17. Recognize the *independent* function of　　5　4　3　2　1
the teaching role.
18. Recognize the *interdependent* function of　5　4　3　2　1
the teaching role.

19. Recognize the *dependent* function of　　　5　4　3　2　1
the teaching role.
20. Assume responsibility for initiating　　　　5　4　3　2　1
teaching appropriate to the learner's needs.
21. Apply the principles of teaching and　　　　5　4　3　2　1
learning in nursing practice.

22. Design a teaching plan which integrates　　5　4　3　2　1
plans of other disciplines.
23. Analyze individual teaching plan based on　5　4　3　2　1
an understanding of the *independent* functions
of the nurse.
24. Analyze individual teaching plan based on　5　4　3　2　1
an understanding of the *interdependent* functions of the nurse.

25. Analyze an individual teaching plan based　5　4　3　2　1
on an understanding of the *dependent* functions of the nurse.
26. Implement the teaching plan designed to　　5　4　3　2　1
improve or maintain health.
27. Initiate action with other health team　　　5　4　3　2　1
members to meet the learning needs of clients.
28. Evaluate the effectiveness of the teaching　5　4　3　2　1
plan based on the understanding of the *inde-*
*pendent* functions of the nurse.
29. Evaluate the effectiveness of the teaching　5　4　3　2　1
plan based on an understanding of the *interde-*
*pendent* functions of the nurse.
30. Evaluate the effectiveness of the teaching　5　4　3　2　1
plan based on an understanding of the *depen-*
*dent* functions of the nurse.

31. Demonstrate an appreciation for the　　　　5　4　3　2　1
cultural and societal factors which affect health
promotion/maintenance, restoration and
rehabilitation.
32. Analyze how personal, social, and cultural　5　4　3　2　1
values influence decision making in providing
care to individuals or groups.
33. Support the individual/group's need to　　　5　4　3　2　1
participate in beliefs and practices meaningful
to their lifestyle.
34. Collaborate with the individual or group in　5　4　3　2　1
identifying alternative actions available to promote, maintain, or restore health consistent
with their cultural values.

35. Utilize a systematic decision-making    5    4    3    2    1
    process to achieve goals with individuals and
    groups.
36. Utilize the principles of change to achieve    5    4    3    2    1
    goals with individuals and groups.
37. Discern the influence of ethical and legal    5    4    3    2    1
    issues on the provision of nursing care.
38. Evaluate the effectiveness of decision    5    4    3    2    1
    making in meeting the needs of individuals or
    groups.
39. Assess communication of clients and    5    4    3    2    1
    families based upon knowledge and techniques
    of interpersonal communication.
40. Use appropriate communication    5    4    3    2    1
    techniques in nursing practice.
41. Utilize knowledge of group dynamics in    5    4    3    2    1
    nursing practice.
42. Communicate effectively through    5    4    3    2    1
    utilization of oral and written methods.
43. Evaluate behavior based on knowledge of    5    4    3    2    1
    human responses and stages of growth
    and development.
44. Evaluate interpersonal relationships with    5    4    3    2    1
    clients.
45. Evaluate interpersonal relationships with    5    4    3    2    1
    peers.
46. Evaluate interpersonal relationships with    5    4    3    2    1
    other health professionals.
47. Involve the client/family in assessing,    5    4    3    2    1
    planning, implementing, and evaluating nursing
    care.
48. Cooperate with other health personnel to    5    4    3    2    1
    promote congruency and continuity of care.
49. Value the contributions of all persons    5    4    3    2    1
    involved in providing health care.
50. Accept responsibility to identify the role    5    4    3    2    1
    of all persons involved in providing health care
    to other health care professionals.
51. Distinguish between nursing role and other    5    4    3    2    1
    health professionals' roles in the health care
    delivery system.
52. Establish effective working relationships    5    4    3    2    1
    with other health team members.
53. Identify issues that impact on the    5    4    3    2    1
    professional nursing role in health care.
54. Appreciate the historical developments    5    4    3    2    1
    which have had an impact on the professional
    nursing role.

55. Relate the significance of the changes          5    4    3    2    1
    effected by nurses and the nursing profession
    to the present and future role of the profes-
    sional nurse.

56. Apply theorectical concepts of nursing and      5    4    3    2    1
    management to own practice.

57. Demonstrate the ability to carry out the        5    4    3    2    1
    nursing process in a variety of settings.

58. Assume total nursing care responsibility        5    4    3    2    1
    for clients.

59. Implement a plan of nursing intervention        5    4    3    2    1
    which is consistent with American Nurses
    Association Standards of Practice.

60. Design plans for directing care given by        5    4    3    2    1
    ancillary personnel.

61. Take necessary action when resources for        5    4    3    2    1
    care are not provided.

62. Evaluate others who give nursing care to        5    4    3    2    1
    promote quality care.

63. Participate in formal activities designed to    5    4    3    2    1
    evaluate the quality of nursing care.

64. Recognize the importance of their future        5    4    3    2    1
    role as leaders.

65. Seek resources to improve own level of          5    4    3    2    1
    practice based on evaluation by self and
    others.

66. Seek current knowledge of the political,        5    4    3    2    1
    social, and economic factors which effect nurs-
    ing practice.

67. Appreciate the importance of                    5    4    3    2    1
    participating in professional organizations and
    community activities.

Thank you for your assistance with this project.

*Do Not* Sign This Questionnaire

Demographic Data:

Have you had experience as a nurse's aid/assistant? __Yes __No
  If yes, length/amount of experience: __months or __years

Are you a Licensed Practical Nurse? __Yes __No
  If yes, length/amount of experience: __months or __years

Have you participated in State Board Review Sessions? __Yes __No

Thank you!

# 19

# Evaluating Prototype Nursing Continuing Education Programs

*Angeline M. Jacobs, DeAnn M. Young,*
*and Felicitas A. Dela Cruz*

*This chapter discusses a Program Evaluation Model that can be used to evaluate nursing education programs. It was tested here on continuning education programs.*

A program evaluation model to assess outcomes of prototype continuing education programs in nursing was developed and applied to two certificated continuing education offerings. The educational programs were a 240-hr hospice nursing course (24 academic units) and a 200-hr (20-unit) program in end stage renal disease nursing, with emphasis on hemodialysis.

## THE HOSPICE EDUCATION PROGRAM

The continuing education program in hospice nursing consisted of six didactic courses, totaling 120 academic hours, and three clinical courses, totaling 360 practicum hours. The curriculum was offered over a period of five academic quarters. The content of the curriculum, based on the hospice philosophy of care, is shown in Table 19.1. The clinical practicum provided for the development of skills in both inpatient and home-care hospice settings. the curriculum, which was designed to meet the needs of the full-time employed registered nurse, required a commitment of 12 hr/week from the student. Didactic courses were offered in the evening, and students employed in hospices used their own agencies for their clinical experience. Students employed in other settings were assigned to hospice agencies participating in the education program as clinical facilities. Academic credit toward the baccalaureate degree in nursing at California State University, Los Angeles, was given for 20 of the 24 units.

Funded by Grants D-10-NU-29098 and D-10-NU-29149, Division of Nursing, U.S. Department of Health and Human Services

**TABLE 19.1** Hospice Courses

| | | |
|---|---|---|
| XN | 442 | Hospice – a Holistic Model of Alternative Care for the Terminally Ill (2 lecture units[a]) |
| XN | 450 | Physical Assessment in Hospice Care (2 lecture units) |
| XN | 342 | Concepts of Loss, Grief, and Support for Hospice Families (2 lecture units) |
| XN | 452 | Symptom Control in Hospice Care (2 lecture units) |
| XN | 344 | Psychosocial Nursing Care of the Hospice Family (2 lecture units) |
| XN | 343 | The Nursing Assessment Process in the Care of Hospice Patients and Families – Clinical Course I (2 clinical units) |
| XN | 345 | Applied Intervention in Hospice Care Nursing – Clinical Course II (4 clinical units) |
| XN | 456 | Stress and the Hospice Nurse (2 lecture units) |
| XN | 441 | Nursing Operation within a Hospice – Clinical Course III (4 clinical units) |

[a]Units are quarter units: 1 lecture unit = 1 hr/week: 1 clinical unit = 3 hr/week.

The program was offered to three cohorts of students. All students were registered nurses with at least 1 year of work experience. Their educational backgrounds varied among diploma (37%), associate (33%), and baccalaureate degrees (27%) (see Table 19.2).

Approximately 37% of the nurses accepted into the program had current or previous hospice experience. Forty-nine students were admitted to the program, and 26 were graduated. An additional three students completed only the didactic portion of the program.

## THE NEPHROLOGY (END STAGE RENAL DISEASE) PROGRAM

This program consisted of eight courses – five didactic, two clinical, and one with both didactic and clinical components. This latter offering was the technical course in initiation, maintenance, and termination of hemodialysis. the curriculum consisted of 20 academic units spread over four academic quarters. Classes were offered in the evenings to accommodate employed students. The amount of time required from the students varied between 8 and 10 hr/week. Of the total 20 units offered in the program, 15 were applicable to the baccalaureate degree at California State University. the nephrology courses are listed in Table 19.3.

Two cohorts of students completed the program; a total of 24 were graduated (Table 19.4). Like the hospice program, all students were registered nurses with at least 1 year of work experience. Twenty-five percent of the matriculants into the program were diploma graduates, and 27% were baccalaureate graduates. About half of the students were currently employed in dialysis units; these students used their work settings for their clinical practicum. the students inexperienced in dialysis were assigned to

**TABLE 19.2** **Educational and Employment Background of Students, Hospice Program**

| Background | Applicants | Matriculants | Graduates (%) |
|---|---|---|---|
| Education | | | |
| Diploma | 24 | 18 | 9 (50) |
| AA | 19 | 16 | 9 (50) |
| BS | 21 | 13 | 7 (54) |
| Masters | 4 | 2 | 1 (50) |
| Totals | 68 | 49 | 26 (53) |
| | | | |
| Prior hospice experience | | | |
| YES | 20 | 18 | 12 (67) |
| NO | 48 | 31 | 14 (45) |
| Totals | 68 | 49 | 26 (53) |

participating dialysis units for their practicum. Students experienced in dialysis had the option to challenge the combined clinical/lecture course in administering hemodialysis by passing a performance examination.

For both the nephrology and hospice program students, there was no significant difference in the number of graduates attributable to either educational or employment experience when a chi-square test of significance was applied to the data.

## ATTRITION

Both programs experienced high attrition – 47% for the hospice program and 45% for nephrology. There were a large number of withdrawals for the combined reasons of health and personal loss, 47% for the hospice and 30% for nephrology. About 13% of the hospice and 20% of the nephrology students experienced academic failure. The most prevalent reason for both groups, however, was the demands of the program, which proved too time-consuming and intensive for full-time employed nurses, most of them with family obligations. This finding has serious implications for the viability of long, extended programs of this type.

## THE EVALUATION MODEL

A major objective of both continuing education programs was to develop and implement a program evaluation model that could subsequently be made available to the nursing community. The program evaluation that was designed consisted of both formative and summative components, based on a model developed at the American Institutes for Research and used by the senior author in several other nursing research studies (Jacobs & Larson, 1976). The model has three major characteristics. First, it is *decision-oriented*: that is, data are collected that assist in making decisions about program modification while the program is in progress, as well as in planning program replication. Second, the evaluation is based on a *program rationale* that makes explicit the dynamics of the cause-and-effect relationships being assessed. This allows for identification of individual program components that should be modified or that deserve consideration when further interventions are planned. Finally, the evaluation emphasizes *impact-referenced* indicators of accomplishment. Program benefits should be openly observable events that are incontrovertible evidence of meaningful improvement.

The program evaluation model (Figure 19.1) illustrates the relationship of process and outcome to ultimate program impact.

- *Program input* includes curriculum objectives, behaviorally stated terminal objectives, and overall project objectives; the student's demographic and experiential characteristics; and the curriculum itself.
- *Process variables* are the activities planned to bring about the curriculum and program objectives, such as recruiting, selection of students, selection of faculty, and instructional strategies.
- *Immediate outcomes* occur as the activities of the program are implemented. For example, course A is completed successfully by $N$ students, $n$ students dropped out, and $N$ students expressed satisfaction or dissatisfaction with the course.
- *Further program input* refers to interventions that are applied as a result of process assessment. For example, in the hospice program, rap sessions were instituted for the first group of students, who were experiencing stress because of the work load, especially the clinical

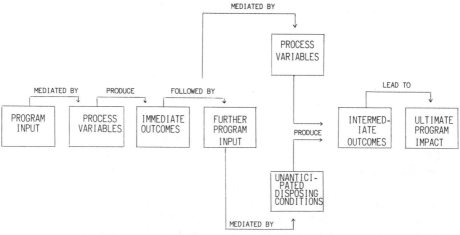

**FIGURE 19.1** Program evaluation model.

experiences. As a result of the feedback from the first group (who experienced high attrition) the clinical practicum for subsequent groups of students was modified, and retention of students improved.

- *Unanticipated disposing or intervening variables* are those events that influence program outcome either positively or negatively. Examples are unanticipated absences of project staff because of illness or unexpected changes in faculty. these events are recorded on process evaluation instruments and are incorporated into the data analysis.
- *Intermediate outcomes* are those that occur relatively close in time and can be measured within the scope of the project; for example; total number of graduates and dropouts, application of learning in employment situations, "ripple effect" on other staff in employing agencies, and benefits or detriments to the graduates.
- *Ultimate program impact* includes those outcomes that are more global and later-maturing; for example, improvement in patient care, long-term collaborative relationships, or other resultant programs. Some of theses occur and can be measured within a project's time frame, but most require a longer maturation time.

**TABLE 19.3 Hospice Courses**

| | | |
|---|---|---|
| XN | 303 | Nursing Technology in Dialysis (4 units,[a] combined clinical and lecture) |
| XN | 346 | Concepts of Loss (1 lecture unit) |
| XN | 372 | Physical Assessment (3 lecture units) |
| XN | 444 | Renal Failure: Pathophysiology and Nursing Management (4 lecture units) |
| XN | 451 | Nursing Assessment of the Nephrology Patient and Family (2 clinical units) |
| XN | 453 | Nursing Intervention (2 clinical units) |
| XN | 486 | Patient Teaching in Nephrology (2 lecture units) |

[a]Units are quarter units: 1 lecture unit = 1 hr/week; 1 clinical unit = 3 hr/week.

**TABLE 19.4 Educational and Employment Background of Students, End Stage Renal Disease Program**

| Background | Applicants | Matriculants | Graduates (%) |
|---|---|---|---|
| Education | | | |
| Diploma | 12 | 11 | 8 (73) |
| AA | 25 | 21 | 9 (43) |
| BS | 18 | 12 | 7 (58) |
| Totals | 55 | 44 | 24 (55) |
| | | | |
| Previous dialysis experience | | | |
| YES | 25 | 21 | 13 (62) |
| NO | 30 | 23 | 11 (48) |
| Totals | 55 | 44 | 24 (55) |

## APPLICATION OF THE MODEL

The same general evaluation design was applied to both educational programs. However, complete data are available only for the hospice education program, as postprogram follow-up data collection for the nephrology program is not complete at the time of this writing.

   The formative evaluation component began with the inception of the projects and continued until the end of the program offerings. Its function was twofold: (1) to aid in the development of the programs and modifications of the offerings between cohorts of students by means of timely and continuous feedback from all program participants and (2) to ultimately shape the programs into the best possible educational offerings for dissemination to the nursing community. The specific activities included in the formative evaluation were as follows:

- A milestone and task audit conducted monthly at the beginning of each project and quarterly toward the end of the project periods.
- Review of teaching strategies for acceptability by students and effectiveness of instruction.
- Collection of anonymous critical incident reports of unanticipated events from students, faculty, clinical facility personnel and project staff.
- Assessment of student progress in each of the courses of the curriculum and comparison of student grades among cohorts of students in each program.
- End-of-course evaluations by students for each course.
- End-of-course evaluations by faculty for each course.
- End-of-course evaluations by the students at the time of their graduation.
- End-of-course evaluations at the end of the project by (a) faculty and (b) participating clinical agencies.

   The summative evaluation utilized a pre/post design, with a nonequivalent control group and with longitudinal follow-up. The control group consisted of two subgroups:
   1. Students who withdrew from the program and thus had comparable data for all three data points – preprogram measurements, some immediate postprogram outcome measures, and outcome data collected at the longitudinal follow-up data point.
   2. Applicants who were not accepted into the program (nonmatriculants). These subjects had only application data (demographics, work experience, goals, etc.) in common with the other subjects and some outcome data collected at the longitudinal follow-up data point.

**TABLE 19.5 Follow-up (6 Months Postgraduation)**

Postprogram employment in field studied
Job promotions
Salary increases
Job satisfaction
Extent of implementation of learnings
Retrospective assessment of satisfaction
  with the program
Professional benefits (or detriments)
  resulting
Personal benefits (or detriments)
  resulting
Supervisor ratings
Agency characteristics that might mediate outcome

The longitudinal follow-up was conducted 6 months after graduation from the programs to determine benefits or negative outcomes (see Table 19.5). At the same time, to provide a common temporal framework, dropouts and nonmatriculants belonging to the graduate cohort were interviewed to determine their employment and educational status relevant to the clinical content of the two programs. Also, personnel from agencies employing the graduates were interviewed concerning benefits or detriments accrued to the agency as a result of their employee's participation in the educational programs.

## INSTRUMENTATION

The pre/post measurement included assessment of the following:

- Knowledge
- Attitudes
- Skills
- Performance in giving patient care: self-rating and supervisor rating
- Patient interviewing skills (videotaped) (Hospice Project)
- Ability to use nursing process and formulate nursing judgments (Nephrology Project)

All instruments were constructed specifically for the projects. The process of instrument construction included the following steps:

- Input from content experts.
- Formating for computer entry, with the help of a system program analyst.

- Field-testing the first version on 20 to 30 subjects who would not be participating in the program.
- Revision of the first version based on item analysis of field-test data.
- Limited tryouts of the revised version on small samples of comparable subjects (5-10).
- Determination of reliability, including measures of internal consistency (usually Cronbach's alpha coefficient) and measures of interrater reliability where applicable (usually Pearson product-moment correlation coefficient).
- Determination of validity, including content validity, by agreement of content experts; discriminative validity; and concurrent validity by correlation with other measures.

## Administration and Scoring

The various instruments used in this evaluation model included questionnaires and rating scales that were completed by the students or their instructors or both, as well as a paper-and-pencil knowledge test. Item scores may be summed to obtain a total score for each instrument.

Following is a brief description of some of the instruments developed. The computer instruments and a description of their development are available in the final report of each project (Jacobs, dela Cruz, & Young, 1986; Young & Jacobs, 1984).

### Knowledge Test

Paper-and-pencil knowledge tests were developed for each of the programs, a 120-item test for the hospice program and a 100-item test for nephrology. About 40% of the items in each test measured recall of factual material, and about 60% tested application of knowledge or problem solving in clinical simulations. The reliability of the tests, using Cronbach's alpha coefficient, was .90 for the hospice test and .72 for the nephrology test.

### Attitude Measurement

In the hospice program, change in student attitudes was measured by pre/post program administration of a 100-item Likert-type scale of value statements, with a reliability coefficient of .97 (Cronbach's alpha). An excerpt from this scale is shown in Figure 19.2. In the nephrology program, two attitude instruments were developed. The first was a Likert-type scale of value statements consisting of 78 items (Cronbach's alpha = .91) and the second a behavioral intentions scale of 45 items (Cronbach's alpha = .78) (Triandis, 1977). An excerpt from the behavioral intentions scale is shown in Figure 19.3. Discriminative validity, using an index of social desirability (Crowne & Marlowe, 1964), indicated that there was no statistical significance between either the values scale or the behavioral intentions scale and the social desirability scale (paired *t*-tests). This suggests that the constructs being measured by the values and behavioral intentions scale are *not* merely social desirability but rather a measure of some other attitudinal constructs.

## Performance Ratings

Rating scales were used in the educational programs to obtain both self-reports and supervisor ratings of performance in critical nursing competencies. In the hospice program, 14 competencies were assessed, including pain management, symptom management, making referrals, providing nutrition, patient/support, and providing bereavement support. The nephrology program performance rating instrument measured 69 spe-

| | Strongly agree | Moderately agree | Slightly agree | Slightly disagree | Moderately disagree | Strongly disagree |
|---|---|---|---|---|---|---|
| 1. If a person with terminal cancer will not accept the recommended treatment (such as radiation or chemotherapy) the cancer team is not responsible for his/her outcome. | ⎯⎯ | ⎯⎯ | ⎯⎯ | ⎯⎯ | ⎯⎯ | ⎯⎯ |
| 2. We should inform the dying patient and family as fully as possible about what symptoms to expect as the disease progresses. | ⎯⎯ | ⎯⎯ | ⎯⎯ | ⎯⎯ | ⎯⎯ | ⎯⎯ |

**FIGURE 19.2** Excerpt from Attitude Instrument, Hospice Likert scale.

After 15 years of dialysis and two unsuccessful transplants, Mrs. S terminates dialysis and 12 days later dies at home.     I:

1. Would ⎯⎯ ⎯⎯ ⎯⎯ ⎯⎯ ⎯⎯ ⎯⎯ ⎯⎯ ⎯⎯ ⎯⎯ would not
   visit Mrs. S as often as she wishes while she is dying.

2. Would ⎯⎯ ⎯⎯ ⎯⎯ ⎯⎯ ⎯⎯ ⎯⎯ ⎯⎯ ⎯⎯ ⎯⎯ ⎯⎯ would not
   view the death as a suicide

Scale = would                                                                 would not

| Always | Almost always | Usually | More often than not | Maybe | Maybe not | Sometimes | Rarely | Never |
|---|---|---|---|---|---|---|---|---|

**FIGURE 19.3** Excerpt from Attitude Instrument, End Renal Disease Behavioral Intention scale.

cific competencies arranged in 14 behavioral groupings, including administering hemodialysis, administering peritoneal dialysis, patient teaching, performing physical assessment, interviewing and counseling patient/ family, providing emotional and spiritual support, providing crisis intervention, making referrals. applying research, and documenting patient care. Both instruments had high interrater reliability, ranging from .80 to .90 (Pearson $r$). Self and supervisor ratings were not statistically different, but supervisor ratings tended to be higher than self-ratings. An excerpt from the nephrology program shows the 6-point rating scale that was used (Figure 19.4).

## Performance Test of Patient Interviewing Skill

This videotaped test was used in the hospice program to make a pre/ post assessment of basic communication skills of the students. The test employed a standardized script, which had a two-track cueing system for the simulated patient's responses. This gave every examinee an opportunity to be tested at each designated observation point. The actor who portrayed the patient was a mental health nursing instructor who used the first track response when an examinee displayed an appropriate skill, the second track when the examinee responded inappropriately. The second track brought the examinee back to the same observation point that the "correct response" led to. The videotape of each student's examination was scored independently by two mental health nursing instructors. The interrater reliability was .61. Excerpts from the test in Figures 19.5 and 19.6 show a part of the script and the observational criteria, respectively.

Circle the number that best fits your
opinion of the individual's competence

| | 5 | 4 | 3 | 2 | 1 | 0 |
|---|---|---|---|---|---|---|
| | Out-standing | | Competent | | Not competent | Not observed |
| A. Administers hemodialysis | | | | | | |
| 1. Prepares equipment, materials, and dialysis baths | 5 | 4 | 3 | 2 | 1 | 0 |
| 2. Computes transmembrane pressure | 5 | 4 | 3 | 2 | 1 | 0 |
| Etc. | | | | | | |

**FIGURE 19.4** Excerpt from Performance Assessment, End Stage Renal Disease.

> I've lost so much weight.
> I looked at myself in a picture the
> other day and now...
> Shake head, quiet, sad expression

Observation IX:
___ Neutral Response

| Observation IX: Positive Response | | Observation IX: Negative Response | |
|---|---|---|---|
| ___ 7. | Reinforces verbalization through words or sounds. | Makes statement which avoids feelings. | 14 ___ |
| | | OR | |
| AND | | Asks question which elicits yes/no. | 15 ___ |
| ___ 8. | Uses silence with position of attending. | OR Extinguishes verbalization through absence or reinforcement. | 16 ___ |
| OR | | | AND |
| ___ 9. | Reaches out to touch. | Uses silence without attending. | 17 ___ |
| OR ___ 12. | Leans toward person. | OR Turns body away or folds arms. | 21 ___ |

**FIGURE 19.5** Excerpt from Patient Interviewing Test.

| | Score | Negative | Score |
|---|---|---|---|
| **Positive** | | | |
| **Verbal** | | | |
| 1. Paraphrases accurately with question | ___ | 13. Paraphrases inaccurately or without a question | ___ |
| **Nonverbal** | | | |
| 12. Leans toward person | ___ | 21. Turns body away from person or folds arms | ___ |

**FIGURE 19.6** Excerpt from Videotaped Performance Test of Patient Interviewing Observational Criteria.

### Skills Inventory

In the hospice program, a self-report inventory of skills was used, including the following 11 skills: pain management, cardiopulmonary assessment, gastrointestinal assessment, urinary catheter insertion, ostomy care, wound care, IV therapy, parenteral feedings. tracheostomy care, symptom assessment, and family assessment. Students were asked to rate their competency in each skill, in both *in-patient* and *home care* settings.

Supervisors also rated the students on the same dimensions. the rating scale was as follows:

1 = I have done this activity and feel competent.
2 = I have done this activity but would have to seek help to feel competent.
3 = I have not done this activity.

The interrater reliability between the self- and supervisor ratings was .80 (percentage of agreement on items). Graduates of the program showed improvement in all skills from pre- to postmeasurement, especially in the home care setting. The paired *t*-tests were statistically significant at the .05 level or better for 14 of the 22 measurements.

## Performance Examination

A performance test was constructed to serve as both a challenge examination and the final exam for the hemodialysis course in the nephrology program. An excerpt from the examination is shown in Figure 19.7. There were 10 critical behaviors that the student had to perform correctly to pass. Criteria for passing the rest of the examination were expressed as percentage of competencies that had to be performed correctly. Students were given copies of the test in advance so that they could use it to prepare themselves. Interrater reliability coefficients have not yet been calculated, but the test had high acceptance among both students and faculty.

Check the
Appropriate Column

|  | Performed correctly | Performed incorrectly | Not performed | Not applicable/ remarks |
|---|---|---|---|---|
| I.   Overriding Critical Behaviors |  |  |  |  |
| A.   Washes hands after any blood-related procedure, etc. (there were 10 critical behaviors) |  |  |  |  |
| III.   Prepares dialysis bath |  |  |  |  |
| A.   Establishes the absence of formaldehyde/ bleach in the machine |  |  |  |  |
| 30.   Measures blood pressure |  |  |  |  |
| 30.1   Uses a cuff which covers 2/3 of the upper part of extremity |  |  |  |  |
| 30.11   Obtains a blood pressure reading that agrees with the instructor's to ± 4 mmHg systolic and diastolic |  |  |  |  |

**FIGURE 19.7** Excerpt from Dialysis Performance Examination.

# EVALUATION RESULTS

The major findings were that the graduates exhibited consistent and significant gains in attitudes, knowledge, and skills and consistently found employment or promotion in hospice or dialysis agencies to a greater extent than did nurses who withdrew from the program. Specific results obtained in the hospice program follow:

## Pre/Postmeasurements

There were significant gains in all of the variables listed in Table 19.6, when pre- and postprogram scores were examined using paired *t*-tests.

## Postprogram Employment

These data are available only for the hospice graduates, as the second group of students in the nephrology program had not graduated. The chi-square for the data presented in Table 19.7 was significant at the .001 level.

## Benefits to Students

Some of the student outcomes for the hospice program are summarized below. The data in Table 19.8 was obtained 6 months after graduation from the program. Graduates more often reported benefits that did dropouts.

**TABLE 19.6** Nursing Gains Resulting from Participation in Hospice Care Program

| Variable | Gain | *t*-Test Significance (*p*) |
|---|---|---|
| Knowledge | 3 (17%) | .01 |
| Attitudes | 26 (42%) | .01 |
| Patient interviewing skills | 15 (28%) | .02 |
| Self-assessment of nursing skills | In all 12 areas | .05 |
| Performance evaluation by supervisors | In all 14 areas | .05 |

**TABLE 19.7** Postprogram Employment in Hospice

| Students | Postprogram employment in hospice | | |
|---|---|---|---|
| | No | Yes | Total |
| Graduates | 7 | 22 | 29 |
| Dropouts | 18 | 6 | 24 |
| Nonmatriculants | 14 | 1 | 15 |
| Totals | 39 | 29 | 68 |

## Benefits to Agencies Employing the Graduates

There were 21 agencies employing the 26 graduates. Benefits were reported by 100% of the agencies and negative impact by 34%. The outcomes were as follows:

More than 70% of the agencies rated the value of the nurse's participation in the program to the agency as "considerable" to "very valuable" on a 4-point scale. Ninety-one percent would agree to participate as a clinical facility in ongoing offerings of the curriculum, and 82% would recommend the program to their employees or to colleagues.

**TABLE 19.8** Student Outcomes from Hospice Program

| Outcome | % Graduates | % Dropouts | Significance of chi-square test |
|---|---|---|---|
| Program helped fulfill goals | 97 | 38 | .001 |
| Program helped cope with stress in care of terminally ill | 83 | 62 | NS |
| Program helped express feelings about loss | 72 | 62 | NS |
| Recognition from supervisors/colleagues | 72 | 30 | .05 |
| Sought as resource | 100 | 67 | .001 |
| Applied learning | 62 | 45 | NS |
| Personal benefit resulted | 100 | 58 | .01 |

**TABLE 19.9** Hospice Program's Impact on Student's Employers

| Outcome | % Agencies |
|---|---|
| Benefits | |
| Acquiring hospice expertise on staff | 72 |
| Resource to other staff | 62 |
| In-service to other staff | 24 |
| Graduate instituted new programs | 21 |
| Graduate serves as liaison to other agencies | 10 |
| Graduate is assuming leadership in planning new hospice | 10 |
| Made agency visible to community | 10 |
| Influenced types of patients admitted by physicians (1 agency) | 3 |
| Negative impact | |
| Lowered productivity of student during program | 14 |
| Stress of program to student necessitated extra support from agency | 14 |
| Backlash of audiotaping visit on patient (1 agency) | 3 |
| Strained relationship with project because of miscommunication (1 agency) | 3 |

## Satisfaction of Students with Program

When asked if they would recommend the program to others, 90% of the graduates and 83% of the dropouts would. (This difference is not statistically significant.) However, the difference between graduates and dropouts was significant in response to the question "Would you do it again?" (chi square, $p = .10$). Ninety-three percent of the graduates would repeat the experience, but only 75% of the dropouts would.

## CONCLUSION

The evaluation model is adaptable to a variety of nursing education programs, and the tools that were developed may be useful in similar programs. Components of the evaluation developed for both the hospice and end stage renal disease courses could be used as they are for similar programs. The general methodology and the process evaluation tools could be modified for programs in any content area. Although these two studies used samples of the whole because the populations were small, the methods are equally relevant to statistical samples in larger programs.

## REFERENCES

Crowne, D., & Marlowe, D. (1964). *The approval motive.* New York: Wiley.

Jacobs, A. M., dela Cruz, F. A., & Young, D. (1986). *Model curriculum for continuing education in nephrology nursing: Final report.* Los Angeles: California State University, Los Angeles.

Jacobs, A. M., & Larsen, J. K. (1976). *Evaluation of WICHE's regional program for nursing research development.* Palo Alto, CA: American Institutes for Research.

Triandis, H. (1977). *Interpersonal behavior.* Monterey, CA: Brooks/Cole.

Young, D., & Jacobs, A. M. (1984). *Model curriculum for continuing education in hospice nursing: Final report.* Los Angeles: California State University, Los Angeles.

# 20

# The Feasibility of Structural Equation Modeling in the Evaluation of Nursing Curricula

## Jean A. Massey and Margaret E. Gredler

*This chapter discusses Structural Equation Modeling, as a statistical method of evaluating instructional events in the classroom and validating instructional objectives.*

The evaluation of nursing curricula has become a priority of increasing importance in the 1980s. The current emphasis on cost-effectiveness in many areas of the health care system has led to the reexamination of procedures and techniques in various aspects of nursing. To the extent that nursing curricula provide the theoretical and practical bases for clinical practice, the effectiveness and efficiency of curriculum and instruction must be addressed early on in the educational process.

Traditional methods of evaluation, however, tend to focus on global measures of outcome variables. Formerly, evaluation typically has focused on program outcomes. Mean achievement scores in relation to course and program performance are often used to measure success of the program (Conley, 1973; Torres & Stanton, 1982). However, findings of moderate or high correlation between end-of-course performance and clinical performance do not provide information about within-course effects. Global measures, in other words, lack the specificity to identify gaps, omissions, redundancies, or inadequate conceptual links between theory and practice.

In order to address the effectiveness and efficiency of both curriculum and instruction in nursing, evaluation must take on a new role. Specifically, methods are needed that can address the curriculum process at all levels. That is, units within courses and specific objectives and classroom events within units of instruction must be evaluated rather than simply end-of-course or end-of-program performance.

Well-designed evaluations, through the identification of within-program strengths and weaknesses, can ultimately improve the cost-effectiveness of the educational process. Redundancies can be eliminated and important prerequisite skills may be identified, thus preventing costly remediation late in the instructional sequence. The purpose of this chapter is to discuss a statistical methodology appropriate for several levels of process analysis and to test a specific application of the technique.

## EVALUATING THE CURRICULUM PROCESS

Approaches to process evaluation have been limited by the lack of statistical techniques that assess the degree of fit between the curricular implementation and the theoretical model. In one example, Charters and Jones (1973) identified four levels of implementation of teaching practices ranging from administrative approval (lowest level) to changes in student behaviors (highest level). Another approach taken by Hall and Loucks (1977) identifies five levels of use of predesigned curricula that range from "mechanical" to "renewal." With both of these methods, like many descriptive checklists, the extent of model fit is a matter of subjective analysis.

In contrast, Bell and Scott (1978) developed the Instructional Sequence Inventory to record classroom activities that matched the events of instruction described by Robert Gagné (1977). Specifically, "introducing the objective," "presenting distinctive stimulus features," "providing learning guidance," and others are essential classroom activities. These activities are implemented in a particular sequence and in somewhat different ways, depending on the type of learning objective. In that study, the observed number of classroom events were summarized under three categories and compared to expected cell frequencies, using chi-square analysis. The highly significant chi square indicated large discrepancies between actual classroom events and prescribed theory. However, such a global measure does not indicate the specific weaknesses to be corrected.

The foregoing studies examined the implementation of specified curricular and instructional events in the classroom. Another aspect of within-course evaluation is that of validating the specific instructional objectives to be taught. Two techniques used in the validation of objectives are the reproducibility coefficient implemented by Cox and Graham (1966) and White and Clark's index (1973).

A reproducibility coefficient may range from 0 to 1.00 and is computed on performance data obtained from a hierarchical set of objectives. A coefficient greater that .90 indicates that a valid hierarchy of skills, from simple to complex, exists. Cox and Graham (1966) investigated the subskills required in children's learning to add two-digit numbers. The initial coefficient was .85, which, after some task reordering, became 0.961. A low reproducibility coefficient, however, indicates merely some difficulty within the set of objectives. Visual examination of student performance data is required to identify specific weak links in the sequence.

White and Clark's index (1973) in contrast, is applied to individual connections between specific skills. Relationships between numbers of students failing pairs of hierarchically linked tasks are examined. However, the technique is difficult to implement and does not provide information about the objectives as a group.

## A DESCRIPTION OF STRUCTURAL EQUATION MODELING

A statistical methodology that may be applied to both the evaluation of instructional events in the classroom and the validation of objectives is structural equation modeling. Briefly summarized, structural equation modeling seeks to explain the effects of theoretically derived variables on one another. The method is an extension of multiple regression and is used to identify structural relationships among ordered variables. Application of the methodology yields path (or effect) coefficients that indicate the strength of particular links or paths between the ordered variables. Similar to beta weights in regression terminology, path coefficients "indicate the direct effect of one variable hypothesized as a cause of a variable taken as an effect" (Pedhazur, 1982, p. 583).

The application of structural equation modeling to the evaluation of curriculum and instruction provides an opportunity for testing process variables. However, use of the methodology requires that the set of variables must be explicitly formulated from theory, including the directions of effects among the variables. Of the three instructional process studies mentioned earlier, (Bell & Scott, 1978; Charters & Jones, 1973; Hall & Loucks, 1977), only the Bell and Scott study derived the variables from a theoretical foundation. Therefore, structural equation modeling is an appropriate methodology for examining the nature of instruction as defined in that study.

Figure 20.1 illustrates the process model for two units of instruction derived from the theoretical approach taken by Bell and Scott (1978). (The model may be extended for the entire length of the course). Specifically, the nature of instruction for each unit should "produce" student achievement at the conclusion of that unit. Further, achievement in subsequent units of the course is influenced both by the nature of instruction for that unit and by prior instruction and achievement (Gallini & Bell, 1983).

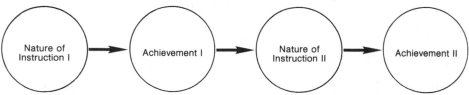

**FIGURE 20.1**   A portion of the instruction process model developed by Gallini and Bell (1983).

The importance of a theoretical foundation for the development of structural models cannot be overemphasized. Hanson (1958) describes the role of theory:

> Causes are connected with effects; but this is because our theories connect them, not because the world is held together by cosmic glue. The world may be glued together by imponderables, but that is irrelevant for understanding causal explanation. The notions behind "the cause of X" and "the effect of Y" are intelligible only against a pattern of theory. (p. 64)

The set of predictor and criterion variables derived from the theory are formulated into types of regression equations known collectively as a structural equation model are then empirically tested and the underlying model is verified or rejected.

## Exogenous and Endogenous Variables

The structural equation model hypothesizes relationships among two general types of variables. They are endogenous and exogenous variables. The endogenous variables are the integral components of the theoretical model. They are influenced by each other, and they, in turn, produce effects later in the model. For example, in attempting to explain achievement in nursing, endogenous variables may include practice setting as well as type of instruction.

In contrast, exogenous variables originate outside the model under consideration. They are important, however, because they influence the endogenous variables. Exogenous variables typically include the traits or characteristics of subjects (1) that originate prior to the proposed sequence of events and (2) are hypothesized to influence those events. In a school setting, potential exogenous variables include self-concept, attitudes toward schooling, prior learning, and others.

The variance of the exogenous variables is determined by factors outside the theoretical model; therefore, an explanation of the variability among these variables is not considered in the analysis. In contrast, the variance of endogenous variables is assumed to be influenced by the exogenous and other endogenous variables in the model (Pedhazur, 1982).

Because the variables in the proposed structural equation model are theoretical constructs, they often are abstract concepts, such as self-concept or motivation. That is, they cannot be directly observed. Thus, the testing of theory is a difficult process. In the structural model, these constructs are referred to as latent variables. They are the hypothetical constructs invented in order to understand the theory (Bentler, 1980).

In order to test the theory, these latent variables are operationalized in the form of variables that may be observed directly or indirectly. The measured variables serve as the indicators of the latent variables. For example, socioeconomic status (latent variable) may be operationalized as "level of parents' income" and "level of parents'education" (measured variables).

## Model Analysis

The data analysis makes use of eight variance-covariance matrices. Four of the matrices provide information about the proposed structural model. They are beta, gamma, phi, and psi. The beta matrix examines the effects of the latent endogenous variables on each other, whereas the gamma matrix is the coefficients of effect of the latent exogenous variables on the latent endogenous variables. Phi is the variance-covariance matrix of the latent exogenous variables, and psi is a variance-covariance matrix of the residuals (Pedhazur, 1982). The other four matrices, theta delta, theta epsilon, lambda-X, and lambda-Y, provide information about how well the measured variables represent the latent variables. Briefly summarized, they provide the goodness-of-fit indices that indicate the reliability of the observed variables.

As indicated earlier, information about the proposed structural relationships among the latent variables is obtained from path (or effect) coefficients. The path coefficients indicate the influence of exogenous on endogenous variables and the influence of endogenous variables on each other.

A commonly used software program to analyze structural equation models is LISREL. This program, developed by Joreskog and Sorbom (1982) generates goodness-of-fit indices, path coefficients, and two coefficients that indicate the reliability of the exogenous and endogenous variables. Referred to as coefficients of determination, each coefficient (one for the exogenous and one for the endogenous variables) is a measure of the strength of several relationships jointly. These coefficients range between 0 and 1.00. The larger the obtained value, the stronger the relationship between particular variables and the greater the degree of reliability of the set of measures (Joreskog & Sorbom, 1982). The coefficients of determination are particularly important in the event that the analysis indicates that the data do not fit the structural model. These provide information as to whether or not the source of the "misfit" may be poorly selected measured variables.

### Goodness-of-Fit Measures

Four goodness-of-fit indices generated by LISREL indicate the degree to which the data fit the structural model. The first goodness-of-fit measure obtained from the LISREL output is chi square. A nonsignificant chi square suggests that the data (measured variables) represent the structural model (latent variables). The greater the reported *p*-value, the more precisely the data represent the theory.

Two other important goodness-of-fit measures are the goodness-of-fit index (GFI) and the adjusted goodness-of-fit index (AGFI). The "GFI is independent of sample size and relatively robust against departures from normality. Unfortunately, however, its statistical distribution is unknown, . . so there is no standard to compare it with" (Joreskog & Sorbom, 1982, p. 141). The AGFI is adjusted for the degrees of freedom in the model and is used to compare one structural model to another. The GFI and the AGFI range from 0 to 1.00. The closer that these indices are to 1.00, the better the fit of the data to the model.

The fourth important measure of fit is the root mean residual (RMR). This measure is used to compare the residuals in different models proposed to explain the same data(Joreskog & Sorbom, 1982). A small obtained value for RMR indicates minimal error in the model. In other words, the larger the RMR, the greater is the model error.

### Individual Effects (Path Coefficients)

The individual estimates in the structural model, known as path coefficients, may be either fixed or free. Prior analysis values are assigned to those paths that represent relationships among variables about which information is available from past studies. In addition, it is occasionally necessary to fix paths to certain values in order the the model and/or individual parameters can be identified. That is, the fixed paths represent nonrandom effects as opposed to the free paths, which represent random effects (Joreskog & Sorbom, 1982).

The fixing and freeing of paths in the data analysis enables the structural model to be more clearly identified, therefore increasing the precision of the conceptualization of the theory (Pedhazur, 1982). In addition, it is "occasionally" necessary to fix paths to certain values in order that the model and/or individual parameters can be identified. LISREL provides estimates for the paths in the model that are freed. These estimates (path coefficients) are then tested for statistical significance, using $t$-tests. Small $t$-values indicate that the path is not significant. A $t$-value of 2.00 or greater is generally accepted as a cutoff for determining statistical significance (Joreskog & Sorbom, 1982; Pedhazur, 1982). Paths with small $t$-values may be deleted from the model. However, as paths are deleted, one must remember that changes in the structural model must be consistent with the conceptualization of the theory being examined (Pedhazur, 1982).

In summary, structural equation modeling provides a mechanism for testing theoretical models. Relationships among major variables are derived from theory and sequenced with the directions of effects specified. The result, a structural model of time-ordered events, is then operationalized in the form of observed variables. The model is then implemented, using the observed variables, and several items of information are obtained. Included are (1) coefficients of determination, which indicate joint relationships between exogenous and endogenous variables; (2) several GOFIs which indicate the fit between the data and the model; and (3) path coefficients, which indicate the strengths of the hypothesized relationships among the variables in the structural model. Further, *t*-values are obtained that show the statistical significance of the path coefficients. A *t*-value of 2.00 is commonly accepted as evidence of a statistically significant path.

## APPLICATION OF THE METHODOLOGY TO PROCESS EVALUATION

One potential application of structural equation modeling to process evaluation is in the analysis of classroom instruction. Specifically, the fit between instructional activities and prescribed theory is an important question to be answered.

A prior issue to be addressed, however, is that of the nature of the instructional objectives; that is, the sequences of instructional objectives to be taught should first be validated. A major purpose of the present study was to test the feasibility of structural equation modeling for the validation of classroom objectives in nursing.

The instructional theory that addresses the design of instructional objectives is Robert Gagné's (1972, 1977) conditions of learning. Briefly summarized, the theory describes several categories or varieties of learning that represent different capabilities that are learned in different ways. For example, learning the definition of "butterfly stroke" belongs to the category of learning referred to as verbal information. The student is required to process the elements in the definition and to develop retrieval cues for later recall (Bell-Gredler, 1986, p. 120).

In contrast, learning to execute the butterfly stroke is a motor skill. Practice with feedback to the learner is essential so that the internal kinesthetic cues that signal correct performance are developed.

Of particular importance to clinical nursing courses, however, is Gagné's (1977) identification of procedures. Specifically, procedures are blends of intellectual skills (such as concept learning and rule learning) and motor skills. An example of a procedure is administering an injection. Among the skills that must be learned are measuring the appropriate amount of the medication (intellectual skill) and drawing up the medication into the syringe (motor skill).

The importance of subjecting the set of hypothesized skills to statistical analysis is that rational determinations may be in error (see, for example, Cox & Graham, 1966). Skills identified through rational analysis may require reorganization and rearrangement.

A second purpose of the present study was to apply structural equation modeling to the validation of objectives that represent a sequence other than a hierarchy of intellectual skills. One disadvantage of prior validation techniques for sequences of subskills is that they are appropriate only for hierarchies, not for procedures (Bell & Massey, 1985/86).

## Methodology and Procedures

The unit of instruction selected for this study is entitled "Determining Heart Rate and Rhythm." A brief analysis indicates that this task includes a set of actions that are performed in a sequential order. Therefore, the task fits Gagnes (1977, p. 260) definition of a procedure. Unlike learning hierarchies, the subskills in a procedure are not folded into the next highest level skill. Instead , at the conclusion of the learning, each skill in the procedure is retained as an identifiable component of the final performance, and all the skills must be performed in the correct sequence.

The analysis of a procedure for the purpose of designing instruction requires first that the particular task be analyzed into the separate steps or links (Gagné, 1977). Each link, however, must be a particular capability. In the procedure of changing a tire, for example, removing the lugs is one step. In the present unit under study, procedural analysis revealed four steps. Specifically, they are (1) to discriminate type of waveform, (2) to measure the intervals using ECG calipers, (3) to classify rhythm as regular or irregular, and (4) to determine atrial and ventricular rates.

The second step in procedural analysis is to identify those steps in the procedure that may be subdivided into part-skills. Since none were found for the unit on determining heart rate and rhythm, the four steps in the procedure became the instructional objectives to be taught.

In the structural equation model the set of four objectives that are the focus of the study are the endogenous variables. According to Gagné's (1977) concept of cumulative learning, the performance of each skill in the sequence should influence the performance of the next skill. The resulting structural model is referred to as a recursive model because the effects are only in one direction (see Figure 20.2).

The next step was to identify the variables outside the hypothesized model (Exogenous variables) that influence skill performance during learning (endogenous variables). Gagné (1977) describes "readiness for learning" in the form of prior learning as an important influence on present learning. Prior learning was therefore designated as the exogenous variable in the proposed model.

Note that in the structural model (Figure 20.2) a dotted line is shown from skill 2, measuring intervals using ECG calipers, to the terminal skill, determining atrial and ventricular rates. the rationale for this path was to determine the separate effects of skill 2 on the terminal skill, in the event of a weak path from skill 3 (classifying rhythm as regular or irregular) to the terminal skill.

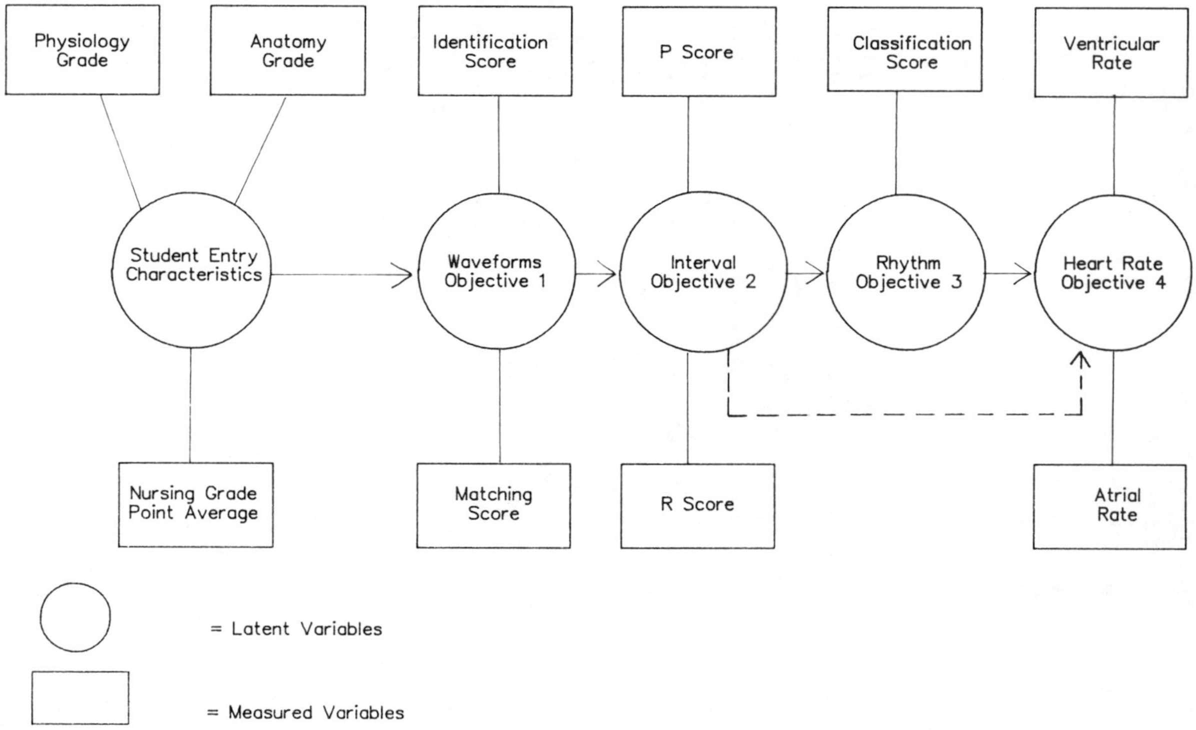

**FIGURE 20.2** Structural Model.

= Latent Variables

= Measured Variables

## Instrumentation

### Latent Variables

The latent variables of the structural model cannot be observed directly. They are conceptual in nature and represent the constructs that the proposed structural model seeks to explain. The latent variables in the model are represented as circles in Figure 20.2. The model is recursive. That is, no variable can be a cause and an effect variable simultaneously. The latent variables were as follows:

1. Student entry characteristics – skills and knowledge the student had prior to enrollment.
2. Waveforms – the identification of the graphic representations of the human heartbeat.
3. Interval – the measurement of the distance between specific waveforms on the ECG using ECG calipers.
4. Rhythm – the classification of the rhythmicity of the human heartbeat.
5. Heart rate – the determination of atrial and ventricular heart rates using the procedure that was taught in the unit of instruction. This is the terminal skill (see Figure 20.2).

### Measured (Observed) Variables

The measured variables represent the operationalization of the latent variables, and they are directly observed. All of the measured variables are continious.

The variables that represent student entry characteristics are: anatomy grade, physiology grade, and nursing grade point average.

Two test scores were obtained for each student to determine ability to identify waveforms on an ECG. The measured variables that represent waveforms are identification score (IDSCORE) and matching score (MSCORE) (see Figure 20.3).

Two scores were obtained for each student to determine ability to measure the distance between specific electrographic waveforms using ECG calipers. the two variables that represent interval are P-to-P interval (PSCORE) and R-to-R interval (RSCORE) (see Figure 20.4).

The classification of heart rhythm was dichotomous – regular or irregular. This classification was based on the P-to-P and R-to-R intervals. One variable classification score (CLASCORE) represented classification (see Figure 20.4).

Determination of heart rates allowed scores to be obtained for each student. This was the terminal skill in the procedure. This skill was represented by two variables: ventricular rate (VHR) and atrial rate (AHR) (see Figure 20.5).

Waveform Matching Test

                                                    Name _____

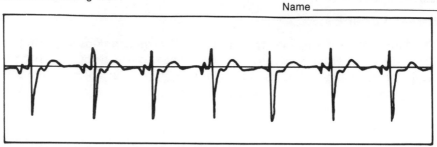

Be sure to count all contractions in this ECG.
How many atrial contractions occur in this ECG strip?
How many ventricular contractions occur in this ECG strip?                Score _____

Waveform Identification Test

                                                    Name _____

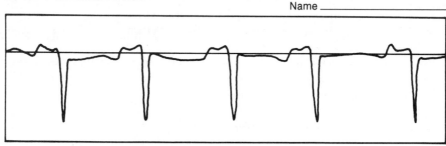

Be sure to count every waveform in the ECG strip.
How many P-waves are in this ECG strip?
How many R-waves are in this ECG strip.                                   Score _____

**FIGURE 20.3** Waveform tests.

Interval and Classification of Rhythm

                                                    Name _____

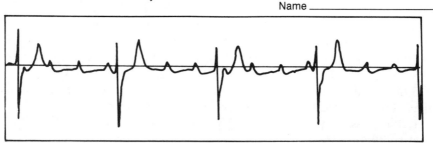

How many small blocks between P-waves in this ECG?        P-to-P score _____
How many small blocks between R-waves in this ECG?        R-to-R score _____
Is the atrial rhythm regular or irregular?                Classification
Is the ventricular rhythm regular or irregular?                score _____

**FIGURE 20.4** Interval and classification test.

Atrial and ventricular Heart Rate

Name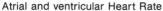

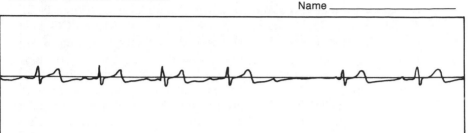

| What is the atrial heart rate? | Atrial rate score _____ |
| What is the ventricular heart rate? | Ventricular rate score _____ |

**FIGURE 20.5** Atrial and ventricular heart rate test.

## Reliability and Validity

The content validity for the items administered to the students was established by three College of Nursing faculty members who taught the course. The faculty stated that all the items were appropriate for the students. The faculty members also completed the items, and a scoring key was made based on the results. If the student's response was the same as the scoring key, then the student received 1 point for that item. The interrater reliability for CLASCORE and VHR was 1.00; the reliability for PSCORE, RSCORE, MSCORE, IDSCORE, and AHR was .667. Based on these results more than one answer for variables with reliabilities of less than 1.00 was accepted.

## Measurement of Variables

Scores for each measured variable were based on whether the student answered the item correctly or incorrectly: 0 for incorrect response and 1 for correct response. For each of the variables except anatomy grade, physiology grade, and nursing grade point average, each student was assigned a score based on the number of items that were answered correctly.

A mastery level of 80% was set for Level I of the unit of instruction (Waveforms). This was the lowest level skill in the sequence of instruction and represented a review of material presented in earlier courses in the curriculum. A mastery level of 60% was set for Level II, Level III, and the Terminal Skill. This content was new to the students.

1. *Anatomy grade* – the grade recorded on the student's transcript for Biology 232 (grade range 1.0-4.0)
2. *Physiology grade* – the grade recorded on the student's transcript for Biology 242 (grade range 1.0-4.0)
3. *Nursing grade point average* – the grade point average of all upper division nursing courses.

4. *IDScore* (WIT) – the score on a test composed of five ECG strips on which student was asked to match the waveforms (range 0-5).
5. *MScore* (WMT) – the score on a test composed of five ECG strips on which student was asked to match the waveforms (range 0-5).
6. *R-to-R score* (RSCORE) – the score obtained by the student in response to the item "How many small blocks between P waves on this ECG?" The student received 1 point for each correct response (range 0-5).
7. *P-to-P score* (PSCORE) – the score obtained by the student in response to the item "How many small blocks between P waves on this ECG?" The student received 1 point for each correct response (range 0-5).
8. *Classification score* (CLASCORE) – the score obtained by the student in response to the following items: "Is the atrial rhythm regular or irregular?" and "Is the ventricular rhythm regular or irregular?" The students answered both questions correctly to receive credit for the item (1 point for correct response and 0 for an incorrect response). These items were asked five times on five different ECG strips (range 0-5).
9. *Ventricular rate* (VHR) – the score obtained by the student in response to the question "What is the ventricular rate?" The student received 1 point for a correct response and 0 for an incorrect response (range 0-5).
10. *Atrial rate* (AHR) – the score obtained by the student in response to the question "What is the atrial rate?" The student received 1 point for a correct response and 0 for an incorrect response (range 0-5).

## Sample

The sample in this study was composed of 40 students enrolled in a senior-level baccalaureate nursing course. The course is a 5-credit-hr elective that has 2 credit-hr of lecture and 3 credit-hr of clinical practice. All of the students enrolled had earned anatomy and physiology grades that were above average, and their nursing grade point averages were also above average.

The unit of instruction was the first unit taught in the course. After content for each objective was presented, the students were given a homework assignment that allowed them to practice the psychomotor and terminal skills in the sequence. The last assessment was taken the following day at the next scheduled class period.

## Results

The structural model was analyzed using LISREL developed by Joreskog and Sorbom (1982). This analysis yields a coefficient of determination, which is an indicator of reliability for the observed variables. The coefficient of determination ranges from 0.00 to 1.00; and the closer to 1.00, the higher the reliability. The coefficient of determination was 0.981 for the observed exogenous variables and 0.919 for the observed endogenous

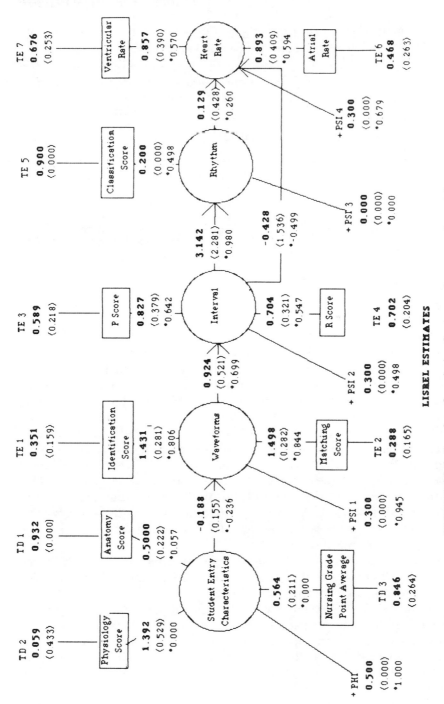

**FIGURE 20.6** Results of analysis of proposed structural model.

**LISREL ESTIMATES**

*Standardized Solution. + Fixed estimates. Chi square = 28.00; $p$ = .518; $df$ = 29. Goodness of fit index = 0.893. Adjusted goodness of fit index= 0.798. Residual = 0.085.

**TABLE 20.1** LISREL Estimates, Standardized
Solutions, and *t*-Values for Latent Variables

| Latent variables | LISREL estimate[a] | Standardized solution | *t*-value |
|---|---|---|---|
| Waveform on | | | |
| interval | 0.924 | 0.671 | 1.774 |
| Interval on rhythm | 3.142 | 0.980 | 1.377 |
| Rhythm on heart rate | 0.129 | 0.260 | 0.301 |
| Interval on heart rate | −0.428 | −0.278 | −0.499 |
| Prerequisite skills | | | |
| on waveform | −0.188 | −0.236 | −1.21 |
| Prerequisite skills[b] | 0.500 | 1.000 | 0.00 |
| Waveform[b] | 0.300 | 0.945 | 0.00 |
| Interval[b] | 0.300 | 0.498 | 0.00 |
| Rhythm[b] | 0.000 | 0.000 | 0.00 |
| Heart rate[b] | 0.300 | 0.679 | 0.00 |

[a] Effect coefficient.
[b] Fixed parameters.

variables. These relatively high coefficients indicate strong relationships between the measured variables and the latent variables.

The goodness-of-fit measures indicate the extent to which the empirical data, in this case student performance on sequenced objectives, fit the structural model, that is, the hypothesized sequenced objectives. The chi square for the model was 28.00, $df = 29$, and $p = 0.518$. This result is not significant, which suggests a good fit between the model and the data. In model testing, a nonsignificant observed chi square is desired because the congruity between the observed variables and the theoretical model reflects "real world" measurement of the constructs. (See Figure 20.6).

Other measures are the GFI and the AGFI which range from 0.00 to 1.00. The GFI and the AGFI were 0.893 and 0.798, respectively. The values indicate a moderately high goodness-of-fit between the empirical data and the structural model.

LISREL analysis generates coefficients of effect (path coefficients) among the exogenous and endogenous variables, standardized solutions, and *t*-values for each coefficient. Table 20.1 illustrates these data for the present model. The exogenous variable, student entry skills, is negatively related to Skill 1, discriminating waveforms (−0.188). A negative relationship also is found for the optional path from Skill 2, measuring intervals to the terminal skill (−0.428). Further, Skill 3, classifying rhythm, does not appear to be directly related to the terminal skill since the path coefficient equals 0.129 and $t = 0.30$. Relationships were observed for the two remaining paths, waveform on interval, and interval on rhythm. However, these paths were not statistically significant; $t = 1.774$ and $t = 1.377$, respectively.

## DISCUSSION AND CONCLUSIONS

A major purpose of the present study was to determine the feasibility of structural equation modeling for the identification of strengths and weaknesses within units of instruction in nursing. Using Gagné's (1972, 1977) theory of learning, a procedural skill, determining heart rate and rhythm, was analyzed rationally into four subobjectives to be taught.

The study indicates that the general model is a good approximation of the essential skills. The goodness-of-fit indices identify a good fit between the data and the latent variables, and the coefficients of determination indicate a high reliability for the sets of endogenous and exogenous variables.

Of major importance, however, are the path coefficients and their associated $t$-values. First, the endogenous variable student entry characteristics (operationalized as prior course grades) does not influence student performance on this unit of instruction. Second, the optional path from Skill 3 to the terminal skill is superfluous and should be deleted. Third, the extremely weak path from Skill 3 to Skill 4 ($t = 0.301$) indicates needed fine-tuning of the model. One possibility is to combine skills 3 and 4 and to teach them as one skill.

The implications for nursing practice are several. First, the methodology provides more information with regard to sequences of objectives than that of prior methods. In addition to goodness-of-fit measures, the viability of each link in the model also is evaluated. Second, global prerequisite skills may be poor indicators of the specific skills required in the clinical setting. Further research should be conducted on the relationships among global academic skills and practitioner skills. Third, fine-tuning the model should indicate the precise mesh of skills that represent the most efficient teaching sequence.

Fourth, continued research in the instructional setting may also shed light on another issue. It is the continued use of $t = 2.00$ as a standard for the retention of model paths. This standard for statistical significance was established in early uses of the methodology. At that time, typical models incorporated global variables, such as socioeconomic status, rather than specific instructional variables. Continued implementations of structural models in restricted time frames with small samples is needed to determine a realistic standard for instructional effectiveness (Bell & Massey, 1985/86). For example, a $t$-value of 1.50 may be found to be a more realistic standard for the validation of classroom instruction, given the above parameters.

In summary, the identification of redundancies and omissions in courses and programs requires an approach that is sensitive to the dynamic nature of course implementation. This study indicates the feasibility of structural equation methodology for these evaluation needs. Stated another way, the methodology contributes to the two major purposes for evaluation identified by Cronbach (1963). One is to understand the ways in which a course or program produces its effects. The other is to provide insights into learning in the educational setting.

## REFERENCES

Bell, M. E., & Massey, J. A. (1985-86). Structural equation modeling: An *Educational Technology System, 14*(4), 347-354.

Bell, M. E., & Scott, C. (1978). An analysis of instruction derived from Gagné's domains of learning. *Journal of Instructional Psychology, 5*(2), 23-26.

Bell-Gredler, M. E. (1986). *Learning and instruction: Theory into practice.* New York : Macmillan.

Bentler, P. M. (1980). Multivariate analysis with latent variables: Causal modeling. *Annual Review of Psychology, 31*, 419-456.

Charters, W. W., Jr., & Jones, J. R. (1973). On the risk of appraising non-events in program evaluation. *Educational Researcher, 2*(11), 5-7.

Conley, V. C. (1973). *Curriculum and instruction in nursing.* Boston: Little, Brown.

Cox, R. C., & Graham, G. T. (1966). The development of a sequentially scaled achievement test. *Journal of Educational Measurement, 3*, 147-150.

Cronbach, L. J. (1963) Course improvement through evaluation. *Teachers College Record, 64*, 672-683.

Gagné, R. M. (1972). Domains of learning. *Interchange, 3*(1), 1-8.

Gagné, R. M. (1977). *Conditions of learning* (3rd ed.). New York: Holt, Rinehart, & Winston.

Gallini, J. K., & Bell, M. E. (1983). Formulation of a structural model for the evaluation of curriculum. *Educational Evaluation and Policy Analysis, 5*, 319-326.

Hall, G. E., & Louchs, S. F. (1977). A developmental model for determining whether the treatment is actually implemented. *American Educational Research Journal , 14*(3), 263-266.

Hanson, N. R. (1958). *Patterns of discovery.* Cambridge: Cambridge University Press.

Joreskog, K. G. & Sorbom, D. (1982). *LISREL V-A general computer program for estimating a linear structural equation system.* Chicago: International Educational Services.

Pedhazur, E. J. (1982). *Multiple regression in behavioral research* (2nd ed.). New York: Holt, Rinehart, & Winston.

Torres, G., & Stanton, M. (1982). *Curriculum process in nursing.* Englewood Cliffs, NJ: Prentice-Hall.

White, R. T., & Clark, R. M. (1973). A test of inclusion which allows for errors of measurement. *Psychometrika, 38*, 77-86.

# 21

# A Reassessment of Instruments for Use in a Multivariate Evaluation of a Collaborative Practice Project

## Gladys Torres

*This chapter discusses five tools – Nurse Job Satisfaction Scale, Patient's Opinion of Nursing Care, Patient's Opinion of Medical Care, Physician's Perception of Quality of Nursing Care, and Nursing Modus Operandi, measures used to judge the effectiveness of a joint nurse-physician collaboration project.*

As functional nursing was being replaced by team nursing to compensate for the nurse shortage of the 1960s, the American Nurses Association was pushing for money to fund an independent study to determine how to "improve the delivery of health care to the American people, particularly through the analysis and improvement of nursing and nursing education" (NCSNNE, 1970, p. 284). To identify changes that would turn nursing into a satisfying lifetime career and stem the mass exodus of nurses from nursing, one of the most significant studies in recent times began. The findings, commonly called the Lysaught Report, contained more than a dozen recommendations for resolving key problems in nursing (NCSNNE, 1970, 1973). One recommendation was to establish national and state joint practice commissions. Two years later, a 16-member National Joint Practice Commission (NJPC), composed of equal numbers of nurses and physicians, was created with the charge to examine the roles of nurses and physicians and suggest how they might be amended to improve the delivery of care.

The NJPC held conferences, published a book of joint practice cases, and eventually put forth the Nurse-Physician Collaborative Practice Model designed to improve patient care by creating a collegial relationship among physicians and nurses (NJPC, 1977; "R.N.-M.D. Conference,"

Acknowledgment is due to Ms. S. Flics, A.D.N., who is coordinating the implementation of the Collaborative Practice Project and the data collection, thus serving as co-investigator.

1973). Five elements were named as essential to this collaborative relationship: primary nursing, an expanded role for nurses in clinical decision making, an integrated patient record, joint reviews of care, and a joint practice committee (Deveraux, 1981b). To test the model, four demonstration sites were selected: a small 86-bed hospital in Maine, a 646-bed general hospital in Oklahoma, a 260-bed community hospital with no house staff in California, and a 350-bed hospital with nursing and medical schools in New York ("Hospitals Named," 1978).

At the end of the 3-year project, a series of conferences was held to report the results. The project was declared a complete success at every site: "Communications improved; physicians began using nurses' notes; and nursing care plans became an important tool for transmitting information. Nurses said they were finding greater satisfaction with their work. Physicians saw that patient care was better and supported use of the joint practice approach in other units," reported Marilyn Notkin, an associate director of the JNPC ("Kellogg to Fund," 1981, p. 2134).

For the most part, however, the results of the joint practice projects have been reported in subjective narratives (Deveraux, 1981a). When, in preparation for a hospital-wide change, a collaborative practice model was proposed for two units – a 34-bed medical unit and a 40-bed surgical unit – the author and a colleague sought to measure the outcomes objectively. The focus of this chapter is on the results of a study that assessed a composite of instruments for their usefulness in evaluating a Collaborative Practice Project. The plan involved looking at the same variables that the JNPC had suggested were affected by the 1978-1981 project: Job satisfaction would be measured with a Nurse Job Satisfaction Scale (developed by the author) and patient satisfaction with an attitudinal rating scale (Hinshaw & Atwood, 1982). A Physician's Perception of Quality of Nursing Care (Ward & Lindeman, 1979) would provide an indirect measure of felt need for medical surpervision. The Rush-Medicus Quality of Care Measure (Ward & Lindeman, 1979) along with other such factors as length of stay would be used to measure the quality of care rendered. The clinical activities of nurses would be measured by the Nursing Modus Operandi Scale (Torres, 1981).

## ADMINISTRATION AND SCORING

With the exception of the Rush-Medicus quality-of-care measure, all instruments are questionnaires that use 5-point, forced choice, Likert-type scales, which are summed to yield interval data; the Rush-Medicus uses a dichotomous scale and yields ratio data. The Rush-Medicus and Nursing Modus Operandi tools are criterion-referenced; the others are norm-referenced.

## MORE ABOUT THE INSTRUMENTS

The Rush-Medicus Quality of Care Measure is an instrument that evaluates nursing care by measuring the nurse's performance of a set of patient care activities. Two concepts underlie the instruments construction: Following the nursing process and meeting patient needs (Ward & Lindeman, 1979).

The tool consists of a master set of 257 criteria grouped within a framework of 28 subcatergories clustered among the six major categories: (1) formulation of a nursing care plan; (2) attention to physical needs; (3) attention to psychosocial, emotional, and mental needs; (4) achievement of nursing care objectives; (5) adherence to hospital procedures; and (6) effectiveness of support from nonnursing sources.

Each of the 257 criteria is stated in objective, measurable terms that elicit a yes or no response. The instrument is administered by a trained observer. A worksheet is used to record responses to criteria selected on the basis of items appropriate to the patient's classification on an acuity rating system. It is recommended that the number of patients observed equal approximately 10% of 1 month's patient census, usually about 20 patients (Ward & Lindemann, 1979). Patients are randomly selected. Data are obtained from a total of eight sources, which are indicated in the provided worksheets and include the patient's record, observations of the patient, personnel, and environment, as well as interviews with the patient and specified personnel (Ward & Lindeman, 1979). The score is derived from the ratio of the number of actual positive responses to the maximum possible positive responses applicable to the situation. For example, "Does cleaning proceed from clean to less clean area of the baby?" would not apply on an adult surgical unit. Computer programs for evaluation of specific patient care aspects by population and level of care (categories 1 to 4), including clinical area, are available from the Rush-Medicus Corporation in Chicago.

The initial version of the Rush-Medicus measure included 900 items. The instrument was used in 19 hospitals. The resulting data were subjected to item analysis, redundancy analysis, cluster analysis, and other computations. Claims for content, construct, and predictive validity have been established by extensive statistical analysis achieving a probability level of <0.001 (Ward & Lindeman, 1979, pp. 510-512).

The Nursing Modus Operandi Scale is a questionnaire that consists of work-related behaviors based on Cerino (1981), who derived a set of behaviors from the New York State Nurses Association's statements of functions for the professional nurse (NYSNA Council on Nursing Education, 1978). On a 5-point scale from Rarely to Almost Always, nurse subjects indicate the frequency with which they perform the 15 direct and indirect care behaviors in their usual practice. The maximum score possible is 210 and reflects a consistent and high level of professional nursing practice.

Construct validity was established by Cerino (1981), who interviewed a large number of staff and supervisory nurses in a Northeast tristate area. Face validity was established by 12 experts in nursing who further validated the identified categories. A Cronbach alpha yielded a reliability coefficient of 0.92, indicating good internal consistency reliability for the scale.

The Physician's Perception of Quality of Nursing Care (Ward & Lindeman, 1979) is a 40-item scale designed to elicit the physician's perceptions of six aspects of nursing: physical care, emotional care, nurse-physician relationships, teaching and preparing for home care, administration, and the degree of satisfaction with the totality of nursing care given his/her patient.

The instrument was developed using a quasi-Delphi (Ward & Lindeman 1979) technique: A group of nurse administrators, nursing faculty, physicians, head nurses, and patients of a municipal hospital were asked to identify what factors were important to good nursing care and give examples of each. Items were drawn from these responses, and the tool was refined by pretesting with personnel on two hospital units. The final questionnaire has five response categories for 36 items and three response categories for 4 items. Scores for this self-administered instrument are computed by assigning a number from 1 to 5 for each of the five choice response options, so that 1 = Never and 5 = Always. The three response questions are assigned a value of 1 for a No, 3 for a Partially, and 5 for a Yes. The score for a given aspect of nursing is the average of the responses to the subgroup of questions used to measure that variable. A value of 3 is assigned to unanswered questions. Information on validity and reliability were not available from its authors (Ward & Lindeman, 1979; B. J. Safford, personal communication, 1984).

The Patient Satisfaction Instrument (Hinshaw & Atwood, 1982) is a 25-item scale that asks patients to rate how strongly they agree or disagree that nurses perform activities in three dimensions of nursing: (a) manual/technical activities and professional knowledge in rendering competent care; (b) relationship/personal characteristics that foster trust and allow constructive client-caregiver interaction; and (c) an ability to teach and to communicate needed information to clients. The scale uses a fifth-grade reading level and takes 10 to 15 min to complete. A high score reflects dissatisfaction with nursing care.

Originally, Risser (cited in Hinshaw & Atwood, 1982) developed the instrument in a series of five clinical and administrative studies carried out over an 8-year period. Hinshaw and Atwood adapted the tool for an inpatient population and used three construct validity techniques: convergent and discriminant strategy, discriminance, and predictive modeling. Each was reported to show acceptable levels of validity. Internal consistency reliability was reported by Hinshaw and Atwood to be as high as 0.91 and 0.90.

The Nurse Job Satisfaction Scale is a 26-item instrument that consists of decriptors, such as "decision-making power" and "variety of work," identified in the literature as important to nurses and relevant to their job satisfaction. The descriptors incorporate factors related to Maslow's (as cited in Bullough, 1974) hierarchy of needs and Herzberg's (as cited in Bullough, 1974) modification of those needs into extrinsic and intrinsic factors (Bullough, 1974; Everly & Falcione, 1976). Instruments used in this study appear at the end of the chapter.

## METHODOLOGY

Prior to data collection three staff development instructors were trained in the use of the Rush-Medicus tool. Interrater reliability was established, with each of the three instructors making independent ratings on five patients. With the exception of the Rush-Medicus instrument, all of the instruments are self-administered questionnaires. Thirty randomly selected patients responded to the satisfaction scales and agreed to data collection on care by a trained observer using the Rush-Medicus tool. Informed consent was obtained from and documented on each patient. Simultaneously, the appropriate questionnaires were distributed to the professional staff along with instruction for the completion and return of the questionnaires to the principal investigator.

Thirty nurses (21 on the surgical unit, 9 on the medical unit) completed the Job Satisfaction and Modus Operandi scales. Thirty-three physicians (8 surgical, 25 medical) completed the questionnaire Physician's Perception of Quality of Nursing Care. The instruments were evaluated for validity and reliability and procedures to increase the rate of return. Return rates for the various instruments are presented in Table 21.1.

**TABLE 21.1 Number of Returned Responses**

| Tool | Unit I<br>40-bed<br>surgical | Unit II<br>34-bed<br>medical | Total |
|---|---|---|---|
| Rush-Medicus Quality of Care | | | |
| Measure | 18 | 28 | 46 |
| Patient Satisfaction Instrument | | | |
| Nursing care | 10 | 20 | 30 |
| Medical care | 10 | 21 | 31 |
| Nurses (no. surveyed) | 26 | 20 | 46 |
| Modus Operandi | 21 | 9 | 30 |
| Job Satisfaction | 21 | 9 | 30 |
| Physicians (no. surveyed) | 200 | 153 | 353 |
| Satisfaction with nursing care | 8 | 25 | 33 |

### TABLE 21.2 Tool Validities and Reliabilities

| Tool | Reliability | Validity (CVI) |
|------|-------------|----------------|
| Rush-Medicus Quality of Care Measure (Interrater) | .89-.98 | |
| Patient Satisfaction Instrument (Cronbach's alpha) | | |
| Nursing care | .9-.93 | |
| Medical care | .93 | .8 |
| Nurses | | |
| Modus Operandi | .92 | .92 |
| Job Satisfaction | .83 | .92 |
| Physicians | | |
| Satisfaction with nursing care | .95 | .78-1.00 |

## RESULTS

The results in terms of the instruments and their validities and reliabilities were gratifying. (See Table 21.2.)

### Instrumentation

Following the initial training session with the Rush-Medicus tool, interrater reliability of three observers yielded a coefficient of 0.89 on one occasion and 0.98 on another. As the known validity of the Nursing Modus Operandi Scale was of a qualitative nature, the author sought to obtain further validation of a quantitative nature by obtaining a content validity index (CVI). Two nurses with extensive experience in nursing education, administration, and utilization review agreed on the relevancy of items and objectives to yield a CVI of 0.92.

The Physician's Perception of Quality of Nursing Care instrument had no data on validity or reliability available. The author calculated a CVI of 0.78 using two medical experts and another CVI of 1.0 using nursing experts experienced in education, administration, and utilization review. A Cronbach alpha was calculated on data gathered from 33 physicians with admitting privileges on the study units. The internal consistency reliability coefficient obtained was 0.95.

It seemed that the three dimensions of nursing activity measured in the Patient Satisfaction Instrument (technical, interpersonal, and communication skills) could also be applied to the physician, so the tool was adapted in this study to measure satisfaction with medical care.

Using two informed consumers, a CVI of 0.80 was obtained. Five items were found not to be relevant to the patient's evaluation of medical care: Three were on the trusting relationship ("Too often the doctor thinks you can't understand the medical explanation of your illness, so he/she just doesn't bother to explain"; "When I need to talk to someone, I can go to the doctor with my problems"; "The doctor should be more friendly than he/she is"). One item was on the technical/professional dimension ("The doctor is often too disorganized to appear calm") and one on the educational ("The doctor asks a lot of questions, but once he/she finds the answers, he/she doesn't seem to do anything"). The internal consistency reliability, as determined by Cronbach's alpha with data obtained from 31 patients, was 0.93.

Face validity of the Nurse Job Satisfaction tool was established by five nurse administrators and five staff nurses. The CVI, computed using two master's-prepared nurses experienced in nursing education and administration, was 0.92. The Cronbach alpha reliability coefficient, calculated using data obtained from 30 nurses, was 0.83.

## Return Rates

Initially the return rate of the nurses' questionnaires was quite good (81%). However, when a coding system was instituted to permit linkage of the battery of tests and the correlation of variables with each other over a period of time, the return rate dropped to 45%. The physicians were even less responsive, with a return rate of 4% for the first unit surveyed and 17% for the second unit surveyed.

## DISCUSSION

Trying to collect and tabulate baseline data on the battery of instruments was revealing in terms of instrument development and problems that can surface during the conduct of research in an institution and in terms of the future of collaborative practice.

## Instrumentation

All of the instruments selected for use in the evaluation of a Collaborative Practice Project proved to have good validity and reliability. Experts considering the questionnaires' individual items and the questionnaires as a whole expressed a high level of agreement on the relevancy of each to their objectives, as evidenced by CVIs ranging from 0.78 to 1.00. They also expressed agreement on the battery of tests and their relevancy to the subsequent study on collaborative practice to yield a CVI of 0.9. The instrument that elicited some questions regarding its appropriateness was the Physician's Perception of Quality of Nursing Care. Some experts felt that physicians were not qualified to evaluate nursing care. They also felt that if physicians were evaluating nursing care, then nurses should evaluate the quality of medical care. When presented with the rationale that patients often comment to their doctors on the quality of care they have received and that doctors observe nurses in action and make judgments on the effect of nursing actions on the therapeutic regiment, it was acknowledged with reluctance that the physician's perceptions could provide an indirect measure or felt need of medical supervision. Consequently, the questionnaire continues to be included in the projected study on collaborative practice.

The tool that requires further refinement is the Patient Satisfaction Instrument as adapted to assess patient satisfaction with medical care. The instrument has 11 items on the trust dimension and seven each on the technical and educational dimensions. To keep the instrument comparable with that on nursing care, five items found to be inappropriate for the physician need to be modified, three on the trust dimension and one each on the other dimensions. Based on evidence that trust and expectancy in the healer and his/her ability, credentials, and demeanor help to engender hope and mobilize energy to improve the health status of the patient (Achterberg, 1985, pp.155-156), it seems that this is an important element to keep in the tool. The climate of current practice, fostering the practice of defensive medicine where informed consent of patients and competence have implications for the cost of health care and the charge of malpractice, supports the need to modify and maintain the items in the educational and technical dimensions.

## Priorities

Implementing the collaborative practice model was a high priority in this institution. Consequently, in an effort to collect some preimplementation data, some questionnaires were distributed to subjects prior to complete development of the methodology and finalization of the whole set of instruments and procedures to be used. This prevented the collection of test-retest data on the instruments for measuring nurse job satisfaction, patient satisfaction with medical care, and physician's perceptions of care.

## Confidentiality

Duane D. Walker (cited in Seybolt & Walker, 1980) asserts that it is crucial to have an outsider administer any satisfaction study so that staff can be assured that confidentiality of their responses will be maintained, and they will feel free to express their ideas with no fear of recrimination. The experience with this study seems to validate Walker's observation.

An attempt to use a coding system that would permit linkage of the battery of tests and correlation of the variables with each other and over time failed with the nurses' questionnaires. Issues of trust, fear of repercussions, and job security emerged and required group discussion for their resolution.

On one unit this led to a good return rate (81%), but the nurses refused to permit the use of codes for fear of being identified with their responses. On the second unit the nurses were to select and administer their own coding mechanism. The result was a 45% rate of return.

## Top-Down

The return rate from the physicians initially was quite sparse, only 4%. Normally a return rate approaching 50% is expected (Polit & Hungler, 1983, p. 317), so it seems probable that resistance was operating in this population. On the second unit the medical director sent a letter reminding his staff that the project was mandated by the executive medical council. The return rate for this unit was 17%. This demonstrates how support from superiors can affect a research effort.

## Role of Resistance

At conferences across the nation on the use of collaborative practice, physicians have reported a reluctance to permit nurses to make judgments about their patients' medical care. At a conference held in New York on April 27, 1982, a physician announced that he did not want a nurse to give an "unordered" aspirin for fear she would give it to a patient who had a peptic ulcer. Similarly, physicians in our study did not want nurses teaching their patients breast self-examination. When joint planning for care was emphasized, the physicians changed their minds. Obviously, many physicians still need to be educated about the modern role of the nurse and what today's nurses can do. The poor physician response rate in this study and their verbal objections to elements of collaborative practice suggest that physician resistance is part of the reason the collaborative practice model has not gathered greater momentum. Today's medical economy, exemplified by the use of the DRG reimbursement system, is undoubtedly another factor.

## Sample Problems

A minor problem occurred during data collection from patients. Since the sample was randomly selected, some subjects turned out to be confused or otherwise unable to cooperate by completing the patient satisfaction tools. Their data will be looked at, but additional subjects who can complete the data set will be randomly selected to replace them.

## CONCLUSION

In the decade of the 1970s much attention was given to the role of the nurse, environmental constraints on professional practice, career dissatisfactions, and burnout as problems contributing to a vicious cycle of turnover and periodic shortages. The Nurse-Physician Collaborative Practice Model was designed to help remedy these problems. It was to create a more collegial relationship among physicians and nurses, elevate the status and satisfactions in nursing, and in turn improve quality of care rendered (Deveraux,1981a). The model was announced, tested with great flare, and then quietly faded from view.

A battery of questionnaires was selected that tested elements of areas that led to the problems the Nurse-Physican Collaborative Practice Model was designed to remedy. The questionnaires were found to have good validity and reliability, thus confirming their usefulness and appropriateness for a study of this nature. Since the tools assessed nursing practice from a variety of perspectives, results using these tools can be used to establish convergent validity with use of the multitrait, multimethod matrix (Waltz, Strickland, & Lenz, 1984). Further refinement of items found not to be relevant in measuring patient satisfaction with medical care would also serve to increase validity and reliability of the tools.

Other variables, including length of patient hospital stay, nurse absenteeism, and nurse crude turnover rates, also reflect quality of care and job satisfaction – that is, the process and outcome of the collaborative practice model – and will be used to supplement the data collected by the questionnaires.

## REFERENCES

Achterberg, J. (1985). *Imagery in healing: Shamanism and modern medicine*. Boston: Shambhala Publications.

Bullough, B. (1974). Is the nurse practitioner role a source of increased work satisfaction? *Nursing Research, 23*(1), 14-19.

Cerino, N. (1981). *The utilization of the baccalaureate graduate in the acute care hospital setting*. Unpublished doctoral dissertation, Columbia University, Teachers College, New York.

Deveraux, P. M. (1981a). Does joint practice work? *Journal of Nursing Administration, 11*(6), 39-43.

Deveraux, P. M. (1981b). Essential elements of nurse-physician collaboration. *Journal of Nursing Administration, 11*(5), 19-23.

Everly, G., & Falcione, R. (1976). Perceived dimensions of job satisfaction for staff nurses. *Nursing Research, 25*(5), 346-348.

Hinshaw, A. S., & Atwood, J. R. (1982). A patient satisfaction instrument: Precision by replication. *Nursing Research, 31*(3), 170-175.

Hospitals named in joint practice demonstration. (1978). *American Journal of Nursing, 78*(5), 778.

Kellogg to fund follow-up sessions on joint practice. (1981). *American Journal of Nursing, 81*(12), 2134-2135.

National Commission for the Study of Nursing and Nursing Education (NCSNNE). (1970). National Commission for the Study of Nursing and Nursing Education: Summary report and recommendations. *American Journal of Nursing, 70*(2), 279-294.

National Commission for the Study of Nursing and Nursing Education (NCSNNE). (1973). *From abstract into action*. New York: McGraw- Hill.

National Joint Practice Commission (NJPC).(1977). *Together: A casebook of joint practices in primary care*. Chicago: NJPC-EPIC.

New York State Nurses Association (NYSNA) Council on Nursing Education. (1978). *Report of the task force on behavioral outcomes of nursing education programs*. Guilderland, NY: New York State Nurses Association.

Polit, D., & Hungler, B. (1983). *Nursing research: Principles and methods* (2nd ed.). Philadelphia: J. B. Lippincott.

R.N.-M.D. Conference on Changing Roles. (1973). *American Journal of Nursing, 73*(1), 20.

Risser, N. (1975). Development of an instrument to measure patient satisfaction with nurses and nursing care in a primary care setting. *Nursing Research, 24*(1), 45-52.

Seybolt, J., & Walker, D. (1980, May 1). Attitude survey proves to be a powerful tool for reversing turnover. *Hospitals*, pp. 77-80.

Torres, G. (1981). *Exploring fear of success among registered nurses*. Unpublished doctoral dissertation, Columbia University, Teachers College, New York.

Waltz, M. A., Strickland, O. L., & Lenz, E. R. (1984). *Measurement in nursing research*. Philadelphia: F. A. Davis.

Ward, M. A., & Lindeman, C. (Eds.). (1979). *Instruments for measuring nursing practice and other health care variables* [Publication Nos. HRA 78-53 (vol.1) & HRA 78-54 (Vol. 2)]. Hyattsville, MD: U.S. Department of Health, Education and Welfare.

# Instrument A: Nurse Job Satisfaction Scale

The following 26 items indicate dimensions of satisfaction with one's job. Please indicate, on a scale of 1 to 5, which best reflects *your feelings* toward your work experience for each item. Please respond to each option presented. CIRCLE the most appropriate number.

1. Importance of work
   significant   1   2   3   4   5   insignificant
2. Responsibility
   much   1   2   3   4   5   little
3. Opportunity to use skills and abilities
   high   1   2   3   4   5   low
4. Ability to be creative
   high   1   2   3   4   5   low
5. Decision-making power
   high   1   2   3   4   5   low
6. Autonomy
   high   1   2   3   4   5   low
7. Variety of work
   varied   1   2   3   4   5   routine/monotonous
8. Interest level
   interesting   1   2   3   4   5   boring
9. Complexity
   great   1   2   3   4   5   simple
10. Work load
    heavy   1   2   3   4   5   light
11. Staffing
    good   1   2   3   4   5   inadequate
12. Working conditions
    good   1   2   3   4   5   bad
13. Tension/pressure
    high   1   2   3   4   5   low
14. On-job stress
    great   1   2   3   4   5   relaxed
15. Recognition for work done
    given   1   2   3   4   5   nonexistent
16. Opportunity for professional development
    high   1   2   3   4   5   low
17. Opportunity for advancement
    good   1   2   3   4   5   poor
18. Relationship with colleagues
    helpful   1   2   3   4   5   competitive

19. Relationship with immediate superior

      supportive    1    2    3    4    5    nonsupportive

20. Relationship with Clinical ADN

      fair treatment    1    2    3    4    5    autocratic

21. Relationship with Director of Nursing

      fair treatment    1    2    3    4    5    autocratic

22. Satisfaction with patient care given

      high    1    2    3    1    5    low

23. Enjoyment of work

      high    1    2    3    4    5    low

24. Status

      respected    1    2    3    4    5    not respected

25. Morale

      good    1    2    3    4    5    poor

26. Motivation to work

      high    1    2    3    4    5    low

Developed by author from material in Bullough (1974) and Everly and Falcione (1976).

# Instrument B: Patient's Opinion of Nursing Care

Please give your honest opinion for each statement on this list by CIRCLING one of the five answers to describe the nurse(s) caring for you:

1. I wish the nurse would tell me about the results of my tests more than he/she does.

| STRONGLY AGREE | AGREE | UNCERTAIN | DISAGREE | STRONGLY DISAGREE |
|---|---|---|---|---|
| 1 | 2 | 3 | 4 | 5 |

2. Too often the nurse thinks you can't understand the medical explanation of your illness, so he/she just doesn't bother to explain.

| STRONGLY AGREE | AGREE | UNCERTAIN | DISAGREE | STRONGLY DISAGREE |
|---|---|---|---|---|
| 1 | 2 | 3 | 4 | 5 |

3. The nurse is pleasant to be around.

| STRONGLY AGREE | AGREE | UNCERTAIN | DISAGREE | STRONGLY DISAGREE |
|---|---|---|---|---|
| 1 | 2 | 3 | 4 | 5 |

4. A person feels free to ask the nurse questions.

| STRONGLY AGREE | AGREE | UNCERTAIN | DISAGREE | STRONGLY DISAGREE |
|---|---|---|---|---|
| 1 | 2 | 3 | 4 | 5 |

5. The nurse should be more friendly than he/she is.

| STRONGLY AGREE | AGREE | UNCERTAIN | DISAGREE | STRONGLY DISAGREE |
|---|---|---|---|---|
| 1 | 2 | 3 | 4 | 5 |

6. The nurse is a person who can understand how I feel.

| STRONGLY AGREE | AGREE | UNCERTAIN | DISAGREE | STRONGLY DISAGREE |
|---|---|---|---|---|
| 1 | 2 | 3 | 4 | 5 |

7. The nurse explains things in simple language.

| STRONGLY AGREE | AGREE | UNCERTAIN | DISAGREE | STRONGLY DISAGREE |
|---|---|---|---|---|
| 1 | 2 | 3 | 4 | 5 |

8. The nurse asks a lot of questions, but once he/she finds the answers, he/she doesn't seem to do anything.

| STRONGLY AGREE | AGREE | UNCERTAIN | DISAGREE | STRONGLY DISAGREE |
|---|---|---|---|---|
| 1 | 2 | 3 | 4 | 5 |

9. When I need to talk to someone, I can go to the nurse with my problems.

| STRONGLY AGREE | AGREE | UNCERTAIN | DISAGREE | STRONGLY DISAGREE |
|---|---|---|---|---|
| 1 | 2 | 3 | 4 | 5 |

10. The nurse is too busy at the desk to spend time talking with me.

| STRONGLY AGREE | AGREE | UNCERTAIN | DISAGREE | STRONGLY DISAGREE |
|---|---|---|---|---|
| 1 | 2 | 3 | 4 | 5 |

11. The nurse should be more attentive than he/she is.

| STRONGLY AGREE | AGREE | UNCERTAIN | DISAGREE | STRONGLY DISAGREE |
|---|---|---|---|---|
| 1 | 2 | 3 | 4 | 5 |

12. The nurse makes it a point to show me how to carry out the doctor's orders.

| STRONGLY AGREE | AGREE | UNCERTAIN | DISAGREE | STRONGLY DISAGREE |
|---|---|---|---|---|
| 1 | 2 | 3 | 4 | 5 |

13. The nurse is understanding in listening to a patient's problems.

| STRONGLY AGREE | AGREE | UNCERTAIN | DISAGREE | STRONGLY DISAGREE |
|---|---|---|---|---|
| 1 | 2 | 3 | 4 | 5 |

14. The nurse gives good advice.

| STRONGLY AGREE | AGREE | UNCERTAIN | DISAGREE | STRONGLY DISAGREE |
|---|---|---|---|---|
| 1 | 2 | 3 | 4 | 5 |

15. The nurse really knows what he/she is talking about.

| STRONGLY AGREE | AGREE | UNCERTAIN | DISAGREE | STRONGLY DISAGREE |
|---|---|---|---|---|
| 1 | 2 | 3 | 4 | 5 |

16. It is always easy to understand what the nurse is talking about.

| STRONGLY AGREE | AGREE | UNCERTAIN | DISAGREE | STRONGLY DISAGREE |
|---|---|---|---|---|
| 1 | 2 | 3 | 4 | 5 |

17. The nurse is just not patient enough.

| STRONGLY AGREE | AGREE | UNCERTAIN | DISAGREE | STRONGLY DISAGREE |
|---|---|---|---|---|
| 1 | 2 | 3 | 4 | 5 |

18. The nurse is not precise in doing his/her work.

| STRONGLY AGREE | AGREE | UNCERTAIN | DISAGREE | STRONGLY DISAGREE |
|---|---|---|---|---|
| 1 | 2 | 3 | 4 | 5 |

19. The nurse gives directions at just the right speed.

| STRONGLY AGREE | AGREE | UNCERTAIN | DISAGREE | STRONGLY DISAGREE |
|---|---|---|---|---|
| 1 | 2 | 3 | 4 | 5 |

20. I'm tired of the nurse talking down to me.

| STRONGLY AGREE | AGREE | UNCERTAIN | DISAGREE | STRONGLY DISAGREE |
|---|---|---|---|---|
| 1 | 2 | 3 | 4 | 5 |

21. Just talking to the nurse makes me feel better.

| STRONGLY AGREE | AGREE | UNCERTAIN | DISAGREE | STRONGLY DISAGREE |
|:---:|:---:|:---:|:---:|:---:|
| 1 | 2 | 3 | 4 | 5 |

22. The nurse is often too disorganized to appear calm.

| STRONGLY AGREE | AGREE | UNCERTAIN | DISAGREE | STRONGLY DISAGREE |
|:---:|:---:|:---:|:---:|:---:|
| 1 | 2 | 3 | 4 | 5 |

23. The nurse is too slow to do things for me.

| STRONGLY AGREE | AGREE | UNCERTAIN | DISAGREE | STRONGLY DISAGREE |
|:---:|:---:|:---:|:---:|:---:|
| 1 | 2 | 3 | 4 | 5 |

24. The nurse always gives complete enough explanation of why tests are ordered.

| STRONGLY AGREE | AGREE | UNCERTAIN | DISAGREE | STRONGLY DISAGREE |
|:---:|:---:|:---:|:---:|:---:|
| 1 | 2 | 3 | 4 | 5 |

25. The nurse is skillful in assisting the doctor with procedures.

| STRONGLY AGREE | AGREE | UNCERTAIN | DISAGREE | STRONGLY DISAGREE |
|:---:|:---:|:---:|:---:|:---:|
| 1 | 2 | 3 | 4 | 5 |

From Risser (1975), adapted by Hinshaw and Atwood (1977).

# Instrument C: Patient's Opinion of Medical Care

Please give your honest opinion for each statement on this list by CIRCLING one of the five answers to describe the doctor(s) caring for you:

1. I wish the doctor would tell me about the results of my tests more than he/she does.

| STRONGLY AGREE | AGREE | UNCERTAIN | DISAGREE | STRONGLY DISAGREE |
|:---:|:---:|:---:|:---:|:---:|
| 1 | 2 | 3 | 4 | 5 |

2. Too often the doctor thinks you can't understand the medical explanation of your illness, so he/she just doesn't bother to explain.

| STRONGLY AGREE | AGREE | UNCERTAIN | DISAGREE | STRONGLY DISAGREE |
|:---:|:---:|:---:|:---:|:---:|
| 1 | 2 | 3 | 4 | 5 |

3. The doctor is pleasant to be around.

| STRONGLY AGREE | AGREE | UNCERTAIN | DISAGREE | STRONGLY DISAGREE |
|:---:|:---:|:---:|:---:|:---:|
| 1 | 2 | 3 | 4 | 5 |

4. A person feels free to ask the doctor questions.

| STRONGLY AGREE | AGREE | UNCERTAIN | DISAGREE | STRONGLY DISAGREE |
|:---:|:---:|:---:|:---:|:---:|
| 1 | 2 | 3 | 4 | 5 |

5. The doctor should be more friendly than he/she is.

| STRONGLY AGREE | AGREE | UNCERTAIN | DISAGREE | STRONGLY DISAGREE |
|:---:|:---:|:---:|:---:|:---:|
| 1 | 2 | 3 | 4 | 5 |

6. The doctor is a person who can understand how I feel.

| STRONGLY AGREE | AGREE | UNCERTAIN | DISAGREE | STRONGLY DISAGREE |
|:---:|:---:|:---:|:---:|:---:|
| 1 | 2 | 3 | 4 | 5 |

7. The doctor explains things in simple language.

| STRONGLY AGREE | AGREE | UNCERTAIN | DISAGREE | STRONGLY DISAGREE |
|:---:|:---:|:---:|:---:|:---:|
| 1 | 2 | 3 | 4 | 5 |

8. The doctor asks a lot of questions, but once he/she finds the answers, he/she doesn't seem to do anything.

| STRONGLY AGREE | AGREE | UNCERTAIN | DISAGREE | STRONGLY DISAGREE |
|:---:|:---:|:---:|:---:|:---:|
| 1 | 2 | 3 | 4 | 5 |

9. When I need to talk to someone, I can go to the doctor with my problems.

| STRONGLY AGREE | AGREE | UNCERTAIN | DISAGREE | STRONGLY DISAGREE |
|---|---|---|---|---|
| 1 | 2 | 3 | 4 | 5 |

10. The doctor is too busy at the desk to spend time talking with me.

| STRONGLY AGREE | AGREE | UNCERTAIN | DISAGREE | STRONGLY DISAGREE |
|---|---|---|---|---|
| 1 | 2 | 3 | 4 | 5 |

11. The doctor should be more attentive than he/she is.

| STRONGLY AGREE | AGREE | UNCERTAIN | DISAGREE | STRONGLY DISAGREE |
|---|---|---|---|---|
| 1 | 2 | 3 | 4 | 5 |

12. The doctor makes it a point to show me how to carry out the doctor's orders.

| STRONGLY AGREE | AGREE | UNCERTAIN | DISAGREE | STRONGLY DISAGREE |
|---|---|---|---|---|
| 1 | 2 | 3 | 4 | 5 |

13. The doctor is understanding in listening to a patient's problems.

| STRONGLY AGREE | AGREE | UNCERTAIN | DISAGREE | STRONGLY DISAGREE |
|---|---|---|---|---|
| 1 | 2 | 3 | 4 | 5 |

14. The doctor gives good advice.

| STRONGLY AGREE | AGREE | UNCERTAIN | DISAGREE | STRONGLY DISAGREE |
|---|---|---|---|---|
| 1 | 2 | 3 | 4 | 5 |

15. The doctor really knows what he/she is talking about.

| STRONGLY AGREE | AGREE | UNCERTAIN | DISAGREE | STRONGLY DISAGREE |
|---|---|---|---|---|
| 1 | 2 | 3 | 4 | 5 |

16. It is always easy to understand what the doctor is talking about.

| STRONGLY AGREE | AGREE | UNCERTAIN | DISAGREE | STRONGLY DISAGREE |
|---|---|---|---|---|
| 1 | 2 | 3 | 4 | 5 |

17. The doctor is just not patient enough.

| STRONGLY AGREE | AGREE | UNCERTAIN | DISAGREE | STRONGLY DISAGREE |
|---|---|---|---|---|
| 1 | 2 | 3 | 4 | 5 |

18. The doctor is not precise in doing his/her work.

| STRONGLY AGREE | AGREE | UNCERTAIN | DISAGREE | STRONGLY DISAGREE |
|---|---|---|---|---|
| 1 | 2 | 3 | 4 | 5 |

19. The doctor gives directions at just the right speed.

| STRONGLY AGREE | AGREE | UNCERTAIN | DISAGREE | STRONGLY DISAGREE |
|---|---|---|---|---|
| 1 | 2 | 3 | 4 | 5 |

20. I'm tired of the doctor talking down to me.

| STRONGLY AGREE | AGREE | UNCERTAIN | DISAGREE | STRONGLY DISAGREE |
|---|---|---|---|---|
| 1 | 2 | 3 | 4 | 5 |

21. The doctor is often too disorganized to appear calm.

| STRONGLY AGREE | AGREE | UNCERTAIN | DISAGREE | STRONGLY DISAGREE |
|:---:|:---:|:---:|:---:|:---:|
| 1 | 2 | 3 | 4 | 5 |

22. The doctor is too slow to do things for me.

| STRONGLY AGREE | AGREE | UNCERTAIN | DISAGREE | STRONGLY DISAGREE |
|:---:|:---:|:---:|:---:|:---:|
| 1 | 2 | 3 | 4 | 5 |

23. Just talking to the doctor makes me feel better.

| STRONGLY AGREE | AGREE | UNCERTAIN | DISAGREE | STRONGLY DISAGREE |
|:---:|:---:|:---:|:---:|:---:|
| 1 | 2 | 3 | 4 | 5 |

24. The doctor always gives complete enough explanations of why tests are ordered.

| STRONGLY AGREE | AGREE | UNCERTAIN | DISAGREE | STRONGLY DISAGREE |
|:---:|:---:|:---:|:---:|:---:|
| 1 | 2 | 3 | 4 | 5 |

25. The doctor is skillful in performing procedures.

| STRONGLY AGREE | AGREE | UNCERTAIN | DISAGREE | STRONGLY DISAGREE |
|:---:|:---:|:---:|:---:|:---:|
| 1 | 2 | 3 | 4 | 5 |

## DO NOT WRITE BELOW THIS LINE

Patient's Hospital Number _____

Date _____

Unit _____

Number of days in hospital this admission _____

Number of hospital admissions _____

From Risser (1975), adapted by Hinshaw and Atwood (1977) and by Torres (1984).

# Instrument D: Physician's Perception of Quality of Nursing Care

Please place an X in the space to the right below the word that best describes how you feel about each question at the left. If you have any additional remarks you would like to make, please use the space "Additional Comment," which is provided at the end of the questionnaire.

|  |  | Always | Usually | Sometimes | Seldom | Never |
|---|---|---|---|---|---|---|
| A. | 1. Did the nurses seem to have an intelligent understanding of your patient's physical status? | | | | | |
| | 2. Were the nurses alert to your patient's physical needs? | | | | | |
| | 3. Did the nurses know their patients? | | | | | |
| | 4. Were you given accurate information concerning your patient? | | | | | |
| | 5. Were nurses competent in carrying out their duties? | | | | | |
| | 6. Were call lights answered promptly? | | | | | |
| | 7. Were your orders for treatments and medications carried out on time? | | | | | |
| | 8. Were you notified promptly of significant changes in your patient's condition? | | | | | |
| | 9. Were adequate precautions taken to prevent patient injuries? | | | | | |
| | 10. Did your patient appear comfortable? | | | | | |
| B. | 11. Did your patient know his nurses? | | | | | |
| | 12. Did the nurses attend to your patient's emotional needs? | | | | | |
| | 13. Did the nurses attend to your patient's religious needs? | | | | | |
| | 14. Were the nurses interested in your patient? | | | | | |
| | 15. Were the nurses sympathetic to your patient? | | | | | |

16. Were the nurses composed?

17. Were the nurses pleasant?

18. Was your patient's room neat and orderly?

19. Did the nurses have time to care properly for your patient?

20. Was appropriate information supplied to your patient's family?

21. Was the patient's family satisfied with the nursing care?

22. Was the patient satisfied with the nursing care he was given?

C. 23. Did the nurses treat you courteously?

24. Were you kept informed of your patient's needs?

25. Was a nurse available when you needed her help?

D. 26. Was the Head Nurse well informed about your patient?

27. Was the charting satisfactory?

28. Were supplies and equipment available when you needed them?

29. Were the supplies and equipment that you used in good condition?

30. Were relationships among nurses harmonious?

31. Did the team seem to work smoothly?

32. Were the personnel in other teams and other departments congenial with the nursing team?

33. Did the staffing seem adequate?

|  | Yes | Partially | No |
|---|---|---|---|

E. 34. Was your patient taught how to care for himself?

35. Was your patient oriented to his surroundings?

36. Were your patient and his family instructed for home care?

37. Were provisions made by the nurse for continued care after discharge (arranging referrals, needed supplies and equipment?)

38. Please indicate which term best describes the nursing care given to
    your patient, _____
    in the last seven days:
    Excellent _____
    Very good _____
    Satisfactory _____
    Only fair _____
    Unsatisfactory _____

Additional Comments:

From Ward and Lindeman (1979).

# Instrument E: Nursing Modus Operandi

Indicate on a scale of 1 to 5 the number which best reflects *reality for you* – what you *actually* think about or do in each case (regardless of what you think nurses "should" do). Please respond to every option presented. Circle the appropriate number to the right of the activity using the following scale:

| 1 | 2 | 3 | 4 | 5 |
|---|---|---|---|---|
| Rarely | Occasionally | Frequently | Usually | Always or Almost Always |

A. Items about Providing Care to Patients

1. When I first meet a patient, I think in terms of formulating a nursing care plan.    1 2 3 4 5

2. In formulating a nursing care plan for the client:
   a. I think of physical, social and environmental factors affecting health status.    1 2 3 4 5
   b. I think mainly of physical factors affecting health status.    1 2 3 4 5

3. In developing a plan of care to achieve patient goals I use the following resources:
   a. health references and literature    1 2 3 4 5
   b. services of other departments, e.g., equipment, aids, supplies, etc.    1 2 3 4 5

4. In developing a care plan I try to anticipate the range of things that can happen in the treatment of the client's actual and potential health problems.    1 2 3 4 5

5. While I decide what needs to be done for the client on the basis of careful thinking, my nursing care plans:
   a are informal and brief    1 2 3 4 5
   b. include the application of current research findings    1 2 3 4 5
   c. are based on my establishing priorities    1 2 3 4 5

6. I make it a point to be present at nursing staff rounds.    1 2 3 4 5

7. I try to figure out more than one way to carry out the patient's care.    1 2 3 4 5

8. I decide what elements of the nursing care plan are most important and carry out the plan of care accordingly.    1 2 3 4 5

9. While carrying out the plan of care I make adaptations in nursing procedures or routines so they will meet the client's needs more appropriately.    1 2 3 4 5

10. I take it on myself to do whatever nursing activities    1   2   3   4   5
are necessary in unanticipated situations even
when I'm not responsible for the client.

11. When I check and recheck the client's condition, I    1   2   3   4   5
take the time to make a systematic and thorough
assessment of relevant data.

12. When teaching a patient I take time to develop an    1   2   3   4   5
explicit teaching strategy.

13. I check to see if what I did for the patient worked    1   2   3   4   5
as I planned it to.

B. Items about Cooperative Interrelationships

   1. I put effort into my interactions with clients so I
     can get:

     a.   as much honest data from them as possible    1   2   3   4   5
     b.   maximum treatment compliance from them    1   2   3   4   5

   2. I work at establishing and keeping a rapport with    1   2   3   4   5
     health team members that permits me to maintain
     a collaborative role with them.

   3. In developing a plan of care to achieve client goals
     I use the following resources:

     a.   allied health personnel (physical therapists,    1   2   3   4   5
        nutritionists, social worker, etc.)
     b.   the client, his/her family and significant others    1   2   3   4   5
     c.   nursing superiors    1   2   3   4   5

   4. While I decide what needs to be done for the client    1   2   3   4   5
     on the basis of careful thinking, my nursing care
     plans are developed in collaboration with nursing
     colleagues.

   5. I involve the client and significant others in carry-    1   2   3   4   5
     ing out his/her nursing care plan.

   6. I do health counseling with my clients that includes:

     a.   providing them with appropriate information    1   2   3   4   5
        and advice
     b.   facilitating their decision-making processes    1   2   3   4   5
     c.   supporting them in decisions made    1   2   3   4   5

   7. I go out of my way to teach clients to assist in    1   2   3   4   5
     their own care.

   8. After teaching a client I check in various ways to    1   2   3   4   5
     make sure the client has learned what he needs to
     know.

   9. I involve other nurses and health care personnel in    1   2   3   4   5
     carrying out patient care activities.

  10. I assist other nurses and health care personnel in    1   2   3   4   5
     carrying out their nursing assignments.

  11. I provide direction to health care personnel in car-    1   2   3   4   5
     rying out delegated nursing activities.

  12. I include the client in checking out if a nursing pro-    1   2   3   4   5
     cedure or treatment worked well.

  13. I participate in nursing staff conferences so as to:

    a.    gain from other nurses and health care person-   1   2   3   4   5
         nel their ideas regarding client needs and ways
         of meeting them

    b.    contribute all I know about the patients' needs   1   2   3   4   5
         and ways of meeting those needs

    c.    maintain good, up-to-date nursing care plans   1   2   3   4   5
         on all the patients in the unit

14. I provide consultations for nurses and/or other
    health care personnel:

    a.    whenever they are requested                1   2   3   4   5
    b.    when I think they are indicated even if no   1   2   3   4   5
         request is made

15. I secure or obtain consultations and referrals when
    needed by:

    a.    following through on requests made by others   1   2   3   4   5
    b.    initiating requests when necessary          1   2   3   4   5
    c.    following through on the requests I make    1   2   3   4   5

From G. Torres (1981).

# PART IV
## Research and Measurement

# 22

# Q-Methodology: New Perspectives on Estimating Reliability and Validity

### Karen E. Dennis

*This chapter describes Q-methodology, a means of collecting quantifiable data on subjective phenomena, such as attitudes, and discusses approaches to assessing its reliability and validity.*

Q-methodology reflects the strengths of quantitative and qualitative methodologies, as they are widely known, in a research tradition that ultimately is neither one. Through Q-methodology Stephenson (1953) gave the scientific community a different way of knowing, a way that is not just a technique but a unique set of premises for studying subjective phenomena. Over the 50-year life span of Q-methodology, researchers have accepted and resisted the approach as they analyzed and critiqued the empirical results. Limited understanding of the striking differences between Q and other research traditions spawns much of the criticism. Since Q-methodology departs from familiar positivistic and ethnographic forms of scientific enterprise, its own tenets must be used to implement and evaluate studies conducted within its domain. Applying the proscriptions of one methodology to the epistemology of another is inconsistent and inappropriate. The study design, data collection, data analysis, and estimations of reliability and validity in Q-methodology are uniquely its own. The purpose of this chapter is to describe Q-methodology and approaches to reliability and validity assessment.

Q-methodology is more than a technique, more than the Q-sort form of instrumentation that is used to gather data. The findings from Q-methodological inquiry extend far beyond a simple rank-ordering of items for which it has been used in nursing research. When implemented to its full potential, Q-methodology statistically derives the dimensions of subjective phenomena as they are intrinsically perceived by the subjects. In addition, it identifies the statistical differences among the dimensions as well as the characteristics of persons associated with each. To realize the full impact of its results, however, the researcher must understand the epistemology of Q and follow Q-technique from inception through interpretation.

The domain of Q-methodology is subjectivity; conceptually, the research may deal with any of a myriad of topics, provided they are self-referent in nature. Q-methodology deals not with statements of facts and establishing truth or falsehood but with statements of problems and exploring the range of meanings (Stephenson, 1984). In a study of the outcomes of nursing care, Q-methodology addresses patients' and/or nurses' subjectivity related to the topic. Q-set might include content such as "Nurses take the rough edges off of things" and "Patients look to nurses as people who care," not the numbers of patients in a nurse's case load or an observer's rating of how easily and frequently the patient gets out of bed.

Q-methodology inherently consists of self-report data, for no outside observor can adequately or accurately reflect the depths of another individual's subjectivity. Moreover, no external standard, whether criterion-referenced or norm-referenced, is used to evaluate the participant's responses. With Q-methodology, a person's subjectivity is not more than or less than someone else's nor above or below a cut score. The inner subjectivity simply "is"; it is the researcher's challenge to explore and understand it.

Q-methodology is important for nurse researchers to consider when studying subjective clinical and educational nursing outcomes such as thoughts, feelings, and desires, beliefs, attitudes, perceptions, and values. Attitudes toward parenting, beliefs about the self, feelings about relationships, perceptions of an educational program, and impressions of nursing care comprise a few very limited examples of the substantive research areas for which Q-methodology could be the method of choice.

## Q-TECHNIQUE DESCRIBED

An overview of Q-technique highlights the study design and provides a basis for exploring new perspectives on reliability and validity estimation. To understand the methodology, however, one must adopt a Q frame of reference and adapt the techniques of the more familiar quantitative and qualitative research traditions to the tenets of Q.

The theoretical framework for the study guides the development of the factorial test blueprint and the subsequent derivation of items. The format resembles the structure of a factorial analysis of variance (ANOVA), but the resultant cells contain items for the Q-set rather than scores of persons. Also like ANOVA tables, the Q-set blueprint may contain multiple levels, depending on the theory and the phenomenon of interest. Table 22.1 depicts a two-way Q-set blueprint drawn from a study evaluating an undergraduate curriculum (Stone & Green, 1975) but restructured to model a factorial format. Each cell contains more than one item, but has the same number of items as all other cells. Therefore, the Q-set is balanced, and the total number of items is a multiple of the basic design. Although most Q-sets contain 40 to 60 items, this range is not rigidly fixed. Some Q-sets number less than 40, but samples larger than than 60 items seldom are necessary. Once the statements are developed, each one is printed on a separate card for subjects' responses in the format of a Q-sort.

Just as a factorial table forms the Q-set blueprint, a factorial table is used for structuring and selecting subjects, known as the P (Person) set. Although this procedure is like the stratification of subjects in quantitative designs, persons participating in Q-studies are selected with the expectation that they will have different perspectives on the topic being studied. Unlike the Q-set, the P-set incorporates relevant person-related characteristics but not necessarily in an equal representation. An example of a P-set that might be used in an approach to curriculum evaluation is provided in Table 22.2.

The size of the P-set reflects the requirement for enough persons to identify the factors that emerge during factor analysis of the Q-sorts. Since fewer than seven factors (often two or three) usually emerge from the data, and since four or five persons give stability to a factor for purposes of identification, very small numbers of subjects are required in comparison to quantitative methodologies. Depending on the complexity of the P-set structure, significant results can be obtained with less than 50, and often 20 or 30 persons.

**TABLE 22.1  Q-Set for a Curriculum Evaluation Study**

| Areas of evaluation | Areas of Development | |
|---|---|---|
| | Professional | Personal |
| Learning objectives and experiences | | |
| Program planning and scheduling | | |
| Teaching styles and methods | | |
| Student-faculty roles and relationships | | |

**TABLE 22.2  P-Set for a Curriculum Evaluation Study**

| Main effects | Levels | |
|---|---|---|
| Role | a) Faculty | b) Student |
| Year | c) First year | d) Second year |
| | e) Third year | f) Fourth year |

## Administration and Scoring

With the derivation of items and the selection of subjects, data collection can begin. To sort the items, subjects use a frame of reference called a condition of instruction. Following through with the example of the curriculum evaluation study, subjects may sort the items according to their perspectives on the entire curriculum, the curriculum for each year, an ideal curriculum, and so forth. When doing the sort, subjects place the items along a specified continuum of significance, such as Most Important to Most Unimportant or Most Relevant to Most Irrelevant, depending on the phenomenon under investigation. Prior to sorting the cards, subjects are told the number of cards they may place in each pile; usually the distribution is flattened-normal. An example of a 9-pile continuum and scoring scale for a 40-item Q-set is depicted in Table 22.3.

An open-ended interview, conducted on completion of the Q-sort, gives subjects an opportunity to discuss the way in which they sorted the items. It also helps the investigator interpret the data once they have been analyzed and provides an approach to the estimation of validity.

## Analysis of Data

Factor analysis is the central form of data analysis in Q, with persons loading on factors rather than items loading on factors. Factors can be derived through centroid factor analysis with hand rotation (Brown, 1980; Stephenson, 1953), or on a computer through principal factoring followed by Varimax rotation. At first, all significant factor loadings are noted, but only the persons who load significantly on just one of the factors are used in further analysis. Each person's significant factor loading is used in a formula that weights the items in his/her Q-sort (Brown, 1980). Weights are aggregated across all persons, with significant loadings on a particular factor to give each item a factor score. When arranged according to their factor-scores, the items create a factor array; there is one factor array for each factor. Each factor array looks like a Q-sort and contains all of the items of the Q-set but in a different order. The order of the items in the factor array is determined by the actual sorts of the persons who loaded significantly on that factor. Factors are examined inductively and given a conceptual interpretation to identify the dimensions (descriptive categories) that elucidate the dynamics of the phenomenon under investigation.

**TABLE 22.3  Q-Sort Continuum**

| Most Unimportant | | | | | | | | Most Important |
|---|---|---|---|---|---|---|---|---|
| −4 | −3 | −2 | −1 | 0 | +1 | +2 | +3 | +4 |
| (3)[a] | (4) | (5) | (5) | (6) | (5) | (5) | (4) | (3) |

[a]Numbers in parentheses indicate the number of cards to be placed in each pile.

These demensions facilitate a general understanding of the phenomenon and may serve as guides to future interventions in the clinical or educational setting.

## RELIABILITY AND VALIDITY

Since Q-methodology incorporates the strengths of both quantitative and qualitative methodologies, approaches to reliability and validity estimation are both quantitative and qualitative in nature. With Q-methodology it is important to remember that reliability and validity reside in the data, not the measure, and that items rather than persons receive scores. Discarding notions of psychometric properties while emphasizing the *concepts* of reliability and validity are essential for maintaining a Q-perspective.

In Q-methodology, reliability is not a matter of true score versus error score variation but of repeatability. Reliability in Q is the consistency with which results are obtained for the same sample of people over time, or across another sample of people drawn from the same population (Fairweather, 1981). The conceptual and statistical procedures used for ascertaining reliability in Q parallel those employed within qualitative and quantitative research traditions, but the implementation and interpretation are different.

Validity is more than a Q-sort achieving the purposes for which it was intended (i.e., the exploration of subjectivity); it also is the accuracy with which the empirical reality of that subjectivity is understood and portrayed. Since there is no outside criterion for a person's point of view, familiar approaches to ascertaining construct or predictive validity are inappropriate and irrelevant. Therefore, approaches to validity in Q more closely approximate those used in qualitative rather than quantitative methodologies.

As with other research traditions, reliability and validity concerns in Q-methodology surface throughout the development, implementation, and analysis stages of the study. Careful attention to the empirical reality of the data obtained strengthens the contributions of Q-methodological inquiry to the body of scientific knowledge on subjectivity.

## Development

### *Validity*

Although reliability is a prerequisite to validity, validity issues are first addressed in the course of item development. Items for the Q-set may be drawn from the literature, modified from extant measures, or derived from interviews with person similar to those who will participate in the study. For example, in a study of patient satisfaction with nursing care, a few hospitalized patients may be interviewed and verbatim comments selected for inclusion in the Q-set. This approach facilitates a natural rather than contrived wording of the items and contributes to an adequate representation of the domain under investigation. The developmental interview, therefore, is one approach to content validity as well as to item derivation.

The estimation of content validity demands caution in Q-methodology because it carries a different meaning from that of the content validity of norm-referenced measures. In Q-methodology one does not seek to *prove* that the items reflect the cells of the test blueprint. Instead expert judges help to ensure that (1) items included in the Q-set constitute an adequate representation of the domain, (2) one cell is not overrepresented to the underrepresentation of another, and (3) the items are relevant to the domain studied. A content validity index can be calculated following usual procedures (Waltz, Strickland, & Lenz 1984) but interpreted without superimposing artificial constraints.

## Implementation

### Reliability

Like norm-referenced measurement, test-retest reliability in Q-methodology can be estimated during the implementation stage, providing the phenomenon is stable. Obtaining data to estimate test-retest reliability in Q resembles procedures established for norm-referenced measures, but the analysis and interpretation are different as depicted in Table 22.4.

With norm-referenced measures, scores of the group at Time 1 are correlated with their scores at Time 2. One correlation coefficient reflects stability of the measure across time for the group of subjects as a composite. In Q-methodology, however, items rather than individuals receive scores; the placement of an item along the continuum during each Q-sort determines its respective scores. Test-retest reliability is estimated for each individual, one at a time. For each person, the scores given to the items at Time 1 are correlated with those obtained at Time 2; there will be as many test-retest reliability coefficients as there are study participants. Results are reported descriptively via mean, median, mode, and range.

### Controlling Threats to Reliability and Validity

Threats to both reliability and validity are evident during the implementation phase of the study and will undermine the results obtained unless given due consideration. All studies need to be explained to participants, but with Q-sorts the explanation of the procedure is particularly critical. Many participants are familiar with questionnaires, rating scales, and various self-report measures used in other types of studies but few have encountered Q-sorts. Therefore, it is important to develop concise yet complete written instructions, and it usually is necessary to show subjects

**TABLE 22.4** Test-Retest Reliability in Norm-Referenced Measures and Q-Methodology

| Norm-referenced measures N = 10 people[a] | | | Q-Methodology N = 10 items[b] | | |
|---|---|---|---|---|---|
| Person No. | Time 1 | Time 2 | Item No. | Time 1 | Time 2 |
| 1 | 3 | 3 | 1 | 1 | |
| 2 | 5 | 4 | 2 | 5 | 4 |
| 3 | 8 | 7 | 3 | 3 | 3 |
| 4 | 2 | 3 | 4 | 2 | 1 |
| 5 | 7 | 8 | 5 | 3 | 3 |
| 6 | 6 | 5 | 6 | 2 | 3 |
| 7 | 3 | 4 | 7 | 4 | 4 |
| 8 | 2 | 2 | 8 | 3 | 2 |
| 9 | 7 | 7 | 9 | 3 | 3 |
| 10 | 8 | 6 | 10 | 4 | 5 |

[a]$r = .91$; [b]$r = .75$.

what to do. A thorough comprehension of the instructions is essential if the subjects are to represent their perspectives accurately and adequately. Both reliability and validity are imperiled if participants do not understand how to respond.

A strength of the pre-set shape of the Q-sort distribution is the inherent requirement that subjects make fine discriminations among items that they otherwise might not make. The limitation on the number of items that subjects may place in each pile meditates against response sets and concerns about social desirability and thus enhances validity of the data. On the other hand, subjects eventually may make mechanical rather than conceptual choices in order to finish the procedure. This serious threat to reliability (repeatability) and validity (accurate reflection of subjectivity) is particularly cogent for patients who may have limited energy resources and tire easily. Instructing participants about the Q-sort process, emphasizing a self-placed approach, and leaving the cards with patients for a 24-hr period enhance responses that are reflective of subjectivity rather than fatigue.

An interview conducted after the subject has sorted the items produces information contributing to the final conceptual interpretation of the factors. It also serves as an important validity check since the veracity of item placement can be ascertained. The researcher is not compelled to believe a subject's Q-sort just because he/she provided it. In Q-methodology it is assumed that subjects feel most strongly about the items sorted at the extreme ends of the distribution. Therefore, it is expected that they will be able to discuss those items clearly and emphatically during the interview. On the other hand, discussions about items sorted toward the neutral zone at the center of the continuum are likely to be somewhat nebulous because feelings about those items are not as strong. Moreover, subjects should not verbally contradict item placement if the Q-sort is a valid representation of their perspectives. That is, subjects should not say an item was "most unimportant" when they placed it in a Most Important category.

## Analysis

### Reliability

With norm-referenced measures, Cronbach's alpha commonly is used to estimate internal consistency reliability. In Q-methodology, the use of Cronbach's alpha is an inappropriate conceptual and statistical application of a norm-referenced technique to methodology and data that are not norm-referenced in nature.

Conceptually, an estimation of internal consistency reliability in Q is not relevant because there is no need to determine homogeneity among the items representing each cell in the Q-set blueprint. To be homogeneous in a norm-referenced sense of the term, each item of a particular cell would need to be placed in the same or contiguous piles on the Q-sort continuum for any degree of "consistency" to be obtained. but that consistency would reflect the investigator's conceptualization of the phenomenon, not necessarily the perspectives of the subjects responding to the items. Of interest on Q is not the design of the items as seen by the investigator but what the subjects *do* with them. The Q-set blueprint is a heuristic guide to make sure the domain under investigation is adequately modeled. Once the items have been developed, the blueprint is "bracketed" or set aside so that it does not constrain an understanding of participants' subjectivity.

Along with conceptual inappropriateness, the use of Cronbach's alpha in Q-methodology poses statistical problems that are obvious on examination of the formula:

$$\text{alpha} = (K/K\text{-}1)\ (1 - [\text{Var Item}/\text{Var Test}])$$

In this formula, K is the number of items; Var Item is the variance of the individual item variances; and Var Test is the variance of the distribution of test scores (Waltz et al., 1984). For any measure, the number of items (K) is determined by the person(s) developing it, but the other parameters are free to vary according to the responses of the study participants. In Q-methodology, however, the test variance also is predetermined on specification of the forced distribution for the continuum. As a result, the only fluctuation or variance left to the discretion of the subjects is the individual item variance. Coefficients resulting from the use of Cronbach's alpha, therefore, reflect statistical artifact rather than internal consistency.

In another approach to reliability that is unique to Q-methodology, factors having at least 4 or 5 persons with significant loadings on them are considered to be fairly stable and thus reliable. This does not mean that the more significant loadings there are, the more reliable the factor is, since more than 4 or 5 persons merely take up space on the factor (Brown, 1980) and add very little to reliability or the conceptual interpretation. On the other hand, factors with less than 4 or 5 persons on them should not be summarily discarded, for even these factors may be conceptually important. An awareness of the number of persons on each factor simply points to one more way of evaluating the reliability of the data.

Still another approach to reliability, which is unique to Q-methodology, involves the conceptual and statistical comparisons of results from replication studies. Like all replication studies, as many aspects of the original Q-study are repeated as possible. Given the dynamic nature of human behavior and circumstances, no study can ever be replicated exactly, regardless of the methods employed (LeCompte & Goetz, 1982). Nevertheless, the same Q-set and P-set, the same approaches to factor analysis of the data are implemented. Once factor arrays for the replication study are derived and interpreted independently, they can be compared conceptually to the factors that evolved from the original study. A case for replication reliability can be made if there are strong conceptual similarities among the factors in the two data sets.

A statistical comparison of the factors from the two data sets also is possible through second-order factor analysis (Adams, 1983; Brown, 1980). As previously described, each factor has an array that contains all of the items in the Q-set assembled in Q-sort in their own right, as if they had been supplied by individuals. If three factors had emerged from both the original and replication studies, for example, there would be six factor arrays submitted to an additional factor analysis with orthogonal rotation. In second-order factor analysis, the factor arrays that are entered into the analysis create and load on new supervectors. Factors that are conceptually similar in the two data sets should load together on the same second-order factor.

Table 22.5 displays the results of a second-order factor analysis from a replicated study of client control during hospitalization (Dennis, 1985) in which conceptually similar first-order factors loaded significantly together on the same supervector. Factors 2 from both data sets (M2 and R2) were characterized by patients' active involvement in making decisions about their care and treatment. These conceptually similar factors loaded significantly together on Second-Order Factor A. In a similar manner, Factor 1 in the major data set (M1) and Factor 3 in the replication data set (R3) were characterized by patients' concerns for role enactment, both their own and their providers'. These factors, which were conceptually similar to each other, loaded significantly together on Second-Order Factor B but were independent and distinct from their conceptually dissimilar counterparts on Second-Order Factor A. That Factor 2 of the replication data set (R2) loaded nearly significantly on both factors supported the conceptual interpretation of being intermediate in stance. In this study, second-order factor analysis statistically substantiated replication reliability and underscored the conceptual comparability of the factors.

## Validity

A prominent concern in the analysis and interpretation of data from ethnographic research is the representation of reality from the perspective of participants rather than from the confines of preconceived, albeit theoretical, notions. LeCompte and Goetz (1982) noted, "ethnographers must demonstrate that the categories are meaningful to the participants, reflect the way participants experience reality, and actually are supported by the data" (p. 17). The same validity goals are critical in Q-methodology.

In an effort to guard against the researcher's own ethnocentrism and perceptual biases, preliminary conceptual interpretation of the factors can be shared with others who are knowledgeable about the substantive area of inquiry and Q-methodology. Input from colleagues may point out investigator biases entering into the interpretation and may facilitate an even greater understanding of the factor structure.

Another approach to reaching validity goals involves the determination of equivalence in meaning between the researcher and the participants (LeCompte & Goetz, 1982). In this approach it is important to ascertain whether the categories (factor arrays in Q) have the same meaning for the subjects that they have for the researcher. For each factor array, returning to a few of the subjects who loaded significantly on it and requesting verification of the investigator's interpretation would be ideal. Alternatively, seeking out other persons like the participants in the study for corroboration of meaning would support interpretative validity.

## SUMMARY

According to Laudan (1977), a research tradition specifies the domain of study and the appropriate methods to be used for investigating the problems and developing the theories within that domain. Inherently, a research tradition also implicates its own ways to estimate reliability and validity. With Q, the domain is subjectivity. The methods are a unique

**TABLE 22.5 Second-Order Factor Analysis[a]**

| First-order factors | Second-order factors (supervectors) | |
|---|---|---|
| | A | B |
| M1 | .31 | .90* |
| M2 | .98* | .20 |
| R1 | .74* | .32 |
| R2 | .59* | .36** |
| R3 | .26 | .80* |

M first-order factors, major data set; R first order factors, replication data set.
[a] Tabled data are factor loadings.
\* Significant loading (>.40).
\*\* Loading approaches significance.

combination and application of quantitative and qualitative research traditions that result in a totally different way of knowing. Approaches to reliability and validity estimations may seem more elusive than the better-known, norm-referenced procedures, but they are not insurmountable barriers. Indeed, from a different perspective, reliability and validity issues pose challenges rather that obstacles to the users of Q.

## REFERENCES

Adams, R. C. (1983). An evaluation of research replication and market segmentation with Q method. *Operant Subjectivity, 6*, 126-139.

Brown, S. R. (1980). *Political subjectivity: Applications of Q- methodology in political science*. New Haven, CT: Yale University Press.

Dennis, K. E. (1985). *A multi-methodological approach to the measurement of client control*. Unpublished doctoral dissertation, University of Maryland, Baltimore.

Fairweather, J. R. (1981). Reliability and validity of Q-method results: Some empirical evidence. *Operant Subjectivity, 5*, 2 - 16.

Laudan, L. (1977). *Progress and its problems: Towards a theory of scientific growth*. Berkeley, CA: University of California Press.

LeCompte, M. D., & Goetz, J. P. (1982). Problems of reliability and validity in ethnographic research. *Review of Educational Research, 52*, 31-60.

Stephenson, W. (1953). *The study of behavior: Q-technique and its methodology*. Chicago: University of Chicago Press.

Stephenson, W. (1984). Perspectives on Q-methodology; Statements of problems. *Operant Subjectivity, 7*, 110-113.

Stone, J. C., & Green, J. L. (1975). The impact of a professional baccalaureate program. *Nursing Research, 24*, 287-292.

Waltz, C. F., Strickland, O. L., & Lenz, E. R. (1984). *Measurement in nursing research*. Philadelphia: F. A. Davis.

# 23

# The Research Appraisal Checklist: Appraising Nursing Research Reports

## Mary E. Duffy

*This chapter discusses the Research Appraisal Checklist, a measure for evaluating nursing research reports.*

Ever since the first person said, "There must be a better way to do this," people have been asking questions designed to improve whatever it is they are doing at any given moment. The purpose of research is to answer such questions in a systematic, detailed manner. Research appraisal, on the other hand, is not directed toward answering such questions per se. Its main focus is on the research process itself and the product or outcome of the research endeavor. Essentially, research appraisal is concerned with the idea of what research is, how it should be conducted, the credibility of the outcome, and the value of it.

The author's review of nursing research texts and articles published between 1979 and 1984 revealed that the appraisal of research usually consists of an evaluation of several major sections in the report. These are the title; the abstract if there is one; the background of the problem, which usually includes a review of the literature and the conceptual framework; the theoretical and/or empirical basis of the study; the methodology, or procedures to carry out the research; the results or findings; the discussion, or interpretation of the findings; the conclusions, which may include recommendations for future research endeavors; and some questions related to the form and style of the report. Although authors may differ in the terminology used to describe the various sections of the appraisal, the major categories remain the same. Authors, however, are not in agreement as to the best method for undertaking the appraisal of a research report.

## PURPOSE

The purpose of the present study was fourfold:

1. To compile a comprehensive, succinct list of relevant criteria to be used in evaluating published research reports.
2. To determine the extent to which these criteria are judged as important components of published nursing research reports.
3. To develop an appraisal checklist of those criteria deemed important in appraising research reports.
4. To conduct a pretest of the instrument to determine empirical evidence of internal consistency, interrater reliability, and construct validity using the contrasted-groups approach.


## BACKGROUND FOR THE DEVELOPMENT OF THE CHECKLIST

The author's review of the topic of research appraisal in the nursing research texts and published articles revealed irregular and uneven treatment of the topic. Several texts, however, made concerted efforts to address the topic in a systematic way. The first (Krampitz & Pavlovich, 1981), devoted three chapters to the discussion of the different types of research critiques. The editors stated in their preface that they did this because there is little written about these critical evaluation skills. The second text (Fox, 1982) contained a chapter devoted to critically evaluating written research reports, citing elements to be included in the evaluation. Seaman and Verhonick (1982) also provided a short section on how to criticize a research report and mentioned specific guidelines that the reader of a research report should consider. Downs (1984) listed specific questions to be asked in doing a research critique and applied them to selected research studies found in the remainder of the book. Polit and Hungler (1984) also provided a chapter on how to evaluate research reports, listing a comprehensive set of questions the reader should ask when appraising the various aspects of the report. Other texts treated the subject in more or less the same fashion as the books mentioned.

Published articles on the subject were few in number. Leininger (1968), in her still timely article on the nature of the research critique, differentiated it from a research review. A research critique is a careful and systematic appraisal of a research study by a critic who uses specific criteria to evaluate the work. In contrast, the research review is a general descriptive account of a study in which the reviewer identifies and summarizes the major characteristics and features of the study. Keeping these distinctions in mind, Leininger asserts, one soon discovers that there are many research reviews but only a limited number of legitimate research critiques. Leininger, however, offered only a few general guidelines for doing a critique, based on her own study of several research reports that met the criteria of an acceptable research critique. These acceptable criteria were not identified in the article.

Fleming and Hayter (1974) provided the reader with more specific guidelines but did not believe that specific step-by-step instructions for the content of a critique should be given because readers differ with regard to their levels of expertise and experience in research. Thus, their guidelines focused on what, in general, a research report should contain. Ward and Fetler (1979) went a step further than their predecessors. They developed an extensive evaluation checklist for research reports, consisting of a number of questions that the reader should ask while reading the report and/or on completion of the reading. Although it was by no means an exhaustive list of questions, they believed that the checklist addressed aspects of a study that should be considered. They concluded that the checklist will have served its purpose if the questions asked help to make readers more constructively critical of research.

Since the checklist seemed to this author to be an improvement over the lists of questions provided by writers on the topic, a brief review of the value of research appraisal checklists was next undertaken. Again, it was found that few authors addressed the topic. Millman and Gowan (1974) and Binder (1981), all non-nurse authors, stated that research checklists can be valuable because they serve as reminders of the many features of a study that should be considered in an appraisal. They also cautioned that the shortcomings of checklists should not be overlooked. Checklists do not provide the criteria with which to judge the elements specified in the checklists. Thus, critics of research must possess some knowledge about the research process on which to base their appraisal of the study. Nor are checklists sufficiently detailed to apply to all types of research reports. These points were particularly important for the present study and were considered in the development of the Research Appraisal Checklist and in the selection of the contrasted-groups validation portion of the pretest.

## INSTRUMENT DEVELOPMENT

In order to compile a comprehensive list of criteria for evaluating published research, the author and a research assistant reviewed all nursing research texts and articles that contained topics on the elements of the research process. These writings were content-analyzed, using the steps specified in Waltz, Strickland, and Lenz (1984). Major categories were first delineated, and the various elements were then categorized under these major headings. An initial total of 49 items emerged. These items were next given to three research colleagues who were asked to determine if the items selected were classified appropriately under the category and representative of the universe of items that could be considered important criteria for appraising research reports. Based on their evaluation, the elements in the categories were judged appropriate. Several items were reworded for greater clarity. Two items on reliability and validity were added to the list. Thus, the revised set of criteria consisted of 51 items, classified under 10 major research categories.

The extent to which these criteria are judged important components of published research reports was assessed by sending the 51 criteria to a stratified random sample of 300 members of the 1983-1984 ANA Council of Nurse Researchers (CNR). These individuals were asked to judge on a 5-point summated rating scale (1, Not Important, to 5, Extremely Important) the extent to which each item could be considered an important criterion for appraising research reports.

The final sample consisted of 156 completed ratings of the CNR membership. Results indicated that 50 of the 51 criteria were judged as either greatly or extremely important criteria. Means ranged from 4.01 to 4.86 on the 5-point scale. Item 4 in the Title category ("Title contains the variables, their relationship with each other, the setting and the target population") received a lower mean (2.86). Written comments indicated that this criterion was redundant of the others in the category. This item was deleted from the list. Criterion 16 ("Significance of the problem is discussed and the research is justified") was judged to be confusing because of the two behaviors required in it. This item was split to make two criteria.

A checklist was developed from the derived criteria, using the criteria as items, because the author wanted to use the resulting Research Appraisal Checklist (RAC) in future research. A quantitative scoring mechanism was developed from the nurse researchers' responses to the criteria. Since differentiation of mean scores was not possible because of the reduced variance in the mean score of the items, the method of determining Items of Consensus was used. The Items of Consensus were determined from the computed frequencies of each of the RAC criteria. Since all but one of the 51 items had been rated in the Greatly Important to Extremely Important category, these scores were examined in detail. Each of the items was classified in terms of how many of the respondents chose the items as very important. For the two items developed from Item 16, containing two behaviors, each was given the rating of the original item. Four categories were used in this classification:

Category 1 – agreement by 90% or more of the sample
Category 2 – agreement by 80% to 90% of the sample
Category 3 – agreement by 70% to 80% of the sample
Category 4 – agreement by less than 70% of the sample

There were 25 items assigned to Category 1, 17 items in Category 2, 6 items in Category 3, and 3 items in Category 4.

Each of the 51 items were then given three anchors: Fully Met (FM), Partially Met (PM), and Not Met (NM). These anchors were next combined with the four categories, resulting in 12 categories. Arbitrary weights were then assigned to each category as follows:

| | | | |
|---|---|---|---|
| Category 1 items that were | FM | = | +4 points/item |
| | PM | = | +3 points/item |
| | NM | = | −4 points/item |
| Category 2 items that were | FM | = | +3 points/item |
| | PM | = | +2 points/item |
| | NM | = | −3 points/item |
| Category 3 items that were | FM | = | +2 points/item |
| | PM | = | +1 point /item |
| | NM | = | −2 points/item |
| Category 4 items that were | FM | = | +1 point /item |
| | PM | = | 0 points/item |
| | NM | = | −1 point /item |

This type of weighting procedure took into account the degree of importance attached to each criterion by the nurse researchers as well as whether the criterion was judged to be fully, partially, or not met by the person appraising a particular research report. (See Table 23.1.)

**TABLE 23.1  Example of Original RAC Format**

| Criteria | Fully Met | Partially Met | Not Met | Comments |
|---|---|---|---|---|
| III. Problem | | | | |
| 8. The general problem of the study is introduced early in the report | +4 | +3 | −4 | |
| 9. Questions to be answered are stated precisely. | +4 | +3 | −4 | |
| 10. Problem statement is clear. | +4 | +3 | −4 | |
| 11. The hypotheses to be tested are stated precisely in a form that permits them to be tested. | +4 | +3 | −4 | |
| 12. Limitations of the study can be identified. | +2 | +1 | −2 | |
| 13. Assumptions of the study can be identified. | +1 | 0 | −1 | |
| 14. Pertinent terms are defined operationally. | +3 | +2 | −3 | |
| 15. Significance of the problem is discussed. | +2 | +1 | −2 | |
| 16. Research is justified. | +1 | 0 | −1 | |
| Category Score | | | | |

Summed scores could then be obtained for each of the RAC categories in the three conditions: Fully Met, Partially Met, and Not Met. The highest possible score that a research report could obtain using this scoring system is 167, indicating that all criteria were fully met. Scores between 117 and 167 denote that the research report was in the Superior range, with more criteria fully met than partially or not met. Scores ranging from 0 to 116 indicate that a report was in the Acceptable range, with some criteria fully met but more criteria that were partially or not met. Any score that fell in the negative range, from 0 to −167, would be considered Not Acceptable. Such a score would indicate that there were more criteria that were not met than fully or partially met.

Each statement criterion has the three anchors, Fully Met, Partially Met, and Not Met, together with the weights derived from the Items of Consensus. Space is also provided beside each criterion for a short comment pertaining to why a particular criterion may not be fully met in a research report. At the end of the RAC, there is a short section for the reviewer to list the major strengths and weaknesses of the report and to make an overall assessment of its merits based on their quantitative judgments. These constructed-response sections of the RAC were included to give reviewers an opportunity for additional statements to appraise the report more clearly. No study of the constructed-response portion of the RAC was done in the pretesting of the instrument.

An empirical trial to test the scoring mechanism was then undertaken with 11 doctoral students in an advanced nursing research course. Each student was asked to appraise one article chosen by the author from a recent issue of *Nursing Research*. Students were also asked for their written comments about using the instrument to appraise the report. All students' comments indicated that the use of the RAC was very helpful and efficient in providing the cues needed to appraise the report systematically. However, two major problems were identified.

1. There was a great deal of confusion over the Fully Met, Partially Met, and Not Met categories and their accompanying weights. Most students had some difficulty deciding what category to use. They said that the numbers in the categories did not differentiate well between the Partially Met and Fully Met categories. They also did not understand why some of the fully Met weights were less for some criteria and more for others. More than half suggested that the actual weightings be deleted from the RAC to eliminate this confusion.
2. The RAC did not allow the reviewer to judge when a criterion was not applicable for a particular study. When encountering this situation, students did not know whether to rate the criterion as Not Met or to omit the rating for that item.

To remedy these problems, the author made some changes in the RAC. First, the weights were removed from the instrument itself so that they would not provide problems for the person using the tool. The weighting system could then be applied after reviewers completed their ratings of a particular report. In place of the weighted categories, a 6-point summated rating scale was used.

## ADMINISTRATION AND SCORING

The revised tool is a rating scale that provides the reviewer of a research article or report criteria to rate on a 6-point scale. The points are distributed in the following manner: a rating of 1 or 2 indicates that the criterion was not met; a rating of 3 or 4 indicates the criterion to be partially met; and a rating of 5 or 6 indicates that the criterion was fully met. The Not Applicable (NA) category is selected if a criterion is not relevant for the study. When the NA category is used for one or more items, as will normally be the case, the reviewer will have to adjust the numerical score for the particular category or categories involved. The evaluator can adjust the Grand Total Score ranges at the end of the RAC by means of the following:

1. Counting the number of times the rating was given.
2. Multiplying the scale values of 2, 4, and 6 by that number to arrive at three numbers.
3. Subtracting the lowest of those three numbers from the highest number in the Below Average range; the second of those numbers from the highest number in the Average range; and the highest of those three numbers from the highest number in the Superior range.
4. Revising the Grand Total Score range scores to reflect this systematic decrease of the NA items. (Duffy, 1985, p. 540)

## ASSESSMENT OF RELIABILITY AND VALIDITY

With these revisions, the RAC was then used to accomplish Purpose 4 of the study: the determination of empirical evidence of internal consistency, interrater reliabilities, and construct validity of the RAC using the contrasted-groups approach. Summated scores were used rather than weighted scores to determine the mean difference scores of the two groups' ratings of the RAC. The revised form of the RAC used in the pretest can be found at the end of the chapter.

### Interrater Reliability of RAC Categories

Prior to the pretest, one nursing research article from a 1981 issue of *Nursing Research* was chosen by the author to serve as the report to be rated in the study. Interrater reliability of the 10 categories containing the 51 items of the RAC by two expert raters was first undertaken. The author and a doctoral candidate research assistant, after discussion and training in the use of the RAC on three other research reports from the same journal, independently rated the research report. As Table 23.2 shows, the Pearson correlation coefficients of the two raters ranged from .50 to 1.00 for the 10 categories. The interrater reliability coefficient for the total RAC was .94. Since these interrater reliabilities were judged to be acceptable, the author proceeded to the next step.

## Pretest

### Sample

Two groups of students judged to have varying degrees of research knowledge and experience were then selected by the author. Group I consisted of 20 (Nursing) students completing the first major course in advanced nursing research. Group II consisted of 24 master's (Nursing) students beginning their first graduate course in the fundamentals of nursing research. Since the author was the primary faculty for both groups, it was decided to test both groups as part of their formal classwork. Permission of the students was secured prior to testing.

### Hypothesis

Based on the premise that differing knowledge and experience with the research process would bring about different ratings of the same research report using the RAC by the two groups of students, the following hypothesis was tested: P.h.D. students' ratings of the research report using the RAC criteria would be closer to an expert's ratings than would beginning master's students' ratings of the same report.

**TABLE 23.2  Research Appraisal Checklist: Interrater Reliabilities (Two Expert Raters)**

| Category | No. of items | Pearson $r$ |
|---|---|---|
| Title | 3 | 1.00 |
| Abstract | 4 | 1.00 |
| Problem | 9 | .50 |
| Literature Review | 6 | .89 |
| Subjects | 6 | .98 |
| Instruments | 5 | .97 |
| Design | 4 | 1.00 |
| Data Analysis | 4 | .94 |
| Discussion | 7 | .91 |
| Form and Style | 3 | 1.00 |
| Total RAC | 51 | .94 |

**TABLE 23.3** Research Appraisal Checklist:
Internal Consistency Reliabilities (Cronbach's
Alpha; *N* = 44)

| Category | No. of items | Alpha |
|---|---|---|
| Title | 3 | .85 |
| Abstract | 4 | .87 |
| Problem | 9 | .65 |
| Literature Review | 6 | .75 |
| Subjects | 6 | .44 |
| Instruments | 5 | .67 |
| Design | 4 | .73 |
| Data Analysis | 4 | .48 |
| Discussion | 7 | .68 |
| Form and Style | 3 | .72 |
| Total RAC | 51 | .91 |

## Internal Consistency Reliability

Prior to testing this hypothesis, internal consistency estimates using
Cronbach's alpha were computed for each of the 10 RAC categories and
the total score of the RAC on all subjects in the two groups (*N* = 44). As
Table 23.3 shows, the alpha ranged from .44 to .87 for the category
scores and was .91 for the total RAC score. All item-total correlations
within the categories and for the total RAC were significant at or beyond
the .05 level. The somewhat low reliabilities, particularly for the Subjects
category (.44) and for the Data Analysis category (.48), may be a statistical
artifact. A review of the item variabilities in these categories revealed that
a majority of respondents rated the items similarly. This lack of variability
in their responses could have resulted in the alpha coefficients being spur-
iously low, especially in these categories. Since the reliabilities were
judged acceptable, testing of the hypothesis was next undertaken.

## Data Analysis

Mean difference scores were next computed by subtracting each group's
summed mean scores on each category and on the total RAC from an
expert rater's category scores and total. The expert rater was a faculty
member with an earned doctorate, experience in teaching graduate level
courses in research, and a published record of research in nursing. These
mean difference scores were then used in the testing of the hypothesis.
A one-directional t-test for independent groups was then computed
between the Ph.D. group mean difference scores and the master's group

mean difference scores, for each category score and for the total score. A .05 alpha level of significance was set. Table 23.4 shows the results of these analyses. Only one significant difference between the two groups was found on scores in the Data Analysis category. Mean difference scores of the categories and the total RAC, however, revealed differences in the predicted direction; that is, there was greater distance in the master's groups mean difference scores from the expert rater's scores than for the Ph.D. group's mean difference scores. This trend was found in 7 of the 10 RAC categories and for the total RAC. The following three categories had approximately equal mean difference scores between the two groups: Title, Problem, and Form and Style.

**TABLE 23.4** Uni-Directional *t*-tests for Two Independent Groups

| Category | Mean | *t*-value | *df* | 1-Tailed Probability |
|---|---|---|---|---|
| Title | 1.5(I)[a] 1.3(II)[b] | .43 | 42 | .34 |
| Abstract | −1.6(I) −2.5(II) | .70 | 42 | .24 |
| Problem | −3.4(I) −3.2(II) | .15 | 42 | .44 |
| LIterature Review | −3.4(I) −3.8(II) | .35 | 42 | .36 |
| Subjects | −4.5(I) −5.6(II) | .91 | 42 | .18 |
| Tools | −9.4(I) −10.4(II) | .97 | 42 | .17 |
| Design | −0.4(I) −2.5(II) | 1.46 | 42 | .08 |
| Data Analysis | −1.8(I) −3.3(II) | 1.64 | 42 | .05 |
| Discussion | −7.7(I) −8.6(II) | .62 | 42 | .27 |
| Form and Style | 1.9(I) 1.3(II) | 1.11 | 42 | .14 |
| Total RAC | −28.8(I) −37.3(II) | 1.26 | 42 | .11 |

*a* Group I, Ph.D. students (*N* = 20).
*b* Group II, M.S. Students (*N* = 24).

## CONCLUSION AND RECOMMENDATIONS

Based on the pretest findings, there is beginning empirical evidence that the RAC is reliable in terms of interrater and internal consistency reliabilities. Content validity has been established. The revisions made during testing of the instrument have resulted in an efficient, comprehensive list of criteria that have been judged systematically by a sample of the nursing profession's researchers as very important criteria to consider in the appraisal of research reports.

The constructed-response portion of the RAC has not been tested. Before using this portion, computation of interrater reliabilities of elements developed through content analysis or subjects' responses into categories is recommended. Since summated scores and not the weighted scores based on the quantitative scoring system discussed in this report were used in the pretest, the weighted scoring system needs to be tested to ascertain if it can satisfactorily differentiate between superior, acceptable and less than acceptable research reports.

Provided raters are trained in the use of the RAC, interrater reliabilities are within acceptable limits. For future use, a glossary of terms related to the criteria needs to be developed in order to assure that interrater reliabilities will continue to be high when used by persons other than the author and her research assistant. Internal consistency reliability estimates of the categories, although acceptable for this study, need to be done on each group that uses the RAC. The reliability coefficient of .94 for the entire tool reflects a high level of consistency within the total RAC.

The contrasted-groups technique was judged appropriate for establishing some empirical evidence of construct validity for this type of instrument. Only one significant difference was found between the two groups on the Data Analysis category. The trend of the mean difference scores being smaller in the Ph.D. group than in the master's group might be a hopeful indication that with larger numbers in the groups, significant differences would emerge in all RAC categories and on the total RAC.

Three possible explanations for the nonsignificant findings that warrant consideration by potential users of the RAC are the following: (1) the groups were not sufficiently differentiated on the variable of interest – previous research knowledge; (2) the study selected for appraisal by subjects in the groups may have been too well reported to permit differences based on previous knowledge about the research process between the groups' ratings on the various criteria to emerge; and (3) a response set bias may have been introduced because the study was carried out as part of a formal course in the students' programs. Further empirical testing of the RAC for construct validity needs to be undertaken before using it as a research instrument. It can, however, be used as an efficient, quantifiable approach to appraise research reports.

## IMPLICATIONS FOR NURSING

Despite the inconclusiveness of the findings of the validity portion of the study, the RAC holds promise for being a reliable, valid measurement tool to assess written research reports. As a data collection instrument, it offers the potential for allowing researchers to critically appraise the state of the art of nursing research. Thus, Leininger's (1968) statement about the larger number of research reviews being done, in contrast to legitimate research critiques, would be corrected.

The RAC should also prove useful to faculty teaching undergraduate and graduate research courses. It provides a comprehensive set of criteria in an easy-to-use format that allows students to appraise the merits of quantitative reports. Such use would also decrease the time faculty spend in scoring such assignments. The quantifiable ratings for each criterion, the subjective overall assessment, and the comments section provide an effective combination that would satisfy both teacher and student. It should be remembered, however, that the RAC is only as good as its user. All of the ratings of the criteria presume previous knowledge about the research process. Thus, the ratings will vary according to the research expertise of the rater.

The nursing profession is continuing to move toward becoming a research-based practice. To maximally incorporate the findings of research into nursing practice, education, and administration nurses at all levels must be able to appraise nursing research in an efficient and accurate fashion. Continued use and refinement of the RAC is an important step in this direction.

## REFERENCES

Binder, D. M. (1981). Critique: Experimental study. In S. D. Krampitz & N. Pavlovich (Eds.), *Readings for nursing research* (pp. 152-160). St. Louis: C. V. Mosby.

Downs, F. S. (1984). *A source book for nursing research* (3rd ed.). Philadelphia: F. A. Davis.

Duffy, M. E. (1985). A research appraisal checklist for evaluating nursing research reports. *Nursing and Health Care, 6,* 538-547.

Fleming, J., & Hayter, J. (1974). Reading research reports critically. *Nursing Outlook, 22,* 172-175.

Fox, D. J. (1982). *Fundamentals of research in nursing* (4th ed.). New York: Appleton-Century-Crofts.

Krampitz, S. D., & Pavlovich, N. (Eds.). (1981). *Readings for nursing research.* St. Louis: C. V. Mosby.

Leininger, M. (1968). The research critique: Nature, function and art. *Nursing Research, 17,* 444-449.

Millman, J., & Gowin, D. (1974). *Appraising educational research: A case study approach.* Englewood Cliffs, NJ: Prentice-Hall.

Polit, D., & Hungler, B. (1984). *Nursing research: Principles and methods* (2nd ed.). Philadelphia: J. B. Lippincott.

Seaman, C. H., & Verhonick, P. J. (1982). *Research methods for undergraduate students in nursing (2nd ed.).* New York: Appleton- Century-Crofts.

Waltz, C., Strickland, O., & Lenz, E. (1984). *Measurement in nursing research.* Philadelphia: F. A. Davis.

Ward, M., & Fetler, M. (1979). What guidelines should be followed in critically evaluating research reports? *Nursing Research, 28,* 120-125.

# Research Appraisal Checklist

Instructions: The Research Appraisal Checklist (RAC) contains 51 criteria which have been ordered under eight major research categories. The RAC is designed to assist you to carefully and systematically assess the worth of a written research report.

   In appraising a research report, you are asked to give only one rating to each criterion. Circle the number you think best describes the degree to which each criterion is met in the research report. The numbers in the rating scale range from "1," meaning "Not Met," to "6," meaning "Completely Met." If you rate a category less than a 5 or a 6, indicating that you believe it to be Partially or Not Met, write a very brief note summarizing your thoughts about that portion of the report. At the end of each category, sum the numbers circled beside the appropriate criteria and place these numbers in the boxes provided at the end of the category.

   After completing the ratings of the 51 criteria, sum the category scores and enter them in the appropriate Total Score box. Then, sum scores for all categories and enter the score in the Grand Total box. Finally, write a brief summary citing the major strengths and limitations of the report.

| CRITERIA | APPRAISAL RATING | COMMENTS |
|---|---|---|

## I. TITLE

1. Title is readily understood.    1 2 3 4 5 6 NA
2. Title is clear.    1 2 3 4 5 6 NA
3. Title is clearly related to content.   1 2 3 4 5 6 NA

> CATEGORY SCORE

## II. ABSTRACT

4. Abstract states problem and, where appropriate, hypotheses clearly and concisely.    1 2 3 4 5 6 NA
5. Methodology is identified and described briefly.    1 2 3 4 5 6 NA
6. Results are summarized.    1 2 3 4 5 6 NA

7. Findings and/or conclusions are
   stated.                                    1  2  3  4  5  6  NA

CATEGORY SCORE

## III. PROBLEM

8. The general problem of the study
   is introduced early in the report.    1  2  3  4  5  6  NA
9. Questions to be answered are
   stated precisely.                         1  2  3  4  5  6  NA
10. Problem statement is clear.          1  2  3  4  5  6  NA
11. Hypotheses to be tested are
    stated precisely in a form that
    permits them to be tested.            1  2  3  4  5  6  NA
12. Limitations of the study can be
    identified.                               1  2  3  4  5  6  NA
13. Assumptions of the study can be
    identified.                               1  2  3  4  5  6  NA
14. Pertinent terms are/can be opera-
    tionally defined.                        1  2  3  4  5  6  NA
15. Significance of the problem is
    discussed.                               1  2  3  4  5  6  NA
16. Research is justified.                 1  2  3  4  5  6  NA

CATEGORY SCORE

## IV. REVIEW OF LITERATURE

17. Cited literature is pertinent to
    research problem.                       1  2  3  4  5  6  NA
18. Cited literature provides rationale
    for the research.                        1  2  3  4  5  6  NA
19. Studies are critically examined.    1  2  3  4  5  6  NA
20. Relationship of problem to previ-
    ous research is made clear.          1  2  3  4  5  6  NA
21. A conceptual framework/
    theoretical rationale is clearly
    stated.                                   1  2  3  4  5  6  NA
22. Review concludes with a brief
    summary of relevant literature
    and its implications to the
    research problem under study.      1  2  3  4  5  6  NA

CATEGORY SCORE

# V. METHODOLOGY
## A. Subjects

23. Subject population (sampling
    frame) is described.           1 2 3 4 5 6 NA
24. Sampling method is described.   1 2 3 4 5 6 NA
25. Sampling method is justified
    (especially for
    nonprobability sampling).      1 2 3 4 5 6 NA
26. Sample size is sufficient to reduce
    Type II error.                 1 2 3 4 5 6 NA
27. Possible sources of sampling error
    can be identified.             1 2 3 4 5 6 NA
28. Standards for protection of sub-
    jects are discussed.           1 2 3 4 5 6 NA

| CATEGORY SCORE |
|---|

## B. Instruments

29. Relevant previous reliability data
    are presented.                 1 2 3 4 5 6 NA
30. Reliability data pertinent to the
    present study are reported.    1 2 3 4 5 6 NA
31. Relevant previous validity data
    are presented.                 1 2 3 4 5 6 NA
32. Validity data pertinent to present
    study are reported.            1 2 3 4 5 6 NA
33. Methods of data collection are
    sufficiently described to permit
    judgment of their appropriateness
    to the present study.          1 2 3 4 5 6 NA

| CATEGORY SCORE |
|---|

## C. Design

34. Design is appropriate to study
    questions and/or hypotheses.   1 2 3 4 5 6 NA
35. Proper controls are included
    where appropriate.             1 2 3 4 5 6 NA
36. Confounding/moderating variables
    are/can be identified.         1 2 3 4 5 6 NA
37. Description of design is explicit
    enough to permit replication.  1 2 3 4 5 6 NA

| CATEGORY SCORE |
|---|

# VI. DATA ANALYSIS

38. Information presented is sufficient
    to answer research questions.      1  2  3  4  5  6  NA
39. Statistical tests used are identified
    and obtained values are reported. 1  2  3  4  5  6  NA
40. Reported statistics are appropri-
    ate for hypotheses/ research
    questions.                         1  2  3  4  5  6  NA
41. Tables and figures are presented
    in an easy-to-understand, informa-
    tive way.                          1  2  3  4  5  6  NA

| CATEGORY SCORE |
|---|

# VII. DISCUSSION

42. Conclusions are clearly stated.    1  2  3  4  5  6  NA
43. Conclusions are substantiated by
    the evidence presented.            1  2  3  4  5  6  NA
44. Methodological issues in study are
    identified and discussed.          1  2  3  4  5  6  NA
45. Findings of study are specifically
    related to conceptual/theoretical
    basis of the study.                1  2  3  4  5  6  NA
46. Implications of the findings are
    discussed.                         1  2  3  4  5  6  NA
47. Results are generalized only to
    population on which study is
    based.                             1  2  3  4  5  6  NA
48. Recommendations are made for
    further research.                  1  2  3  4  5  6  NA

| CATEGORY SCORE |
|---|

# VIII. FORM & STYLE

49. Report is clearly written.         1  2  3  4  5  6  NA
50. Report is logically organized.     1  2  3  4  5  6  NA
51. Tone of report displays an unbi-
    ased, impartial, scientific attitude. 1  2  3  4  5  6  NA

| CATEGORY SCORE |
|---|

GRAND TOTAL: _____

# FINAL SUMMARY OF MAJOR STRENGTHS AND LIMITATIONS

STRENGTHS:                              LIMITATIONS.

Enter Grand Total Score in the Appropriate Category:

_____ Superior          (205-306 Points)
_____ Average           (103-204 Points)
_____ Below Average     (0-102 Points)

# 24

# Measuring Knowledge of Research Consumerism

## Cheryl B. Stetler and E. Ann Sheridan

*This chapter discusses the knowledge of Research Consumerism Instrument, a measure testing for the basic level of understanding of the research process necessary to be a "consumer" of nursing research.*

The purpose of this study was to create a reliable and valid criterion-referenced tool to measure the variable "knowledge of research consumerism." Impetus for its development came from interest in research utilization (Stetler, 1985) and related refinement of the Stetler/Marram model for applicability of research findings to practice (Stetler, 1984; Stetler & Marram, 1976; Van Servellan & Stetler, 1986). In this model, there are three critical components:

Validation (Phase I) – the potential consumer applies knowledge of research principles and methods to perform a traditional research critique on the studies involved.

Comparative Evaluation (Phase II) – the consumer applies special criteria to evaluate the desirability and feasibility of applying study findings to a nursing practice situation.

Decision Making (Phase III) – a judgment is made by the consumer regarding use or nonuse of the reviewed research.

Inherent within this model are the assumptions that a nurse must possess basic knowledge of the research process in order to complete Phase I, a prerequisite to the ultimate use of findings in practice; and that Phases II and III require a level of knowledge specific to the utilization process (Haller, Reynolds, & Horsley, 1979; Stetler, 1984). The continuum in Figure 24.1 depicts this conceptualization in terms of the multicomponent variable "knowledge of research." Consumerism is thus seen as requiring a lower level of knowledge than Production; and within the Consumerism end of the continuum, the ability understand and appraise (i.e., Phase I or performance of a traditional critique) is seen as requiring a lower level of knowledge than the direct evaluation of applicability of findings to practice (i.e., phases II and III. For this project, only the lowest level, or Phase I, of Consumerism was of concern. A criterion-referenced approach was chosen for tool development because interest was not in comparing nurses with one another but rather in measuring what a nurse does or does not know about the research process.

The initial review of nursing literature did not provide a tool to measure the variable of interest. Recently, however, a related test has been published by Thomas and Price (1984) that may be of interest to those needing to measure knowledge of research. In the nonnursing literature, a number of studies were found that measured research knowledge. However, either the target audience was graduate students, where a higher level of knowledge, including advanced statistics, was the focus; or the tool had a norm-referenced focus; or there did not appear to be evidence of the tool's reliability or validity (Hastings, 1972; Rosenblatt & Kirk, 1981; Scott, 1971). The steps described in the following sections were therefore undertaken to develop a criterion-referenced tool to measure Phase I, Consumerism.

## METHOD

### Purpose and Domain

The defined purpose of this research tool is to measure cognitive understanding of the research process relative to predetermined standard. More specificially, it was developed to measure the most basic level of knowledge of research that enables a nurse to read, understand, and assess the scientific soundness of published research. A competent consumer at this level would be able to recognize research terminology, interpret the meaning of research concepts and methods within a study, and critically appraise a study's major strengths, to weaknesses, and findings. The global objective for this criterion-referenced tool was defined as follows: Given a series of multiple choice questions regarding selected

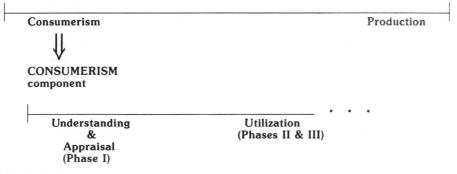

FIGURE 24.1 Knowledge of research.

dimensions of the research domain, and given abbreviated reports of hypothetical research with a series of related multiple choice questions regarding selected dimensions of the research domain, the nurse will answer a predetermined percentage of items correctly. The first component of this objective would provide for measurement of the cognitive functions of knowledge and interpretation; the second component would cover measurement of the higher-order cognitive functions of problem solving/evaluation (Professional Examination Service, 1981).

In defining the variable's domain, it became obvious through a review of the literature that no standardized content regarding basic knowledge of nursing research was available. For example, in surveys about research coursework in undergraduate programming, agreement was not found as to either (1) the role of graduates of various educational levels relative to research or (2) content required in related courses (Bogal-Allbritten, Marcum, & Raspberry, 1982; Shelton, 1979; Thomas & Price, 1980). Within the framework of Phase I Consumerism, a decision was therefore made to define the domain of content through use of a current textbook on nursing research. After a review of many such references, Polit & Hungler's *Nursing Research: Principles and Methods* (1983b) was selected.

Based on the organization of this textbook, seven subdomains were identified (see Figure 24.2). This covered material on all chapters except those dealing with advanced statistics, computerization, and preparation of a research proposal. The latter were considered relevant to the Production component of the knowledge continuum and therefore not appropriate for the domain of interest. For each subdomain, a description, general objective, and series of knowledge statements were then developed (see Table 24.1).

## Item Generation

Within the *Instructor's Manual* by Polit and Hungler (1983a), a series of multiple choice questions had been developed for each chapter. These 207 items, each focusing on an isolated concept or limited content within a subdomain, became the original pool for Part I of the tool. This part primarily addressed that component of the objective regarding knowledge and interpretation. For Part II, the investigators created three hypothetical research abstracts and multiple choice items for each abstract. These 30 items crossed all seven subdomains and were designed primarily to measure that component of the objective regarding problem solving/ evaluation.

## RELIABILITY AND VALIDITY

To begin testing this tool, a two-step process was undertaken: (1) subjective validation by a panel of nurse experts and (2) objective validation through test administration.

## Subjective Validation

Six nurse faculty who met the criterion of currently teaching research in a baccalaureate program were employed by the investigators as content experts. All had at least a master's degree in nursing. Two held doctorates, two were doctoral candidates, and one was enrolled in a doctoral program. All were located at schools in the New England region.

The first task of the judges was to assess content validity for the original pool of items. To accomplish this, judges were given standard instructions and provided with subdomain specifications. Each judge then independently rated each of the 237 items for its relevancy and congruency:

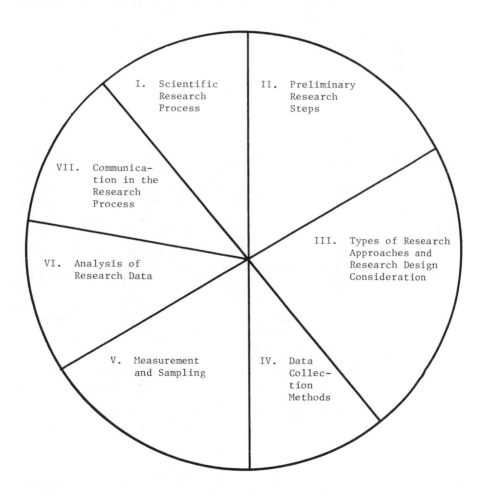

**FIGURE 24.2** Domain of nursing: research principles and methods.

1. Relevancy to the overall domain of Research Consumerism, Phase I, as operationalized by the following question:

    How important is this question in terms of the basic concepts and principles necessary to read and appraise published research at a beginning level?

    Not at All                                    Extremely
    Important ____ ____ ____ ____ ____ Important

2. Congruency of each item with its subdomain as operationalized by the following question:

    How representative is this question to the content and objective described for this subdomain?

    Not at All                                    Highly
    Representative ____ ____ ____ ____ ____ Representative

    Both scales thus provided data for calculation of interrater agreement regarding the content validity of each item (Rovinelli & Hambleton, 1977).

3. Technical construction: To enhance validity, judges were also asked to rate the technical construction of each item and validate the "correct" response.

    Technically, how good is this question as constructed?

    Very Poor ____ ____ ____ ____ ____ Excellent

## TABLE 24.1 Sample of Subdomain Specifications

| Subdomain III<br>Types of Nursing Research Approaches<br>and Research Design Considerations | |
| --- | --- |
| Description: | The description and characteristics and use of experimental, quasi-experimental, preexperimental, nonexperimental, and additional types of research, and descriptions of how studies can be designed to maximize quality and interpretability of results. |
| Objective: | Given a series of multiple choice questions, the nurse who functions as a consumer of research at a beginning level (Phase I) will understand and apply general knowledge of various types of nursing research approaches and research design considerations to the review and appraisal of published studies. |
| Knowledge statements: | |
| K-1 | Characteristics of and differences in experimental, quasi-experimental, preexperimental, and nonexperimental research design (particular reference to control of independent variable). |
| K-2 | graphic representation of designs. |
| K-3 | Internal and external validity and threats to same. |
| K-4 | Strengths and weaknesses of various research designs. |
| K-5 | Causal and correlational relationships. |
| K-6 | Distinction between types of nonexperimental studies (e.g., expost facto, prospective, retrospective). |
| K-7 | Purposes of various types of research (survey, evaluation, needs assessments, historical, case studies, secondary analysis, methodological, and cross-sectional). |
| K-8 | Control of extraneous variables. |

4. Correct response:
   Is the answer clearly the right answer?
   ____ Yes      ____ No

Data from the six judges were analyzed to obtain a per-item mean and standard deviation for the relevancy, congruency, and technical construction factors. Based on the following criteria, the pool of 237 items was then reduced to 126, or 53% of the original: (1) a mean of $\geq 3$ on all factors; (2) standard deviation of $\leq 1$ on all factors; and (3) a clearly correct answer. This left 102 items in Part I and 24 items in Part II (see Table 24.2.)

After instructions were written for test takers, the tool was pretested with nine newly graduated baccalaureate nurses to further enhance its reliability and validity.

## Administration and Scoring

The instrument is a test that is administered to the examinee via paper and pencil. Items are scored as either correct or incorrect. Percentage scores are derived for Parts I and II and the total test based on the percentage of correct responses.

Because this is a criterion-referenced test, a passing, or cut, score had to be set. The method used to determine this standard of performance was a modification of the Angoff (1971) standard-setting method; that is, a cut score was defined as that score expected from the person whose knowledge is on the borderline between the acceptable and unacceptable level of knowledge, as measured by the test. In order to determine this standard, the six experts were assembled to, first, individually judge the probability, in terms of a percentage, that borderline test-takers would answer any given item correctly. Individual judges rated each item using the approach noted in Table 24.3. With the instruction that the use of no more than three contiguous percentages are allowed for ultimately setting the cut score, the judges were then told as a group to discuss the individual ratings. One or more of the judges subsequently adjusted the rating for items where contiguity had not initially been present. Once these final individual ratings were established, a "master" was defined by calculating the average percentage of the six probability judgments for each item and then determining the mean probability (i.e., cut 6 or passing score) across all items for each part and for the test as a whole. The resulting cut scores were 62.7% for Part I, 64.3% for Part II, and 63.5% for the total test.

## Objective Validation

In order to assess objective validity, the 126-item instrument was administered to two types of subjects: (1) members of the target group (i.e., students or newly graduated nurses with a baccalaureate education who have had research content) and (2) registered nurses who have had no research coursework or no such course within the past 5 years. The former group will henceforth be referred to as the Instructed Group and the latter as the Uninstructed Group.

Data were collected (a) from two Uninstructed Groups of nurses [one from a large teaching center ($N = 31$) and the other from an RN- entry BSN program ($N = 5$)] and (b) from five Instructed Groups of student nurses at four schools on nursing in the New England region ($N = 129$). The large Uninstructed Group consisted of the following educational mix: 6.5% ADN, 25.8% diploma, 64.5% BSN, and 3.2% MA.

Because of the lack of consensus regarding content of instruction in research (Thomas & Price, 1980), data from the separate schools of nursing were not automatically combined. In addition, there was concern that differences would be found if (a) the test was administered at different times postcoursework or (b) research was taught in a discrete course versus integrated throughout other nursing content. The two Uninstructed Groups were thought to also be potentially different as the smaller group was currently enrolled in baccalaureate coursework and could conceivably be exposed to research concepts. The first step in data analysis was therefore to determine whether significant differences existed among the various Instructed Groups and the Uninstructed Groups, as well as between the Instructed Groups and the Uninstructed Groups.

**TABLE 24.2 Item Retention per Content Validation Process**

| Section | Original No. of items | No. items retained | Percentage of items retained |
|---|---|---|---|
| Subdomain I | 31 | 11 | 35 |
| Subdomain II | 28 | 14 | 50 |
| Subdomain III | 38 | 15 | 39 |
| Subdomain IV | 45 | 13 | 29 |
| Subdomain V | 28 | 22 | 79 |
| Subdomain VI | 24 | 20 | 83 |
| Subdomain VII | 13 | 7 | 54 |
| Abstract I | 10 | 7 | 70 |
| Abstract II | 10 | 10 | 100 |
| Abstract III | 10 | 7 | 70 |
| Totals | 237 | 126 | 53 |

**TABLE 24.3 Standard Setting**

Basic question:
"What percentage of minimally competent nurses that are Phase I Consumers of Research will answer this item correctly?"
Response scale: 0   15   30   45   60   75   90

Table 24.4 provides information on the mean score (percentage of items correct) for all groups relative to the total test. A one-way ANOVA was significant at the .000 level ($F = 19.770$; $df = 6/158$). Post hoc comparisons using Scheffe's Test revealed significant differences in the expected direction at a probability level at or below .05 between all but one of the Instructed Groups and the larger ($N = 31$) Uninstructed Group. The one exception was that group of students (Group 5) for whom research concepts were integrated throughout a number of nursing courses. Only one of the Instructed Groups (Group 4) was significantly different from the smaller ($N = 5$) Uninstructed Group; again Instructed Group 5 (Integrated) was not significantly different. Significant differences were also found among several of the Instructed Group comparisons: for example, 1 versus 2 and 5, and 2 versus 4. Instructed Group 5 (Integrated Coursework) was henceforth eliminated as it was not significantly different from either Uninstructed Group but was significantly different from three other Instructed groups. Uninstructed Group 7 was also eliminated as it was not consistently different from the Instructed Groups and could not therefore be combined with Uninstructed Group 6; in addition, the $N$ was considered too small to continue to treat it separately. Instructed Groups 1, 2, 3, and 4 were therefore treated separately in all comparisons with Uninstructed Group 6. As the probability of a Type I error would thus be increased, the level for significance was reset at .025.

Analyses to determine objectively based validity, conducted at the test and/or item level, are described below.

**TABLE 24.4** Group Comparisons and Mean Correct Percentage Scores on Total Test

| Groups | $N$ | Mean | S.D. | Significantly Different Groups |
|---|---|---|---|---|
| Instructed 1 (at 3 months)[a] | 20 | 73.90 | 9.54 | #2, #5, #6 |
| Instructed 2 (at 3 months) | 47 | 62.30 | 13.02 | #1, #4, #6 |
| Instructed 3 (at 3 months) | 22 | 66.59 | 8.61 | #1, #4, #6 |
| Instructed 4 (immediately postcourse) | 10 | 84.00 | 12.16 | #2, #3, #5, #6, #7 |
| Instructed 5 (at 3 months; integrated) | 30 | 55.23 | 7.01 | #1, #3, #4 |
| Uninstructed 6 | 31 | 54.00 | 7.49 | #1, #2, #3, #4 |
| Uninstructed 7 | 5 | 61.60 | 7.13 | #4 |

$F = 19.770$; $df = 6/158$.
[a] The time of a group's testing, postcourse, is shown within parentheses.

## Decision Validity

In order to obtain information regarding the overall test, a type of construct validation known as decision validity was utilized (Hambleton, 1979). This type of validation involves a comparison regarding the number of subjects who were correctly classified as a master or nonmaster within each precondition (Instructed or Uninstructed). Analyses were done for Part I, Part II, and the total test; the matching cut group that were classified as masters and nonmasters is presented in Tables 24.5, 24.6, and 24.7. A chi square analysis that compared the Uninstructed and Instructed groups indicated that differences were significant in two cases for the total test; that is, in the comparison between Instructed Group 1 and the Uninstructed Group and in the comparison between Instructed Group 4 and the Uninstructed Group. Part I comprised 81% of the total test; significant between-group differences found in Part I were thus identical to results for the total test. For Part II, only one of the four comparisons was significant.

**TABLE 24.5** Decision Validity: Proportion of Mastery/Nonmastery Classification for the Total Test

| Precondition of instruction | Classification | |
|---|---|---|
| | Mastery | Nonmastery |
| Instructed Group #1* | 25% | 75% |
| Instructed Group #2 | 6% | 94% |
| Instructed Group #3 | 9% | 91% |
| Instructed Group #4** | 50% | 50% |
| Uninstructed Group | 0% | 100% |

Chi-square was based on raw numbers.
*$p \leq .014$ for difference between Instructed and Uninstructed Groups.
**$p \leq .002$ for difference between Instructed and Uninstructed Groups.

**TABLE 24.6** Decision Validity: Proportion of Mastery/Nonmastery Classification for Part I

| Precondition of instruction | Classification | |
|---|---|---|
| | Mastery | Nonmastery |
| Instructed Group #1* | 35% | 65% |
| Instructed Group #2 | 9% | 91% |
| Instructed Group #3 | 14% | 86% |
| Instructed Group #4** | 60% | 40% |
| Uninstructed Group | 0% | 100% |

Chi-square was based on raw numbers.
*$p \leq .002$ for difference between Instructed and Uninstructed Groups

**TABLE 24.7 Decision Validity: Proportion of
Mastery/Nonmastery Classification for Part II**

| Precondition of instruction | Classification | |
|---|---|---|
| | Mastery | Nonmastery |
| Instructed Group #1 | 15% | 85% |
| Instructed Group #2 | 11% | 89% |
| Instructed Group #3 | 5% | 95% |
| Instructed Group #4* | 60% | 40% |
| Uninstructed Group | 0% | 100% |

Chi-square was based on raw numbers.
*$p \leq .002$ for difference between Instructed and Uninstructed
Groups.

## Item Validity

Three analyses were conducted to obtain information on item difficulty
and item discrimination:

1. *Item difficulty*, the $p$ level or proportion of correct responses per item.
   This was calculated and a comparison made between the various
   Instructed Groups and the Uninstructed Group. A z, or critical ratio,
   test was to be used for this comparison (Brunig & Kintz, 1977; Colton, 1974); but for programming reasons. a chi-square had to be utilized with raw numbers. Results ranged from .00 to 23.58 and, as
   might be expected, varied across items and from group to group
   comparison. For example, a significant chi-square was found for 44
   (or 35%) of the items in at least one of the four group comparisons;
   and in 29 (or 23%) of the items, there were two or more significant
   chi-squares among the four group comparisons.
2. *Item discrimination*, as measured by the Criterion Groups Difference
   Index (CGDI). The CDGI was calculated by subtracting the proportion of nurses in the Uninstructed Group with a correct response
   from the proportion of correct responses in each Instructed Group.
   As with item difficulty, results varied across items and from group
   to group comparison. In this case, 54 (43%) of the items had a *positive* CGDI of .20 or greater in at least two of the four group
   comparisons.
3. *Item discrimination*, as measured by $K_{max}$ (Waltz, Strickland, & Lenz,
   1984). In this type of discrimination, a comparison per item is made
   in terms of mastery classification per total test versus mastery classification per item (i.e., correct or incorrect response). All subjects
   were therefore merged into one group for this analysis as pretesting
   status was of no significance. (This included the additional subjects
   from eliminated groups that could not be used in the primary analysis; the total $N$ was therefore 165.) Fifty percent of the items had
   $K_{max}$ of .20 or greater.

## Assessment of Reliability

KR20, a special case of Crombach's alpha, was used to assess the internal consistency of the instrument because answers were dichotomously scored as correct or incorrect. Although this reliability measure is not recommended for criterion-referenced tests, with the inclusion of the uninstructed subjects it was assumed that sufficient variability would exist so that spurious results due to statistical artifact would not occur. Again, all tested subjects were used to increase the $N$ to 165. Results were as follows: Part I, .826; Part II, .575; and Total, .854.

## Tool Refinement

Based on the decision validity and reliability data, it was felt that sufficient evidence existed to warrant further testing of the Knowledge of Research Consumerism Instrument. However, a measurement tool of 126 items was judged to be too lengthy, and steps were therefore taken to begin item reduction. Since no clear rules exist to facilitate this decision-making process, criteria were set that would err in the direction of retaining items, including both strong discriminators and marginal discriminators. The following three-step process was used:

1. A liberal level or criterion of acceptability was established for each individual type of item analysis: For Item Difficulty, the chi-square comparison had to be significant at .025 probability level or less; for Item Discrimination/Criterion Groups Method, the CGDI had to be positive and at least .20; for Item Discrimination/K Method, the $K_{max}$ had to be .20 or greater.

2. A single rating of acceptability was then assigned to each item for each category of item analysis where four group comparisons had been made, that is, for Item Difficulty and for Item Discrimination/ CGDI, where four group comparisons per item had been calculated. An item/validity category was given an acceptable rating if at least 2 of the 4 group comparisons met the criterion for acceptability cited above.

3. An item was retained if either of the following criteria were true: if two of the three final criteria of acceptability were achieved – Strong item; or if one of the three final criteria of acceptability were achieved – Marginal item. Through this process, 36 items will be eliminated from the instrument. This includes one of the three abstracts (No. 3) and all related items, even though four of these items would have been retained based on the single-item criteria.

In addition, 23 items have been noted that would increase reliability if deleted from the test. Many of these items were rated as marginal or unacceptable. The original 126 items are listed at the end of the chapter.

Because of its potential accessibility to students, the correct answers are not shown. They can be obtained for the total test from the authors or, for Part I, by referring to the Polit and Hungler *Instructor's Manual* (1983a).

## DISCUSSION

Preliminary results for the Knowledge of Research Consumerism, Phase I Instrument, support its further development. However, methodological limitations in terms of potential intervening variables are recognized and concomitant modifications are being made in further testing:

1. *Knowledge of statistics*: Because of the relationship between research and principles of statistics, individuals who have had the coursework in the latter may perform better than nurses without such coursework. Statistical comparisons will therefore be made with this variable. Thomas and Price (1984) found some support for this hypothesis.
2. *Instructor background*: Differences existed among the instructors of the BSN subjects (e.g., completed doctorate vs. doctoral student) and length of time as research course instructor. Such variables may impact on outcomes and therefore should be considered in future analyses.
3. *Research course content/method*: As indicated previously, the content of a specific research course may vary from school to school, depending on the instructor's course design, for example, sampling, statistics, or instrumentation may or may not be emphasized. Such differences could account for differential scores per subdomain. Focus on Consumerism versus Production could also affect competency outcomes, and use of the Polit and Hungler (1983b) textbook is yet another factor. (It should be noted that the Instructed Groups that performed most competently were those taught by one of the investigators. One potential explanation is that bias was thereby introduced, although course design was not changed due to this project. Other factors in this instance that may be relevant are the ones cited above, that is, this instructor has a doctorate, has taught research for 1½ years, and uses the Polit and Hungler textbook.)

Other steps that are planned for future testing include the following:

1. Calculation of reliability by a test-retest procedure, using only instructed subjects.
2. Pre- and posttesting of subjects in relation to research coursework.
3. Exploration of an empirically set cut score.
4. Accumulation of validity data and related item refinement.

In closing this discussion, the relatively low scores achieved by some of the Instructed Groups (Table 24.4) should be of interest to both nursing faculty in educational programs and to administrators in service settings. These data are the result of pilot testing; however, they are consistent with the extensive data reported by Thomas and Price (1984 p. 8): In field testing, the mean score for undergraduate students on the Form B (the easier form) 50-item knowledge test was 27.29 (SD, 6.85); for graduate students, on the Form B test, the mean was 31.34 (SD, 7.82). Of equal interest is Thomas and Price's finding, again similar to these results, that students in programs where research was integrated did significantly less well than their counterparts with a separate research course.

Given such data, researchers, educators, and administrators must continue to explore empirically the role of research within nursing. The content and methodology of courework, per level of education, as well as expectations for performance of various levels of graduates in the practice setting must thus be examined; and if research is to make realistic impact on nursing practice, then a revision in either educational methodology, as suggested by Stetler(1983), may be necessary.

# REFERENCES

Angoff, W. (1971). Scales, norms and equivalent scores. In R. L. Thorndike (Ed.), *Educational measurement (pp.508-600)*. Washington, DC: American Council on Education.

Bogal-Allbritten, R., Marcum, C., & Raspberry, H. (1982). *Research coursework in the baccalaureate nursing curriculum: A nationwide survey.* (ERIC Document Reproduction Service No. ED 222 112)

Bruning, J., & Kintz, B. (1977). *Computational handbook of statistics* (2nd ed.) Glenville, IL: Scott, Foresman.

Colton, T. (1974). *Statistics in medicine*. Boston: Little, Brown.

Haller, K., Reynolds, M., & Horsley, J. (1979). Developing research-based innovation protocols: Process, criteria, and issues. *Research in Nursing and Health, 2,* 45-51.

Hambleton, R. (1979). *Test score validity and standard setting methods*. Unpublished project report.

Hastings, G. (1972). Independent learning based on behavioral objectives. *The Journal of Educational Research, 65,* 411-416.

Mallick, M. (1983). A constant comparative method for teaching research critiquing to baccalaureate nursing students. *Image: The Journal of Nursing Scholarship, 15,* 120-123.

Polit, D., & Hungler, B. (1983a). *Instructor's manual for nursing research: principles and methods* (2nd ed.). Philadelphia: J. B. Lippincott.

Polit, D., & Hungler, B. (1983b). *Nursing research: Principles and methods* (2nd ed.). Philadelphia: J. B. Lippincott.

Professional Examination Service. (1981). *Three levels of cognitive behavior* (adapted from B. S. Bloom & H. Levine). New York: Professional Examination Service.

Rosenblatt, A., & Kirk, S. (1981). Cumulative effect of research courses on knowledge and attitudes of social work students. *Journal of Education for Social Work, 17,* 26-34.

Rovinelli, R., & Hambleton, R. (1977). On the use of content specialists in the assessment of criterion-referenced test item validity. *Tijdschrift voor Onderwijresearch, 2*, 49-60.

Scott, O. (1971). Relative effects of four types of assignment on competence in research consumership. *The Journal of Educational Research, 65*, 183-189.

Shelton, B. (1979). Research components in baccalaureate programs in nursing. *Journal of Nursing Education, 18*, 22-33.

Stetler, C. (1983). Nurses and research: Responsibility and involvement. *NITA: The Journal of the National Intravenous Therapy Association, 6*, 207-212.

Stetler, C. (1984). *Nursing research in a service setting, Massachusetts General Hospital, Department of Nursing*. Reston, VA: Reston Publishing.

Stetler, C. (1985). Research utilization: Defining the concept. *Image: The Journal of Nursing Scholarship, 17* 40-44.

Stetler, C., & Marram, G. (1976). Evaluating research findings for applicability in practice. *Nursing Outlook, 24*, 559-563.

Thomas, B., & Price, M. (1980). Research preparation in baccalaureate nursing education. *Nursing Research,29* 259-261.

Thomas, B., & Price, M. (1984). *Thomas-Price inventory of nursing research: Instructor's manual*. St. Louis: Mosby Systems.

Van Servellen, G. Marram, & Stetler, C. (1986). Utilization of research: Critiquing research for practice. In A. M. Lieske (Ed.), *Clinical nursing research (pp. 231-242)*. Rockville, MD: Aspen Systems.

Waltz, C., Strickland, O. & Lenz, E. (1984). *Measurement in nursing research*. Philadelphia: F. A. Davis Co.

# Knowledge of Research Consumerism Instrument

Instructions: This questionnaire is designed to assess your current level of knowledge about nursing research. It consists of two sections:

Part I: A series of multiple choice questions that focus on various aspects of research.

Part II: Abstracts of two research studies, each followed by a series of multiple choice questions about the content of the abstracted study.

For each question in Part I and Part II, select the ONE BEST answer (a, b, c, or d,) and indicate your choice on the answer sheet provided. Please use a No. 2 lead pencil and *completely* fill in the circled number on the answer sheet that corresponds to the *letter* which you believe indicates the right answer. Please answer ALL of the test questions.

## PART I

1. The majority of studies at midcentury focused on
   a. consumer satisfaction
   b. clinical problems
   c. health promotion
   d. educational issues
2. Inductive reasoning is the process of
   a. verifying assumptions that are part of our heritage
   b. developing scientific predictions from general principles
   c. empirically testing observations that are made known through our sense organs
   d. forming generalizations from specific observations
3. Empiricism refers to the process of
   a. making generalizations from specific observations
   b. deducing specific predictions from generalizations
   c. gathering evidence rooted in objective reality
   d. verifying the assumptions upon which the study was based
4. The concept of generalization refers to
   a. the ability to go beyond the specifics of the situation at hand

*Note.* All items in Part I of this instrument were taken from the following source: Polit, D., & Hungler, B. (1983a). *Instructor's manual for Nursing research: Principles and Methods* (2nd ed.). Philadelphia: J. B. Lippincott. All abstracts and items in Part II were developed by C. Stetler and A. Sheridan.

    b.   the confidence that a researcher has in the outcomes of the investigation

    c.   whether the study has been linked to a theory

    d.   the belief that all phenomena have antecedent causes

5. The purpose of an operational definition is to
   a. assign numerical values to variables
   b. specify how a variable will be defined and measured
   c. state the expected relations between the variables under investigation
   d. designate the overall plan by which the research will be conducted

6. Of the following, the most appropriate example of an attribute variable is
   a. maternal-infant bonding
   b. method of teaching
   c. nurse-client teaching
   d. blood type

7. The dependent variable(s) in the study "Is the job performance of nurses affected by salary or perceived job autonomy?" is (are)
   a. job performance
   b. salary
   c. perceived job autonomy
   d. both salary and perceived job autonomy

8. The overall plan developed by the researcher to obtain answers to the questions being studied is called
   a. analysis of data
   b. operationally defining the variables
   c. problem statement
   d. research design

9. Individuals who participate in a study are referred to as the
   a. data
   b. target population
   c. subjects
   d. probability statistics

10. Representativeness in a sample refers to
    a. how well the sample reflects the characteristics of the population in terms of the variables being studied
    b. the possibility of a particular person from the population being included in the study
    c. the use of random procedures in selecting sample units
    d. the sampling technique employed to obtain subjects from the population

11. The following are all examples of descriptive statistics except
    a. criterion measures
    b. frequencies
    c. means
    d. percentages

12. Developing a research problem from a theory or conceptual framework requires the logical reasoning process of
    a. critical thinking
    b. deduction
    c. induction
    d. conceptualization

13. Which of the following statements best describes the problem statement "To what extent do health policies influence the health of American citizens?"
    a. acceptable as stated
    b. not a research problem because it addresses a moral issue
    c. not acceptable as stated because it lacks an independent variable
    d. not acceptable because of the vagueness of the concepts

14. A primary source for literature review may be defined as
    a. a description of an investigation written by the researcher who con- ducted the study
    b. a summarization of relevant research that has been conducted on the topic of interest
    c. a thesaurus that directs the reader to subject heading germane to the topic
    d. any retrieval mechanism that helps to locate articles on the area of interest

15. Sources for literature review include all the following *except*
    a. bibliographies
    b. books
    c. computer searches
    d. personal experience

16. A set of logically interrelated propositions is associated with
    a. statistical model
    b. conceptual framework
    c. theory
    d. schematic model

17. The power of theories lies in their ability to
    a. capture the complexity of human nature by the richness of the opera- tional definitions associated with the variables
    b. minimize the number of words required to explain phenomena and thereby eliminate semantic problems
    c. prove conclusively that relations exist among the phenomena studied
    d. specify the nature of the relations that exist among phenomena

18. The overall purpose of a theory is to
    a. make scientific findings meaningful and generalizable
    b. explain relations that exist among variables as well as the nature of the relation
    c. stimulate the generation of hypotheses that can be empirically tested
    d. summarize accumulated facts

19. The building blocks for theory are
    a. concepts
    b. empirical testing
    c. hypothesis
    d. models

20. The major similarity between theories and conceptual frameworks is that both
    a. use concepts as their building blocks
    b. use the deductive reasoning process almost exclusively
    c. contains set of logically interrelated propositions
    d. provide a mechanism for developing new propositions from the original propositions

21. A research hypothesis
    a. is a set of logically interrelated propositions
    b. is usually more general in scope than the problem statement
    c. predicts the nature of the relation between two or more variables
    d. predicts the absence of a relation between two or more variables

22. The following are all purposes of the research hypothesis *except*
    a. proving the validity of a theory
    b. extending human knowledge
    c. linking the abstract and conceptual with the concrete and observable
    d. providing direction to the research design

23. A research hypothesis predicts the nature of the relationship between
    a. the functional and causal nature of the variables
    b. a theoretical framework and observable phenomena
    c. a presumed cause and a presumed effect
    d. statistical testing and the assumption of innocence

24. Deductive hypotheses are almost always
    a. testable
    b. researchable
    c. complex
    d. directional

25. The term randomization may be defined as
    a. assignment of subjects to a group in such a way that neither the subject nor the researcher knows who is receiving treatment
    b. each subject having an equal chance of being selected for any group
    c. the assurance that systematic bias will be present in the selection of subjects into groups
    d. the matching of subjects' attributes that are likely to affect the outcome

26. Which of the following must be present in quasi-experimental research?
    a. a comparison group
    b. manipulating a variable
    c. matching of subjects
    d. randomization

27. The term internal validity refers to
    a. the elimination of competing explanations that could account for any observed differences
    b. making an inference that the experimental intervention resulted in any observed differences
    c. the nonequivalence of groups before the treatment
    d. the occurrence of events external to the treatment that could affect the manipulation

28. Which of the following research designs is *weakest* in terms of the researcher's ability to establish causality?
    a. experimental
    b. ex post facto
    c. preexperimental
    d. quasi-experimental

29. In an ex post facto study, compared to an experimental study, the researcher forfeits control of
    a. the independent variable(s)

b.   the dependent variable(s)
c.   the criterion variable(s)
d.   the attribute variable(s)

30. A study that followed, over a 20-year period, users and nonusers of oral contraceptives to find long-term effects would be called a
    a.   prediction study
    b.   retrospective study
    c.   prospective study
    d.   descriptive correlational study

31. If a researcher wanted to describe the frequency with which nursing students performed breast self-examination, the study would be classified as
    a.   descriptive correlational
    b.   prospective
    c.   retrospective
    d.   univariate descriptive

32. Which of the following types of nonexperimental research would probably require the longest data collection period?
    a.   descriptive correlational
    b.   prospective
    c.   retrospective
    d.   univariate descriptive

33. In survey research, the approach that typically yields the highest response rate is
    a.   personal interviews
    b.   telephone interviews
    c.   home-delivered questionnaires
    d.   mailed questionnaires

34. One of the advantages of the case study method is the
    a.   ease with which the data can be analyzed
    b.   facility with which the findings can be generalized
    c.   objectivity that can be maintained by the researcher
    d.   in-depth nature of the data collected

35. Data collected before the institution of a treatment are sometimes referred to as
    a.   posttest data
    b.   baseline data
    c.   case study data
    d.   secondary data

36. How many hypotheses can be tested in a two-factor design?
    a.   1
    b.   2
    c.   3
    d.   4

37. The most effective method of controlling extraneous variables is by
    a.   analysis of covariance
    b.   matching
    c.   randomized control group
    d.   repeated measures design

38. Suppose a researcher conducted a study using clients in a rehabilitation facility as subjects. The researcher does the study again. However, for the sec-

ond study, clients in a general hospital became the subjects. This process refers to the concept of

a. counterbalancing
b. precision
c. variability
d. replication

39. Research projects that collect data at one point in time are referred to as
    a. cohort studies
    b. cross-sectional studies
    c. cross-sequential studies
    d. panel studies

40. A researcher used hemoglobin levels as an index of the likelihood that a person would develop a pressure sore. Hemoglobin levels are classified as what type of physiological measure?
    a. physical
    b. chemical
    c. microbiological
    d. cytological

41. The concept of objectivity for physiological measures refers to the
    a. lack of interactions that generally accompanies their use
    b. unobtrusive nature of their presence
    c. precision with which they measure the target concept
    d. agreement of two independent observers of the observed measurement

42. Which of the following topic areas would be most conducive to study by observational methods?
    a. attitude toward preventive health practices
    b. knowledge of the danger signals of cancer
    c. interactions in a psychiatric crisis center
    d. effectiveness of support groups for drug abusers

43. When the researcher uses a self-report technique but specifies neither the questions nor the response alternatives in advance, the interview is referred to as
    a. standardized
    b. structured
    c. unstructured
    d. face-to-face

44. A data-collection technique that quantifies a person's attitude along a bipolar dimension is called a
    a. cafeteria checklist
    b. checklist
    c. graphic rating scale
    d. rank-order question

45. A major purpose of a pretest is to
    a. detect inadequacies in an interview schedule/questionnaire
    b. obtain some preliminary results on the research problem
    c. assess the adequacy of the research design
    d. evaluate whether a structured or unstructured schedule is preferable

46. On a 7-point Likert scale, the response "undecided" would be scored as
    a. 0

    b.   1
    c.   4
    d.   7

47. On a 20-item Likert scale with 5 response categories, the range of possible scores is
    a.   0 to 100
    b.   20 to 80
    c.   20 to 100
    d.   0 to 50

48. Which of the following scaling procedures is an example of a cumulative scale?
    a.   Thurstone scale
    b.   Likert scale
    c.   Guttman scale
    d.   Semantic Differential scale

49. Which of the following techniques *cannot* be administered by mail?
    a.   critical incidents technique
    b.   Delphi technique
    c.   sentence completion techniques
    d.   psychodrama

50. Suppose a researcher wants to forecast future priorities for research in obstetrical nursing. The participants will be nurse midwives. Which of the following techniques would most probably be employed?
    a.   content analysis
    b.   projective technique
    c.   Delphi procedure
    d.   Thematic Apperception Test

51. The technique that is least susceptible to response set bias is
    a.   interviews
    b.   Delphi procedure
    c.   questionnaires
    d.   projective measures

52. A bias that may be present in the use of records is known as
    a.   acquiescence bias
    b.   extreme response bias
    c.   selective deposit bias
    d.   social desirability bias

53. Another term for universe is
    a.   sample
    b.   population
    c.   true scores
    d.   set of rules

54. The level of measurement that classifies and ranks objects in terms of the degree to which they possess the attribute of interest is
    a.   nominal
    b.   ordinal
    c.   interval
    d.   ratio

55. Religion is measured on the
    a.   nominal scale

b. ordinal scale
c. interval scale
d. ratio scale

56. The most primitive and least precise level of measurement is
    a. nominal
    b. ordinal
    c. interval
    d. ratio

57. Keeping a record of the fluid intake, in ounces, of a postsurgical patient is an example of which level of measurement?
    a. nominal
    b. ordinal
    c. interval
    d. ratio

58. Which level of measurement permits the researcher to add, subtract, multiply, and divide?
    a. nominal
    b. ordinal
    c. interval
    d. ratio

59. The difference between a true score and an obtained score is referred to as
    a. internal inconsistency
    b. discriminability
    c. response sampling
    d. error of measurement

60. One source of measurement error is
    a. response set bias
    b. inefficiency
    c. speed
    d. absence of validity

61. The Spearman-Brown prophecy formula is applied after using
    a. K-R 20
    b. split-half technique
    c. Cronbach's alpha
    d. multitrait-multimethod matrix

62. Cronbach's alpha is used to determine which of the following instrument attributes?
    a. internal consistency
    b. stability
    c. criterion validity
    d. construct validity

63. The aspect of reliability for which interobserver reliability is appropriate is
    a. stability
    b. internal consistency
    c. equivalence
    d. criterion related

64. If a Cronbach's alpha was computed to be 0.80, this coefficient would represent
    a. the true variability in scores
    b. the observed variability in scores

    c.   the variability associated with random error
    d.   the proportion of true to obtained variability

65. A perfect correlation between two variables would be represented by a coefficient of
    a.   0.00
    b.   −1.00
    c.   2.00
    d.   100.00

66. The type of validity that employs only logical rather than empirical procedures in its assessment is
    a.   content
    b.   concurrent
    c.   predictive
    d.   construct

67. Suppose a researcher were interested in assessing the adequacy of an instrument to measure the theoretical conceptualization of territorial space. The type of validation procedure would most probably be
    a.   content
    b.   concurrent
    c.   predictive
    d.   construct

68. Which of the following terms does not belong with the other three?
    a.   content validity
    b.   criterion-related validity
    c.   predictive validity
    d.   concurrent validity

69. Sampling may be defined as the
    a.   set of elements used for selecting the sample
    b.   process of selecting a subset of the population to represent the entire population
    c.   aggregation of subjects who meet a designated set of criteria for inclusion in the study
    d.   technique used to ensure that every element in the population has an equal chance of being included in the study

70. Bias in sampling refers to
    a.   systematic overrepresentation or underrepresentation of some segment of the population on the attribute of interest
    b.   lack of heterogeneity in the population on the attribute of interest
    c.   sample selection in nonprobability-type sampling designs
    d.   the margin of error in the data obtained from samples

71. Strata are incorporated into the design of which of the following types of samples?
    a.   systematic
    b.   purposive
    c.   quota
    d.   simple random

72. The type of sampling design that is most likely to obtain a representative sample is
    a.   stratified random
    b.   snowball

    c.   purposive

    d.   quota

73. Which of the following types of samples is considered to be the weakest in sampling design?

    a.   accidental

    b.   quota

    c.   purposive

    d.   systematic

74. Suppose a nurse researcher subdivided a list of nurses obtained from the Board of Registration in Nursing according to type of nursing position held and then randomly selected 50 nurses from each position listed. The type would be

    a.   stratified random

    b.   cluster

    c.   systematic

    d.   simple random

75. If the bulk of scores from a test occurred at the upper end of the distribution, the distribution would be described as

    a.   normal

    b.   bimodal

    c.   positively skewed

    d.   negatively skewed

76. A parameter is a characteristic of

    a.   a population

    b.   reliability

    c.   a sample

    d.   validity

77. The standard deviation is an index of

    a.   bivariate relationships

    b.   central tendency

    c.   skewness

    d.   variability

78. The measure of variability that takes into account the actual score values is the

    a.   mean

    b.   median

    c.   range

    d.   standard deviation

79. The degree of relationship between two variables is best expressed by a:

    a.   correlation coefficient

    b.   mean

    c.   standard deviation

    d.   univariate statistic

80. The most appropriate measure of central tendency to use with the variable "pulse rate" is the

    a.   mode

    b.   median

    c.   mean

    d.   correlation coefficient

81. Which of the following is an example of a bivariate descriptive statistic?

    a.   frequency distribution
    b.   mean
    c.   semiquartile range
    d.   correlation coefficient

82. One of the characteristics of a normal distribution is that
    a.   it is bimodal
    b.   68% of the values are within two standard deviations from the mean
    c.   semiquartile range
    d.   correlation coefficient

83. The symbol $\bar{x}$ represents:
    a.   the sum of
    b.   the mean
    c.   the number of cases
    d.   an individual score

84. The symbol $\Sigma$ represents:
    a.   the sum of
    b.   the mean
    c.   the number of cases
    d.   an individual score

85. The use of inferential statistics permits the researcher to
    a.   generalize to a population based on information gathered from a sample
    b.   describe information obtained from empirical observation
    c.   interpret descriptive statistics
    d.   none of the above

86. The standard deviation of a sampling distribution is called a
    a.   sampling error
    b.   standard error
    c.   variance
    d.   parameter

87. A major factor that affects the standard error of the mean is
    a.   point estimation
    b.   confidence limits
    c.   sample size
    d.   value of the mean

88. For which of the following levels of significance is the risk of making a Type I error greater?
    a.   0.10
    b.   0.05
    c.   0.01
    d.   0.001

89. A 95% confidence level is associated with how many standard deviation units?
    a.   1.96
    b.   2.36
    c.   2.58
    d.   depends on sample size

90. If a researcher calculates a $t$-statistic to be $-2.2$ and the tabled $t$-value (for $df = 60$ and the level of significance of 0.05) is 2.0, the researcher would
    a.   conclude that an error in calculation had been made

b.   accept the null hypothesis
c.   reject the null hypothesis
d.   use a different level of significance

91. A statistical procedure that is used to determine whether a significant difference exists between any number of group means is the
    a.   *t*-test
    b.   analysis of variance
    c.   correlation coefficient
    d.   Mann-Whitney U-test

92. How many null hypotheses would there be for a study with 40 subjects, using a two-way ANOVA?
    a.   2
    b.   3
    c.   5
    d.   10

93. If a researcher wanted to determine whether observed proportions differ significantly from expected proportions, the statistic would be a(n)
    a.   *t*-test
    b.   correlation coefficient
    c.   analysis of variance
    d.   chi-square

94. When both the independent and dependent variables are measured on a ratio scale, the appropriate test statistic is a (n)
    a.   *t*-test
    b.   ANOVA
    c.   chi-square
    d.   Pearson's *r*

95. Suppose a researcher hypothesized that a relationship existed between nurses' leadership behavior and job satisfaction. Correlational analysis revealed an *r* = .60 that had a *p*-value beyond the 0.001 level. The researcher may conclude all of the following *except*
    a.   the greater the leadership behavior of the nurse, the higher the degree of job satisfaction
    b.   the data analysis demonstrated that the research hypothesis was correct
    c.   a statistically significant relationship exists between nurses' leadership and job satisfaction
    d.   high levels of leadership behavior caused high job satisfaction

96. The answer to whether the researcher went "beyond the data" in the study would be found in which section of the research report?
    a.   introduction
    b.   methods
    c.   results
    d.   discussion

97. The medium through which the findings of research would be communicated to the broadest audience is the
    a.   dissertation
    b.   journal article
    c.   results
    d.   discussion

98. The person who critiques a published research report should strive to
    a.  consider that all flaws have equivalent value
    b.  focus only on the inadequacies inherent in the study
    c.  judge the merits of the study based on the researcher's background
    d.  remain as objective as possible
99. All of the following aspects of a study would be evaluated in the methods section *except*
    a.  underlying assumptions
    b.  subject selection
    c.  description of instruments
    d.  rationale for research design
100. "Does the research control for threats to the internal and external validity of the study?" would be asked in which section of a research report?
    a.  introduction
    b.  methods
    c.  results
    d.  discussion
101. Which of the following journals would most likely contain the highest number of primary sources for a research literature review?
    a.  *American Journal of Nursing*
    b.  *Nursing '82*
    c.  *Nursing Outlook*
    d.  *Nursing Research*
102. In a dissertation or technical report, a copy of the data collection instrument would be included in which of the following sections?
    a.  introduction
    b.  methods section
    c.  appendix
    d.  bibliography

# PART II
## Abstract 1*
## The Effect of Relaxation Training on Postoperative Pain and Vomiting

Relaxation training has been theorized to decrease abdominal tension (a cause of postop pain ) as well as to reduce anxiety (a correlate of postoperative vomiting). A two-group, posttest only design, with random assignment, was used to determine if postoperative pain and vomiting differ in adult cholecystectomy patients in two treatment conditions.

All cholecystectomy patients in a small community hospital operated on in July and who agreed to participate were included. Data were collected on pain, through the use of a self-report scale, and on vomiting. Information regarding the latter was retrieved from the patient's chart and measured in terms of quantity

*Fictitious study

of vomitus. Seven patients received relaxation training and seven other patients received the unit's standard preoperative teaching, which did not include relaxation.

The mean scores were analyzed through analysis of variance. Results indicated statistically significant, positive effects ($p = .01$) for pain but not for vomiting.

103. The independent variable in this study was
    a. pain
    b. vomiting
    c. relaxation training
    d. standard preoperative teaching
104. The type of research design utilized was
    a. nonexperimental
    b. preexperimental
    c. experimental
    d. ex post facto
105. The type of sample selected was
    a. probability
    b. nonprobability
    c. stratified
    d. randomized
106. The use of random assignment increased the study's
    a. generalizability
    b. internal validity
    c. variance
    d. reliability
107. the operational definition of vomiting can be considered weak due to a question of
    a. intervening variables
    b. true definition of vomiting
    c. reliability of charts
    d. reliability of vomitus
108. Analysis of variance enabled the researcher to
    a. randomize to a complete population
    b. describe characteristics of the subjects
    c. draw inferences for a hypothetical population
    d. randomize for a hypothetical population
109. The results of this study should be generalized to
    a. all postoperative patients
    b. all cholecystectomy patients
    c. all patients with relaxation training
    d. no other group of patients

## Abstract 2*
## Bereavement Crisis Intervention for Mothers Upon the Loss of a Child

It has been suggested that grief or bereavement is an acute stage of anxiety caused by the precipitating factor of the death of a person with whom one is emotionally involved.

This grief in turn causes specific behavior and feelings in affected individuals. These reactions can be lessened by the presence of a strong support system or exacerbated by the presence of psychiatric illness.

In order to test a nursing intervention designed to facilitate coping, the following hypothesis was tested: There is no difference in the change of self-report of depression by mothers who received crisis intervention and mothers who receive no such treatment.

Fifty mothers whose children died in a large teaching center in the midwest were enrolled in the study. The first 25 mothers whose children died after the study was initiated were placed in the treatment group; the second 25 were merely interviewed to obtain the needed data.

An Adjective Scale for Depression (ASD) was used at two points in time. With the ASD, subjects were asked to indicate their current level of depression on a series of 5-point scales. Split-half reliability coefficients for this tool are .35 for males and .29 for females.

The crisis treatment consisted of a series of support group sessions conducted by a psychiatric nurse clinician, according to a standardized protocol. In addition, individual follow-up sessions were held with each mother, again according to a recommended protocol.

A $t$-test was used to analyze the difference in the change scores between the two groups. The results indicated no significant differences but there was a trend ($p = .08$) in the expected direction. No significant differences were found between the two groups for age, education, or marital status. However, past psychiatric illness was found to be significantly related to the level of depression across the total sample.

110. The variables of depression and crisis intervention can be considered which of the following?
    a.   a model of bereavement intervention
    b.   an example of critical thinking
    c.   concepts relevant to a theory of bereavement
    d.   a framework for probability testing
111. Of potential concern to a reviewer of this study would be which of the following?
    a.   relevance of the bereavement theory to patient care
    b.   consent process used to obtain subjects
    c.   qualifications of the bereavement group leader
    d.   focus of the study on death of children

---

*Fictitious study

112. What type of hypothesis was used?
    a. null
    b. research
    c. alternative
    d. retrospective
113. Past psychiatric illness was measured as a means of
    a. testing the stated hypothesis
    b. manipulating the independent variable
    c. providing a control group
    d. controlling an intervening variable
114. The reliability coefficient of .29 indicates
    a. an acceptable level of consistency for the tool
    b. an unacceptable level of consistency for the tool
    c. an acceptable level of relevancy for the tool
    d. an unacceptable level of relevance for the tool
115. The statement that "there was a trend ($p = .08$) in the expected direction" should be interpreted as indicating
    a. that crisis intervention most probably does decrease depression
    b. that crisis intervention most probably does not decrease depression
    c. that the researcher has accepted the results of inferential testing
    d. that the researcher has not accepted the results of inferential testing
116. A standardized protocol was utilized by the psychiatric nurse clinician in order to control for
    a. the precise definition of the independent variable
    b. randomization
    c. the subject's extraneous characteristics
    d. the subject's relevant characteristics
117. An alternative method of measuring depression that would control for a socially desirable response would be
    a. a checklist for subjects with only yes/no response alternatives
    b. use of a Galvanic Skin Response
    c. observation and rating of subject behavior by a nonparticipant observer
    d. observation and rating of subjects by a fellow subject
118. This is an example of what type of research design?
    a. experimental
    b. quasi-experimental
    c. ex post facto
    d. descriptive correlational
119. What level of measurement is the Adjective Depression Scale?
    a. nominal
    b. at least ordinal
    c. at least ratio
    d. Guttman

## Abstract 3*
## The Relationship of a Social Support Network to the Perception of Health Status

A researcher hypothesized that clients with a strong support network would describe themselves as being healthier than clients with a weak support network. To test this hypothesis the first 100 residents of a housing complex for the elderly, who were attendees at a mobile health clinic held each week, were asked to rate themselves on a 7-point scale regarding their current physical health status (1 = very poor health and 7 = excellent health) and their system of support. (A 10-item Likert-like scale was used to measure the quality of individual support networks).

The self-ratings of descriptions of physical health were normally distributed for the sample as a whole: 3% excellent, 14% very good, 23% good, 21% neither good nor poor, 21% poor, 14% very poor, 4% extremely poor. These were then classified into three categories: 17 (17%) of these clients were classified as having a high level of health, 44 (44%) with moderate level, and 39 (39%) with low level of health. When the data were reviewed, it was also found that the clients ranged in age from 65 to 75 years; there were 45 females and 55 males.

The groups were compared according to health ratings and support systems. The means and standard deviations are as follows:

### Level of Support

| Health Status | Mean | Standard Deviation |
| --- | --- | --- |
| Low | 7.1 | 7.4 |
| Moderate | 11.9 | 4.5 |
| High | 23.3 | 3.2 |

In this sample, a Pearson $r$ was used to describe the relationship of the ratings on health status and intensity of support network: $r = .76$, $p < .05$.

120. The type of sample selected for this study is referred to as
    a. stratified sample
    b. random sample
    c. convenience sample
    d. cluster sample
121. The Pearson $r$ of .76 is best interpreted as
    a. a measure of the differences between the responses of men and women
    b. a significant relationship between intensity of support network and health status rating
    c. a relatively weak relationship between a self-report of health status and assessment of support network
    d. an indication that the hypothesis is poorly supported by the data collected

---

*Fictitious study

122. The study is best described as
    a. descriptive-correlational
    b. ex post facto
    c. quasi-experimental
    d. experimental
123. In which category of level of health status was the highest degree of variability in the scores on social support found?
    a. high
    b. medium
    c. low
    d. not reported
124. What type of instrument is the health status measurement?
    a. structured interview schedule
    b. summated rating scale
    c. graphic rating scale
    d. critical incident
125. The hypothesis in this study is best described as
    a. statistical hypothesis
    b. directional hypothesis
    c. null hypothesis
    d. not a hypothesis as stated
126. If this study were to be read and considered for inclusion in a review of literature, which of the following is most appropriate?
    a. State: "It was found that clients with strong support networks are healthier than their counterparts with weak support networks."
    b. State: "This study found a positive relationship between the health status of elderly clients and support networks."
    c. State: "A difference was observed between men and women in their reports of health status and support networks."
    d. The findings are so inconclusive that the study should not be included in the review.

# PART V
# Future Directions

# 25

# Future Directions for Improving the Quality of the Measurement of Outcomes for Education and Research in Nursing

## Nan B. Hechenberger

The purpose of this chapter is to discuss the where, why, and how of its title; that is, (1) *Where* are we now with regard to measuring outcomes for education and research in nursing, (2) *Why* do we need to improve on the state of the art, and (3) *How* can we bring about the needed improvement? In an attempt to assess the present state of the art of the measurement of outcomes in nursing, 191 articles published in the three leading nursing research journals between January 1980 and September 1981 were reviewed by Waltz and Strickland (1981). Fewer than one-third of the articles published in the three journals during the specified time period focused on some aspect of outcome measurement, and 81% of those investigated clinical rather than educational outcomes. This, the authors believed, is reflective of the amount of importance placed on educational research in nursing. They state that it should be noted that nurse educators are just as accountable for their practice as educators as are nurses in clinical settings. Research on the outcomes of strategies and programs employed in nursing education is needed to improve practice in that area, and the results should be widely disseminated in the research literature to encourage replication and application of those educational strategies for which there is evidence of effectiveness. Interestingly, a cursory review and categorization of the projects presented at the Measurement of Clinical and Educational Outcomes in Nursing Conference in 1985 indicated that approximately 60% were clinically oriented, and approximately 40% were concerned with outcomes for education and research in nursing.

The environment for nursing education during the next decade and a half mandates improved measurement of both instructional and administrative outcomes. Just as the prospective payment system requires practitioners of health care to develop a data base for practice-related decisions and activities, so the changing demographic, economic, social, and political conditions are giving an entirely new character to the administration of nursing education programs. From now on, the administration of these programs will reflect a more conscious effort to plan the course of their development, to reflect a more conscious effort to plan the course of their development, to relate process to outcome, and to seek an optimum return both quantitatively, from limited resources. Nursing faculties will need to work differently, better, more systematically, and, most likely, longer and harder to fulfill the tripartite mission of teaching, research, and service. The time is now for a good healthy dose of corporate discipline to be imposed upon the academy!

We hear from our counterparts in nursing practice and we read in both the professional literature and the public media that the prospective payment system, with its concomitant diagnosis-related groupings, has created chaos and upheaval in the health care industry. At the same time we are told by proponents of the system that provides incentives to manage scarce resources so that health care costs can be reduced. From a quantitative point of view, we know that patient days in acute care facilities are down even when admissions remain stable because patients are being discharged sooner. This results in an overall lower occupancy rate in hospitals and a decrease in revenues generated. The impact on the nursing job market is presently a negative one.

For the first time in at least 30 years, schools of nursing must respond to environmental conditions in a buyer's market rather than in a seller's market. Declining enrollments, deteriorating facilities, smaller state appropriations, fewer federal dollars, and more competition for private dollars imply a different approach to the recruitment, retention, and graduation of nursing students and to the overall administration and governance of schools of nursing. Just as hospitals experience a decline in overall occupancy even though admissions remain stable, schools of nursing experience a drastic decline in full-time equivalent students even though admissions remain stable because of the dramatic shift from full-time to part-time study. This results in less revenue generated and impacts negatively at some point on the job market for nursing faculty. Now is the time for thoughtful educators and academic executives who are farsighted statesmen to confront the challenges that face us.

The need for strategic planning and data-based decision making is now crucial if schools of nursing are to survive, compete, and forge ahead in educating health care professionals, contributing to the generation and transmission of new nursing knowledge and providing services to the community and the profession itself. The chief academic officer in a school of nursing will no longer survive, not will the school itself, with the old "seat of the pants" approach to administration. The administrator's repertoire must now include a firm grounding in administrative/organizational theory, financial management, organization developement, marketing, public relations, and strategies for fund raising. In an area of cost control and limited resources, we are faced with balancing the need to cut costs, and therefore programs, on the one hand, and the need to generate more income, on the other. The ability depends in large part on the quantity and quality of information available for decision making. The presence of a comprehensive master plan for program evaluation is vital to the generation of data necessary for rational goal-oriented decision making. In addition, an ongoing program of institutional research should generate such information as (1) projections of enrollment results based on new marketing procedures that reduce the error between projected and actual enrollment, (2) program reviews of academic offerings that show the cost-effectiveness of each program and department, (3) measures of student attitudes and performance to determine the holding influence of the institution, (4) marketing and accounting strategies to determine whether support services such as the media center, research center, and student services are cost-effective, (5) facility utilization results to gauge the needed investment in renovation and maintenance, (6) plans for generating dollars to balance the budget and provide needed funding for new equipment and maintenance when there are not sufficient funds to cover such expenditures, and (7) fund-raising strategies related to specific operational goals, endowment, or capital campaign needs (Ringle & Savackas, 1983). Outcome measurement is a vital component of both program evaluation and institutional research. However, very few nursing educators/administrators are even now beginning to develop this concept systematically.

## DEVELOPMENT OF A PLAN FOR NURSING ORGANIZATION DEVELOPMENT

A recent example of the "management revolution" at the University of Maryland School of Nursing can be seen in the development and implementation of a strategic plan that is part of an overall organization development program that has been in place since 1979. Previous organization development outcomes include (1) a management development program for academic administrators, (2) an assessment of the organizational climate in the school of nursing and development of administrative strategies to reduce organizational barriers to the effective use of people, (3) reorganization of the administrative structure in the school of nursing, (4) development and implementation of a master plan for program evaluation, and (5) a prescriptive faculty workload plan with a system for faculty and administrator evaluation. Following the assessment of the organizational climate and implementation of administrative strategies to cope with areas identified as problematic, a field test of a technique designed to measure the effects of the administrative interventions was conducted.

An analysis of the results indicated (1) a significance reduction in perceived blockages and (2) that the magnitude of specific changes could be moderately predicted prior to the second data gathering. These results seemed to argue well for the tested methodology as an administrative evaluation tool (Hechenberger & Bausell, 1982).

The latest phase in the organization development program is the strategic plan. The plan includes a mission statement that identifies the school as an integral part of a university academic health center with a unique role in combining the missions of the university and the goals of a professional discipline. The mission of the School of Nursing is to provide leadership in nursing through scholarship, research, and evaluation. Identification and development of areas of practice and nursing care delivery systems that anticipate and are responsive to societal needs through the development of research and teaching programs is the primary focus.

In addition to the mission statement, the plan describes what the school will have by the year 1990 through the development of 11 goals listed in priority order. For each goal there is a series of performance standards that describe the conditions necessary to exist to justify that the School of Nursing goals have been met. Further, each performance standard has been broken down into operational objectives, each with an allocation of responsibility and time frame for initiation.

The goal with the highest priority rating was "a climate and environment that facilitates and supports faculty research and scholarship activities." Examples of performance standards for this goal include (1) the number of faculty of self-supporting research grants has increased, (2) appropriate equipment for research activities has been made readily accessible and available to faculty, and (3) on the average, the equivalent of 20% of the total salaries of senior faculty has been secured from external funding. There is a total of 15 performance standards for this goal, with a total of 47 operational objectives involving 160 people over a period of 6 years in its implementation.

The second highest priority rating was assigned to the goal "Programs are planned and decisions made that are justified on the basis of evaluation data from a variety of sources." Among the performance standards developed for the goal were the following: (1) the master plan for evaluation and marketing analysis have been implemented, and (2) organizational and program priorities including those within programs have been established. In order to meet the latter standard, criteria were developed to prioritize the 18 program offerings at the master's level. Five criteria were related to faculty (e.g., "Programs given priority status are provided by outstanding faculty whose research and publications make a unique contribution to the profession"); 7 criteria were related to students (e.g., "Programs given priority status are those that attract large numbers of highly qualified and diversified applicants"); 10 criteria were related to the program itself (e.g., "Programs given priority status are those that are of higher quality, as evidenced by evaluative data, than are the same or similar programs offered by competitors"); 2 criteria were related to resources (e.g., "Programs given priority status are those that the University of Maryland School of Nursing has unique and/or outstanding specific resources to offer that are not generally available elsewhere"), and 9 criteria were related to costs (e.g., "Programs given priority status are those that can justify their cost on the basis of relevance, need, and demand"). Faculty were asked to use a professional judgment in rating the extent to which each criterion was achieved within the particular specialty program. They were asked to rate the extent of achievement of the current program of each criterion on a scale of 1 (Not at All) through 9 (Completely). In addition, they were asked to use available data and examples to provide the rationale for their judgment.

The academic administrator responsible for each program presented the data to all of the school of nursing academic administrators (deans, chairmen, directors) at one of the three administrative retreats scheduled annually. Following these presentations and discussion thereof, a Delphi technique was employed in an attempt to obtain data that reflected the majority view of the academic administrators with regard to what program(s) should be eliminated and what program(s) should be given priority in the reallocation of scant resources. Although the ultimate decision-making responsibility in this regard rested with the School of Nursing Executive Committee [dean, associate deans (two), and assistant deans (two)], the collective view of the academic administrators group was considered an important input into the process.

Each member of the academic administrators group was asked by mail to complete a series of rankings of the specialty tracks in the master's program. The mailing included a set of instructions for how the rankings should be done, and the completed rankings were returned by mail to dean's office and analyzed by staff in the Office of Evaluation. Responses were tabulated and summarized. Since we were interested in majority views, frequency distributions and the mode served as a basis for the decision regarding when the majority view was reflected in the data. A summary of the findings from the first series of rankings was returned to the group by mail. Each individual in the group was asked to consider the information in the summary and to then complete and return by mail a second series of rankings. In order to preserve anonymity, each individual was asked to keep a copy of his/her own completed rankings so that they could readily be compared with the summary data provided at the time of the second series of rankings. The process was terminated at the completion of the third series of rankings when the resulting data clearly reflected a majority view of the group.

The specialty tracks were ranked in two ways: for elimination from the masters program (from 1, first to be eliminated, to 18, last to be eliminated) and for priority when master's program resources are reallocated (from 1, first priority, to 18, last priority). When the data were analyzed, the first three specialty tracks targeted for elimination from the master's program were the last three targeted for elimination. A marketing analysis is currently underway to further refine and expand the information available for making critical program decisions.

## CONCLUSION

Clearly, administrators in schools of nursing need to be planners, organizers, delegators, and evaluators. They need to be acutely aware of trends in the health care industry and the trends in higher education in order to conceptualize and implement the appropriate strategies to keep nursing education programs relevant in today's society. They need to understand their own roles in their own organizations and how they relate to others both inside and outside their own institutions. They need second-level administrators to whom they delegate major program responsibility and whom they hold accountable for productivity in that program. They need administrators and faculty who understand that nursing education is in a transition period, that the decisions made today will determine not only what the future will be but whether, in fact, there will be a future. Some schools of nursing will survive the present resource crisis and some will not. surviving schools will be those whose faculties understand the importance of strategic planning and whose administrators make it their number-one priority.

Since good academic planning requires sound data-based decision making, the importance of outcome measurement and program evaluation in nursing education is evident. The present state of the art of the measurement of outcomes *must* be improved through the inclusion of measurement and evaluation content in graduate programs in nursing, in postdoctoral and fellowship programs in nursing, and in continuing education and faculty development programs. In addition, the concept of "mentorship" in this area is important if the necessary appreciations, understandings, and measurement skills are to be transmitted from the current experts in the field to those who are novices. A network of measurement and evaluation specialists should evolve that will spawn future generations of nurses interested and informed about the measurement of nursing outcomes. Most important, wide dissemination of the outcomes of such activities through paper presentations at professional meetings and publications in the nursing literature is imperative. It is hoped that through projects such as this nursing will "come of age" in the measurement of nursing outcomes for education and research for the enhancement of nursing science.

# REFERENCES

Hechenberger, N. B., & Bausell, B. R. (1982). Measuring the effects of administrative intervention: A technique: *Evaluation and the Health Professions, 5*, 469.

Ringle, P. M., & Saveckas, M. L. (1983). Administrative leadership. *Journal of Higher Education, 54*(6), 649-661.

Waltz, C., & Strickland, O. (1982). Measurement of nursing outcomes: State of the art as we enter the eighties. In W. E. Field (Ed.), *Measuring outcomes of nursing practice, education, and administration: Proceedings of the First Annual SCCEN Research Conference, December 4-5, 1981* (pp. 47-62). Atlanta: Southern Council on Collegiate Education for Nursing, Southern Regional Education Board.

# Appendix:
# Measurement of Clinical and Educational Nursing Outcomes Project

## PROJECT PARTICIPANTS AND TOPIC AREAS

| PARTICIPANT | TOPIC AREA |
| --- | --- |
| Lois Ryan Allen, R.N., Ph.D.<br>Widener University<br>Chester, Pennsylvania | Attitude Toward Computer-Assisted Instruction |
| Jean M. Arnold, R.N., Ed.D.<br>Rutgers University<br>Newark, New Jersey | Diagnostic Reasoning Protocols for Nursing Clinical Simulations |
| Patricia M. Bailey, R.N., Ph.D.<br>University of Kentucky<br>Lexington, Kentucky | Comparison of Ideal Values of Nurse Faculty and Values Taught |
| Betsy M. Barnes, R.N., M.S.N., CCRN<br>Lander College<br>Greenwood, South Carolina | Student Performance Evaluation Form – The Nurse as Teacher with Basic Knowledge |
| Elizabeth A. Barrett, R.N., Ph.D.<br>The Mount Sinai Medical Center<br>New York, New York | Measuring Quality of Nursing Care for DRGs Using The HEW-Medicus Nursing Process Methodology – a Pilot Study |
| Clarissa Beardslee, R.N., Ph.D.<br>University of Pittsburgh<br>Pittsburgh, Pennsylvania | Evaluation of the Advanced Clinical Nursing Component of a Graduate Program in Nursing in Preparing Students for "On-the-Job" Functioning |

Doris R. Blaney, R.N., Ph.D.,
F.A.A.N.
Indiana University
Gary, Indiana

Development and Psychometric
Analysis of a Scale to Measure
Attitude Toward Cost-Effective-
ness in Nursing

Patricia Bohachick, R.N., Ph.D.
University of Pittsburgh
Pittsburgh, Pennsylvania

Level of Physical Activity
Questionnaire

Marion E. Broome, R.N., M.N.
Medical College of Georgia
Augusta, Georgia

Development and Testing of an
Instrument to Measure Children's
Fears of Medical Experiences

Linda Brown, R.N., Ph.D.
University of Chicago
Chicago, Illinois

Information Processing and Actions
Taken by Nurses in Response to
Advanced Information Technology

Kathleen Buckwalter, R.N., Ph.D.
Iowa University
Iowa City, Iowa

Development and Testing of the
Iowa Self-Assessment Inventory

Shirley Mitz Caldwell, R.N., Ed.D.
Vanderbilt University
Nashville, Tennessee

Family Well-Being Assessment:
Conceptual Model, Reliability,
Validity and Use

Shirley A. Carter, R.N., Ed.D.
University of Delaware
Newark, Delaware

Quantification and Analysis of
Selected Intervening Variables
Affecting Course Outcomes

JoAnn H. Collier, R.N., M.S.
University of Akron
Akron, Ohio

Impact of Computer-Assisted Deci-
sion Making in an Existing
Diabetes Patient Education
Program

Carol Collison, R.N., Ph.D.
University of South Carolina
Columbus, South Carolina

Family Functioning as Conceptualized from a Systems Perspective

Nancy S. Creason, R.N., Ph.D.
University of Illinois
Urbana, Illinois

Operational Definitions of State-
ments of Nursing in the PES
(Problem, Etiology, Signs, and
Symptoms) Format

Linda Cronenwett, R.N., Ph.D.
University of Michigan
Chelsea, Michigan

Child Care Activities Scale

Ann D. Crutchfield, R.N., M.S.
Kennesaw College
Marietta, Georgia

Nursing Competencies Related to
Assessment

Gail C. Davis, R.N., Ed.D.
Texas Christian University
Fort Worth, Texas

Measurement of the Clinical Outcomes of the Patient with
Chronic Pain

Mary E. Duffy, R.N., Ph.D.
University of Texas
Austin, Texas

The Research Appraisal Checklist:
Development and Validation of
an Instrument to Appraise
Nursing Research Reports

Sandra R. Edwardson, R.N., Ph.D.
University of Minnesota
Minneapolis, Minnesota

Revision and Testing of the
Haussman and Hegyvary
Outcome Measure for Myocardial
Infarction

Lillian Eriksen, R.N., D.S.N.
University of Wyoming
Laramie, Wyoming

Patient Satisfaction with Nursing
Care: A Magnitude Estimation
Approach

Sr. Mary Jean Flaherty, R.N., Ph.D.
The Catholic University of
   America
Washington, D.C.

Grandmother Functioning Scale

Martha J. Foxall, R.N., Ph.D.
University of Nebraska
Omaha, Nebraska

Evaluation of Measurements to
Assess Family Response to
Chronic Illness

Linda Holbrook Freeman, R.N.,
   M.S.N.
University of Louisville
Louisville, Kentucky

Evaluation of Assertive Behavior in
Registered Nurses Following a
Continuing Education Program

Lorraine Gentner, R.N., Ph.D.
Baylor University
Dallas, Texas

A Proposal for the Development of
a Tool to Measure Loneliness

Valerie D. George, R.N., Ph.D.
Cleveland State University
Cleveland, Ohio

Measuring the Sense of Coherence

Louise M. Givens, R.N., M.S.N.
Children's Hospital National Medi-
   cal Center
Washington, D.C.

Clinical Competencies and Adjustment Levels of Nurse Orientees

Davina Gosnell, R.N., Ph.D.
Kent State University
Kent, Ohio

Development of a Reliable and
Valid Instrument to Assess
Persons' Potential Risk for
Pressure Scores

Carol Gramse, R.N., Ph.D.
State University of New York
Stony Brook, New York

Assessment of Validity and Reliability of a Measure of Women's
Health Beliefs Using the Multitrait Multimethod Approach

Elsie Gulick, R.N., Ph.D.
Rutgers College of Nursing
Newark, New Jersey

Development of the Self-Administered ADL Scale for Persons with Multiple Sclerosis

Blossom Gullickson, R.N., M.S.
St. Olaf College
Northfield, Minnesota

Development of a Simulated Clinical Performance Examination

Ann Gunnett, C-N.P., M.S.N.
University of Maryland
Baltimore, Maryland

Improving Measurement of Student Clinical Performance

Cathie Guzzetta, R.N., Ph.D.
The Catholic University of
    America
Washington, D.C.

Development of a Protocol for Validating Nursing Diagnosis

Winifred B. Hagan, R.N., M.S.N.
The Hospital of the Albert
    Einstein College of Medicine
Bronx, New York

Nursing Staff Behaviors and Acutely Ill Older Adult Outcomes in a 24-Hour Reality Orientation Program

Donna Hawley, R.N., Ed.D.
Wichita State University
Wichita, Kansas

Development of a Questionnaire That Identifies Persons Who Have Symptoms Consistent with Fibrositis

Kathryn Hegedus, R.N., D.N.Sc.
The Children's Hospital
Boston, Massachusetts

Examination of Clinical Performance

Sharron Humenick, R.N., Ph.D.
University of Wyoming
Laramie, Wyoming

The MICAM: The Maturation Index for Colostrum and Mature Milk

Helen M. Jenkins, R.N., Ph.D.
George Mason University
Fairfax, Virginia

Clinical Decision Making Measured by the Clinical Decision Making in Nursing Scale

Joan M. Johnson, R.N., Ph.D.
University of Wisconsin
Oshkosh, Wisconsin

Assessment of Students in Relation to Curriculum Objectives and Correlated with Other Data

Colette Jones, R.N., Ph.D.
University of Maryland
Baltimore, Maryland

An Instrument to Measure the Perception of Both Fathers and Mothers Regarding Their Infants' Characteristics

Sarah Keating, R.N., C-P.N.P.,
    Ed.D.
Russell Sage College
New York, New York

The Measurement of Client Outcomes in Home Agencies

Marguerite Kinney, R.N., D.N.Sc.     Development of a Protocol for Vali-
University of Alabama                 dating Nursing Diagnosis
Birmingham, Alabama

Imogene King, R.N., Ed.D.            A Criterion-Referenced Measure of
University of South Florida           Goal Attainment
Tampa, Florida

Margaret Kostopoulos, R.N.,          Reliability and Validity of the Regis-
   M.S.N., C.N.A.                     tered Nurse Performance
Doctor's Hospital of Prince           Evaluation
   Georges County
Lanham, Maryland

Janet W. Krejci, R.N., M.S., C.N.S.  Attributions of Chronic Pain
St. Michael Hospital                  Patients
Milwaukee, Wisconsin

Ursel Krumme, R.N., Ph.D.            Measurement of Baccalaureate Stu-
Seattle University                    dents Nursing Process Competen-
Seattle, Washington                   cies: A Nursing Diagnosis
                                      Framework

Therese G. Lawler, R.N., Ed.D.       Measuring Socialization to the Pro-
East Carolina University              fessional Role
Greenville, North Carolina

Helen Lerner, R.N., Ph.D.            Questionnaire Identification of
Lehman College                        Social and Intellectual
Bronx, New York                       Stimulation Available to Young
                                      Children in Their Home

Dona J. Lethbridge, R.N., Ph.D.      The Childbirthing Decision Aid
University of New Hampshire
Durham, New Hampshire

Margaret Louis, R.N., Ph.D.          Nursing Instrument to Test New-
University of Nevada                  man's Conceptual Framework
Las Vegas, Nevada

Maragret Lunney, R.N., M.S.N.        The Concept of Nursing Diagnosis:
Hunter College – Bellevue             Dimensions and Issues
New York, New York

Francine R. Margolius, R.N.,         Coping of a Child and Family Dur-
   M.S.N.                             ing Hospitalization
Medical College of South Carolina
Charleston, South Carolina

Beverly J. McElmurry, R.N., Ed.D.
University of Illinois
Chicago, Illinois

A Multidimensional Measure of
Health in Older Women

Elizabeth McFarlane, R.N., D.N.Sc.
The Cathlic University of America
Washington D.C.

Determinants of Cardiovascular
Patients Compliance with Prescribed Health Regimens

M. Denise McHugh, R.N., M.S.
University of Wisconsin
Oshkosh, Wisconsin

Nursing Assessment: Data Specified
on Nursing Assessment Formats

Elaine McIntosh, R.N., M.S.N.
Tennessee Department of Health
    and Environment
Nashville, Tennessee

Women's Learning Needs Assessment Tool

Susan C. McMillan, R.N., Ph.D.
University of South Florida
Tampa, Florida

Reliability and Validity of Selected
Measures of Chemotherapy-
Induced Nausea and Vomiting

Michelle Miller, R.N., M.S.
St. Michael Hospital
Milwaukee, Wisconsin

Professional Practice Climate in
Nursing

Barbara Mims, R.N., M.S.N.,
    C.C.R.N.
Parkland Memorial Hospital
Lewisville, Texas

Development of a Clinical Performance Examination for Critical
Care Nurses

Linda Moody, R.N., Ph.D.
University of Florida
Gainesville, Florida

Nursing/Health Policy Survey

Ann Morgan, R.N., M.S.N.
University of Maryland
Baltimore, Maryland

Measurment of the Impact of a
Continuing Education Physical
Assessment Course on Nursing
Practice in a Selected Community
Hospital

Doris E. Nicholas, R.N., Ph.D.
Howard University
Washington, D.C.

Measurement of Helping Outcomes
in Nursing

L. Claire Parsons, R.N., Ph.D.
University of Virginia
Charlottesville, Virginia

Development of a Nurse Neuro-
logic Assessment Tool

Mary Lou Peck, R.N., Ph.D.
Russel Sage College
New York, New York

Application of the Bondy Scale and
Videotapes to Measure Short-
Term Skill Development of
Student Nurses

Shirley Pisarek, R.N., M.S.N.  
Veterans Administration Medical Center  
Hampton, Virginia

Perceptual Adaptation Differences in Medication Teaching

Marjorie Ramphal, R.N., Ed.D.  
Columbia University  
New York, New York

Urinary Incontinence

Olive J. Rich, R.N., Ph.D.  
Temple University  
Philadelphia, Pennsylvania

Maternal Tasks in Taking on a Second Child

Judy Richter, R.N., Ph.D.  
University of Northern Colorado  
Greeley, Colorado

Reliability and Validity of the Lifestyle Assessment Questionnaire

Karen Robinson, R.N., M.S.  
Veterans Administration Medical Center  
Fargo, North Dakota

Denial and Anxiety in Second-Day Myocardial Infarction Patients

Joanne Scungio, R.N., Ph.D.  
University of Alabama  
Birmingham, Alabama

Parental Coping of Childhood Cancer

Ann Sheridan, R.N., Ed.D.  
Massachusetts General Hospital  
Boston, Massachusetts

Development of a Criterion-Referenced Tool to Measure Knowledge of Research Consumerism Phase I

Judith Shockley, R.N., M.S.N.  
University of Texas  
San Antonio, Texas

Advanced Placement Examination in BSN Programs: Development of Domain-Referenced Instruments

Bonnie Ketchum Smola, R.N., Ph.D.  
University of Dubuque  
Dubuque, Iowa

Refinement and Validation of a Research Tool to Measure Leadership Characteristics of Baccalaureate Nursing Students

Janet R. Southby, R.N., D.N.Sc.  
U.S. Army Nurse Corps  
Washington, D.C.

Attitudes about and Expectations of Graduate Nursing Education

Jacqueline Stemple, R.N., Ed.D.  
West Virginia University  
Morgantown, West Virginia

Self-Care Professional Role Orientation: Instrument Development

Nancy A. Stotts, R.N., Ed.D.  
University of California  
San Fransisco, California

Testing a Wound Assessment Instrument

Cheryl B. Stetler, R.N., Ph.D.
Massachusetts General Hospital
Boston, Massachusetts

Development of a Criterion-Referenced Tool to Measure Knowledge of Research Consumerism Phase I

Sarah S. Strauss, R.N., Ph.D.
Medical College of Virginia Hospitals
Richmond, Virginia

Information References and Information Seeking in Hospitalized Surgery Patients

Jean Stremmel, R.N., M.S.
University of Maryland
College Park, Maryland

Measurement of the Impact of a Continuing Education Physical Assessment Course on Nursing Practice in a Selected Community Hospital

Jane P. Taylor, R.N., M.S.
University of Delaware
Newark, Delaware

Clinical Testing to Measure Cognitive Behavioral Changes in Nursing Students

Gladys Torres, R.N., Ed.D.
Brooklyn Veteran Administration Center
Brooklyn, New York

Multivariate Evaluation of a Collaborative Practice Project: Preliminary Impressions

James P. Turley
University of South Florida
Tampa, Florida

Measurement of Time as Tempo

Sandra Underwood, R.N., M.S.N.
Chicago State University
Chicago, Illinois

Measuring the Instructional Validity of Computer-Based Instruction in the Development of Higher Level Cognitive Skills in Nursing

Gwen van Servellen, R.N., Ph.D.
University of California
Los Angeles, California

The Individualized Care Index – Test of Discriminate Validity

Peggy L. Wagner, R.N., M.S.N.
St. Michael Hospital
Milwaukee, Wisconsin

Exhaustion of Adaptive Potential: Measurement in the Clinical Setting

Clarann Weinert, R.N., Ph.D.
Montana State University
Bozeman, Montana

Revision and Further Development of a Social Support Measure: The Personal Resource Questionnaire

Mary Wierenga, R.N., Ph.D.
University of Wisconsin
Milwaukee, Wisconsin

Measurement of Diabetes Well-Being

Janie Wilson, R.N., Ph.D.                    Clinical Evaluation of Students in a
San Antonio College                             Management Course
San Antonio, Texas

Constance Ziegfeld, R.N., M.S.               Nursing Knowledge of Principles of
Johns Hopkins                                   Chemotherapy Management: A
Baltimore, Maryland                             Criterion-Referenced Evaluation

Kenneth Zwolski, R.N., M.S., M.A.            Development of a Tool for the
Columbia University                             Measurement of Ability to
New York, New York                              Formulate Nursing Diagnoses

# Index